Medical

Management

of

Atherosclerosis

Clinical Guides to Medical Management

Consulting Editor

BURTON E. SOBEL, M.D.
Medical Center Hospital of Vermont
University of Vermont
Burlington, Vermont

Medical Management of Heart Disease, edited by Burton E. Sobel
Medical Management of Rheumatic Musculoskeletal and Connective Tissue Diseases, edited by Jan Dequeker, Gabriel Panayi, Theodore Pincus and Rodney Grahame
Medical Management of Atherosclerosis, edited by John LaRosa

Additional Titles in Preparation

Medical Management of Liver Disease, edited by Edward L. Krawitt
Medical Management of Pulmonary Diseases, edited by Gerald S. Davis, Theodore W. Marcy, and Elizabeth A. Seaward
Medical Management of Kidney and Electrolyte Disorders, edited by John F. Gennari

Medical

Management

of

Atherosclerosis

edited by

John C. LaRosa
Tulane University Medical Center
New Orleans, Louisiana

MARCEL DEKKER, INC.   NEW YORK · BASEL · HONG KONG

ISBN: 0-8247-0149-6

The publisher offers discounts on this book when ordered in bulk quantities. For more information, write to Special Sales/Professional Marketing at the address below.

This book is printed on acid-free paper.

MARCEL DEKKER, INC.
270 Madison Avenue, New York, New York 10016
http://www.dekker.com

Current printing (last digit):
10 9 8 7 6 5 4 3 2 1

PRINTED IN THE UNITED STATES OF AMERICA

Clinical Guides to
Medical Management

The Clinical Guides to Medical Management are designed to provide practitioners, both generalists and specialists, with the information needed to identify and respond optimally to recognition of cardinal signs and symptoms of disease and to translate even the most recent advances in biomedical research into improved clinical care for their patients. Macrovascular disease, including coronary, cerebral, and peripheral vascular disease, is an ideal topic for these volumes because of the ubiquitous nature of atherosclerosis in our society and the value of medical interventions. Much recent press regarding the management of vascular disease has focused on dramatic interventions including angioplasty, stents, and surgical procedures, all of which have made positive contributions and prolonged lives. However, the underlying need for such interventions is the remarkably high prevalence and insidious nature of atherosclerosis, a condition that must be attacked by medical means and lifestyle modification, and over long intervals if the sequelae that have been such a cogent focus are to be markedly attenuated. The implementation of such long-term approaches requires active, dedicated, and knowledgeable participation in the care of patients in populations by dedicated practitioners armed with current information and committed to translating new knowledge into improved clinical care.

This book, with its objectives and approach so eloquently described in Dr. Lenfant's foreword, addresses pathophysiology of atherosclerosis; interventions including lipid lowering, normalization of elevated systemic arterial blood pressure, smoking cessation, and other lifestyle modifications; the use of hormone replacement therapy and antithrombotic regimens; prevention through clinical interventions, public health programs, and, potentially, gene therapy; and the economics involved in reducing the toll from atherogenesis. Dr. LaRosa and the contributors to his book provide relevant current information in a remarkably thorough and readable format entirely consistent with the overall objectives of the Clinical Guides program. This text will undoubt-edly benefit its readers and, even more importantly, their patients.

Burton E. Sobel, M.D.

Foreword

In a wonderful book titled *A Short History of Cardiology* (1), James Herrick included a chapter on "The Coronary Artery and Its Diseases." This chapter is introduced by a quote from Leonardo da Vinci:

> The heart in itself is not the beginning of life, but is a vessel made of dense muscle, vivified and nourished by the artery and vein, as are other muscles.

Then the chapter begins:

> In the last few decades, in all discussions concerning the heart, the coronary artery has assumed a position of ever increasing importance.

Of course, Herrick had good reason to make this assertion as he was the person who, in 1912, presented to the Association of American Physicians a landmark contribution on, "Certain Clinical Features of Sudden Obstruction of the Coronary Arteries."

Believe it or not, for years, Herrick expressed deep disappointment because almost no one grasped the significance of this contribution!

Most interesting is the fact that arteriosclerosis was not even part of the discussion of the time. Yet for nearly two thousand years, anatomists and clinicians had known that arteries could be obstructed by a material that became known as "atheromatous" matter.

In the earlier part of the twentieth century, the role of cholesterol and lipoprotein in the development of arteriosclerosis became recognized by the medical community, and, eventually, by the public as attested by a 1950 *Saturday Evening Post* article titled, "Are you eating your way to arteriosclerosis?"

Many researchers and clinicians became fascinated by the study of coronary arteriosclerosis and its treatment. They were driven by the fact that coronary artery disease was the leading cause of death in the United States, as in many other countries. The last two or three decades have revealed a great deal of practical information of great public health importance and value—if put to use!

Dr. John LaRosa has been a major contributor to our current knowledge about the prevention and treatment of arteriosclerosis. Over the years, he has championed the importance of making certain that the medical community and the public know about coronary arteriosclerosis and use the knowledge to their benefit.

This book is one more weapon in Dr. LaRosa's crusade. It is hard to think of many other clinical researchers who could present what we know in a more convincing way. Physicians, even specialists, will be well served by reading this book, and thus, the patients will benefit.

Claude Lenfant, M.D.
Bethesda, Maryland

1.   Published by Charles Thomas. Springfield, IL, 1942.

Preface

Coronary artery disease has long been viewed as an anatomical problem requiring anatomical solutions. As a result, attention has been directed at invasively correcting specific anatomic lesions identified by angiography. The process of atherogenesis, however, cannot be altered by these anatomical interventions. The purpose of this volume is to review the evidence that identifies certain characteristics as predictive of the progression of atherosclerosis, and examine the evidence which demonstrates that changing those risk factors in fact lowers the risk of subsequent progression. In essence, the aim of the book is to review what can be done medically, rather than anatomically, to prevent, arrest, or reverse atherosclerosis, particularly in the coronary arteries.

Chapters 1–5, authored by me, Dr. Joseph Witztum, Dr. Henry Black and Dr. William Elliot, Dr. Thomas Kottke, and Dr. Neil Stone, respectively, focus on coronary risk factors and the evidence that intervention can prevent atherosclerosis. These chapters also outline specific methods for reducing these risk factors.

Chapter 6, by Dr. Robert Knopp, provides a discussion of the surprisingly profound effects of gonadal hormones, particularly estrogens, on the process of atherosclerosis.

In Chapter 7, Dr. Bertram Pitt discusses various pharmacological interventions, in addition to lipid lowering, blood pressure lowering, and hormone therapies.

Chapter 8, by Dr. Robert Vogel, summarizes some of the methods by which prevention of atherosclerosis can be introduced into clinical practice.

In Chapter 9, Dr. David Cohen deals with the cost-effectiveness of these interventions and the factors that render them more or less appealing in an environment in which resources are clearly finite.

Chapter 10 provides a glimpse into the future of genetics and gene therapy, and the potential for enormous changes in our thinking about the therapies of atherosclerosis as the information based in human genetics becomes more extensive and more available for therapeutic application.

Chapter 11 is a review by Dr. William Roberts of the current thinking about the correlations of pathological findings in the coronary arteries with clinical events. Among other things, this chapter emphasizes the important concept that atherosclerosis is a diffuse, and not an isolated disease, the manifestations of which cannot be adequately treated by focusing on only a few lesions.

This book provides a thorough review of currently available interventions that slow the progression of coronary atherosclerosis, as well as a look at the possible future of such interventions. Because many of these medical interventions are not being widely applied, even though they are solidly based in science, it is my hope that this book will serve as a reference and guide for physicians who want to do everything medically possible to help patients with coronary atherosclerosis avoid future coronary morbidity and mortality.

I want to thank all the authors for their hard work and patience in the editing process. I want to particularly thank Ms. Mary Beth Romig for her excellent administrative and editorial assistance. I hope that the book's impact will justify the hard work of all of these individuals.

John C. LaRosa, M.D.

Introduction

Not long ago, atherosclerosis was viewed as a patchy, slowly developing disease. Clinical symptoms were produced when isolated atheromatous lesions grew large enough to block blood flow or at least slow it enough that local clotting occurred, forming an occluding thrombus. Thus, vessels that appeared in angiography to be less than 50% occluded on angiogram were felt to be "hemodynamically insignificant," i.e., of little immediate threat, since blood flow was not significantly compromised. For more occluded areas, anatomically directed interventions such as coronary bypass surgery or angioplasty were regarded as virtually curative. As a result, millions of patients underwent corrective anatomical procedures with little attention paid, either before or after the procedure, to intervention on risk factors such as smoking, hypertension, and hypercholesterolemia.

These concepts began to change as a result of newer approaches to the examination of pathological specimens (1) and, more recently, intravascular ultrasound studies of "normal" coronary artery segments in patients with angiographically demonstrated coronary atherosclerosis (2). Such studies demonstrate that atherosclerosis is indeed a diffuse, rather than a patchy, disease. Terms such as "single-vessel disease" are misleading if they are taken to imply that the remainder of the vasculature, particularly in the coronary vessels, is normal.

More recently, it has become clear that the initiating events in the development of atherosclerosis, before there is evidence of atheromatous changes, are the result of alterations in endothelial function leading to decreased synthesis of vasodilators like nitric oxide, decreased synthesis of anticoagulants like tissue plasminogen activator, and increased synthesis of vasoconstrictors such as endothelin, as well as chemoattractants capable of attracting circulatory monocytes and other inflammatory cells (3). Such endothelial dysfunction may be triggered by a variety of factors, including such common risk factors as hypercholesterolemia, cigarette smoking, hypertension, hyperinsulinemia, and hypoestrogenemia (4,5).

Circulating monocytes, attracted by dysfunctional endothelium, are attached to endothelium and transformed into macrophages. These macrophages ingest minimally oxidized low-density lipoprotein (LDL) and probably other cholesterol-rich lipoproteins as well. Eventually, they will become saturated with cholesteryl ester, which they cannot catabolize, and form what are known histologically as "foam" cells—cells with large numbers of cholesteryl ester–containing cytoplasmic vacuoles. Oxidized lipoproteins, or their breakdown products, are cytotoxic, and as these cells are lysed, their cytoplasmic cholesteryl ester forms an extracellular cholesterol pool beneath the endothelium. The overlying and surrounding dysfunctional endothelium, along with smooth muscle cells and macrophages, form an atherosclerotic plaque (5,6). Eventually the plaque becomes larger and more fibrous. Different stages of this atheroma may be associated with different clinical syndromes, ranging from unstable angina to transmural myocardial infarction (1). The key processes resulting in occlusion of the vessel, however, do not appear to be solely related to the size of the atheroma, but rather to the friability of the cellular cap over the extracellular cholesteryl ester pool; the degree of surrounding inflammation, as reflected in the number of macrophages; the propensity for clotting; and abnormal vasospasm in the area of active atheroma (7).

Vascular occlusion, then, is not related simply to the size of the atheroma but also its activity. It should not be surprising, then, that almost 70% of myocardial infarctions occur in the distribution of coronary vessels that on angiography are "hemodynamically insignificant," i.e., < 50% occluded (8).

There is no evidence that anatomical interventions can or should be used on such lesions. Rather, we must consider interventions that take into account atherosclerosis as a diffuse disease of endothelium triggered by a number of risk factors. On the other hand, the presence of sufficiently high levels of circulating cholesterol-rich lipoproteins in the plasma does appear to be necessary for the development of disease. Both laboratory and population studies indicate that without hypercholesterolemia, other risk factors, including hypertension and diabetes, correlate much less strongly with atherosclerosis (9,10). This may be because the pathophysiological pathway to severe atherosclerosis is the development of an extracellular cholesterol pool. The level of circulating cholesterol necessary to promote atherogenesis, however, is much lower than what is considered "normal" in Western populations, probably because normal is confused with average. Atherogenesis can be supported by cholesterol levels as low as 160 mg/dl (4.0 mmol/L) (11,12).

None of this means that anatomical interventions are not of value. Indeed, coronary bypass surgery, particularly in patients with severe lesions in the left main coronary artery or with numerous severe lesions requiring multiple bypasses, has been demonstrated to be life-preserving (13). Given the limited nature of angioplasty, it is not surprising that it has not been demonstrated to affect subsequent morbidity or mortality. Anatomical procedures, however, must be considered temporary (and expensive) maneuvers to correct an immediate problem and provide symptom relief without attacking the underlying atherogenic process that created the problem.

The purpose of this volume is to review the evidence that identifies certain characteristics as predictive of future progression of atherosclerosis, to examine the evidence which demonstrates that changing those risk factors in fact lowers the risk of subsequent atherosclerotic events, and to identify for practicing physicians the best ways of successfully intervening to prevent atherosclerotic progression. Although it is thought that the process of atherosclerosis is similar in all vascular beds, most of the data have been gathered in patients with coronary atherosclerosis. As a result, coronary disease will form the predominant focus of these discussions.

Currently recognized risk factors and interventions, of course, do not explain all the factors that initiate or support the development of atherosclerosis. It is likely that in the future we will have better, more selective means for identifying and treating patients who are at risk, and for more effectively lowering risk in those who have already had a clinical event. These discussions do, however, represent a state-of-the-art review of currently accepted interventions.

John C. LaRosa

REFERENCES

1. Roberts WC. Qualitative and quantitative comparisons of amounts of narrowing by atherosclerotic plaques in the major epicardial coronary arteries of necropsy in sudden death. Am J Cardiol 1989; 64:423–328.
2. Mintz GS. Painter JA, Richard AD, Kent KM, Satler LF, Popma JJ. Atherosclerosis in angiographically "normal" coronary artery reference segments: an intravascular ultrasound study clinical corrections. J Am Coll Cardiol 1995; 5:1479–1485.
3. Luscher TF, Tanner FC, Tschudi MR, Noll G. Endothelial dysfunction in coronary artery disease. Annu Rev Med 1993; 44:395–418.
4. Vita JA, Treasure CB, Nabel EG, et al. Coronary vasomotor response to acetylcholine relates to risk factors for coronary artery disease. Circulation 1990; 81:491–497.
5. Wissler RW. Important points in the pathogenesis of atherosclerosis. In: Gotto AM, ed. Atherosclerosis. Kalamazoo, MI: Upjohn Company, 1992.
6. Davies, SW, Wedzicha JA. Hypoxia and the heart. Br Heart J 1993; 69(1):3–5.
7. Fuster V, Badimon L, Badimon JJ, et al. The pathogenesis of coronary artery disease and the acute coronary syndromes. N Engl J Med 1992; 326:242–250, 310–318.
8. Falk E, Shah PK, Fuster V. Coronary plaque disruption. Circulation 1995; 92:657–671.

9. Alexander RW. Theodore Cooper Memorial Lecture. Hypertension and the patho-
    genesis of atherosclerosis. Oxidative stress and the mediation of arterial inflam-
    matory response: a new perspective. Hypertension 1995; 25:155–161.
10. Ruderman NB, Schneider SH. Diabetes, exercise and atherosclerosis. Diabetes Care
    1992; 15(suppl 4):1787–1793.
11. Roberts WC. Atherosclerotic risk factors: are there ten or is there only one? Am
    J Cardiol 1989; 64:552–554.
12. St. Clair RSW. Atherosclerosis regression in animal models. Current concepts of
    cellular and biochemical mechanisms. Prog Cardiovasc Dis (1983; XXVI:109–131.
13. Yusef S, Zucker D, Peduzzi P, et al. Effect of coronary artery bypass graft surgery
    on survival: overview of 10-year results from randomised trials by the Coronary
    Artery Bypass Graft Surgery Trialists' Collaboration. Lancet 1994; 344:563–570.

Contents

Contributors

Henry R. Black, M.D. Roberts Professor and Chairman, Department of Preventive Medicine, Rush Medical College, Rush University, Chicago, Illinois

Bartolome Bonet[*] Northwest Lipid Research Clinic, and Department of Medicine and Department of Obstetrics and Gynecology, University of Washington School of Medicine, Seattle, Washington

Antonio Cabrera, M.D., Ph.D.[†] Department of Medicine, Mayo Clinic and Foundation, Rochester, Minnesota

David J. Cohen, M.D., M.Sc. Assistant Professor, Cardiovascular Division, Department of Medicine, Beth Israel-Deaconess Medical Center, and Harvard Medical School, Boston, Massachusetts

William J. Elliott, M.D., Ph.D. Associate Professor, Department of Preventive Medicine, Rush Medical College, Rush University, Chicago, Illinois

Ronald B. Goldberg, M.D. Professor of Medicine, Chief, Division of Diabetes and Metabolism, Diabetes Research Institute, University of Miami School of Medicine, Miami, Florida

Paul N. Hopkins, M.D., M.S.P.H. Associate Professor of Medicine, Division of Cardiology, Cardiovascular Genetics Research Clinic, University of Utah School of Medicine, Salt Lake City, Utah

---

Current affiliations:
[*] Urbanización Monteprincipe, Centro de CC Experimentales y Técnicas, University of San Pablo, Madrid, Spain
[†] Research Unit, Hospital de la Candelaria, Santa Cruz de Tenerife, Canary Islands, Spain

Steven C. Hunt, Ph.D. Professor of Medicine, Division of Cardiology, Cardiovascular Genetics Research Clinic, University of Utah School of Medicine, Salt Lake City, Utah

Robert H. Knopp, M.D. Professor of Medicine and Director, Northwest Lipid Research Clinic; University of Washington School of Medicine; and Chief, Endocrinology, Metabolism and Nutrition, Harborview Medical Center, Seattle, Washington

Thomas E. Kottke, M.D., M.S.P.H. Professor, Department of Medicine, Mayo Clinic and Foundation, Rochester, Minnesota

John C. LaRosa, M.D., F.A.C.P. Chancellor, Tulane University Medical Center, New Orleans, Louisiana

Miriam A. Marquez, Ph.D.[‡] Department of Medicine, Mayo Clinic and Foundation, Rochester, Minnesota

Bertram Pitt, M.D. Professor, Department of Internal Medicine, University of Michigan Medical School, Ann Arbor, Michigan

William C. Roberts, M.D. Executive Director, Baylor Cardiovascular Institute, Baylor University Medical Center, Dallas, Texas

Orlando Rodríguez, M.D. Instructor of Medicine, Cardiovascular Division, Beth Israel-Deaconess Medical Center, and Harvard Medical School, Boston, Massachusetts

Neil J. Stone, M.D. Professor of Clinical Medicine, Department of Cardiology, Northwestern University School of Medicine, Chicago, Illinois

Robert A. Vogel, M.D. Herbert Berger Professor of Medicine, Associate Chairman for Clinical Affairs, and Head, Division of Cardiology, Department of Medicine, University of Maryland School of Medicine, Baltimore, Maryland

Roger R. Williams, M.D. Professor of Medicine, Division of Cardiology, and Director, Cardiovascular Genetics Research Clinic, University of Utah School of Medicine, Salt Lake City, Utah

Joseph L. Witztum, M.D. Professor of Medicine, Division of Endocrinology and Metabolism, Department of Medicine, and Co-Director, Specialized Center of Research in Atherosclerosis, University of California, San Diego, La Jolla, California

---

[‡] *Current affiliation*: School of Public Health, University of Puerto Rico, San Juan, Puerto Rico

Lily Wu, Ph.D. Associate Professor of Pathology and Medicine (Cardiology), Cardiovascular Genetics Research Clinic, University of Utah School of Medicine, Salt Lake City, Utah

Xiaodong Zhu, M.D. Senior Research Fellow, Department of Medicine, Northwest Lipid Research Clinic, and University of Washington School of Medicine, Seattle, Washington

Medical

Management

of

Atherosclerosis

1
Lipid Lowering

John C. LaRosa
Tulane University Medical Center, New Orleans, Louisiana

I. INTRODUCTION

The central role that circulating lipids, particularly cholesterol, play in the pathogenesis of atherosclerosis is reviewed (1). Given that central role, it is not surprising that circulating cholesterol, triglycerides, apoproteins, and the lipoproproteins with which they are associated have all been identified as risk factors for atherogenesis, particularly in the coronary arteries.

The overall purpose of this book is to review the medical therapies that are effective in preventing the progression of atherosclerotic disease, particularly in the coronary arteries. The best treatment, however, is still prevention. For that reason the role of circulating lipids in the identification of those at high risk of developing coronary atherosclerosis will be reviewed, as will the evidence that lipid lowering is of benefit in preventing or delaying the initial onset of coronary disease.

For purposes of orientation, an overview of the clinically salient aspects of lipid and lipoprotein metabolism and their relationship to atherogenesis is the first order of business.

II. LIPOPROTEIN METABOLISM

A. Lipoproteins

Lipoproteins are large, spherical, macromolecules with a core of water-insoluble neutral lipid, triglyceride, and esterified cholesterol, surrounded by a

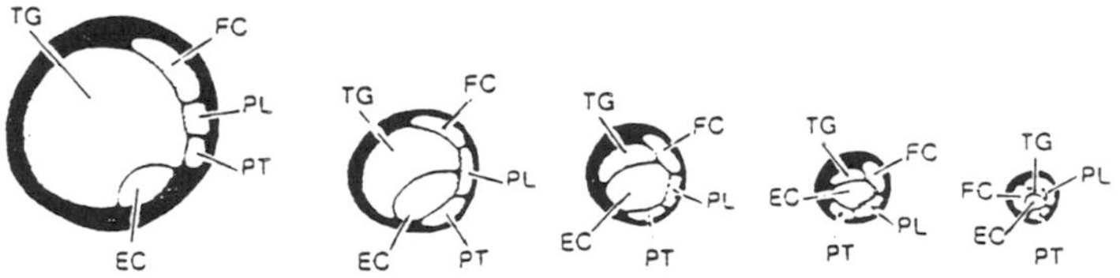

	CHYLOMICRONS		VLDL	IDL	LDL	HDL
Electrophoretic Mobility	Origin		Prebeta (Alpha-2) Globulin Region	Beta to Prebeta	Beta	Alpha
Hydrated Density	<1.006		<1.006	1.006-1.109	1.019-1.063	1.063-1.21
Diameter (A°)	750-12,000		500-700	300-500	225	100-150
Lipids (%)						
Cholesterol	5		20	40	50	25
Triglycerides	90		60	20	7	5
Phospholipids	3		14	22	22	26
Protein	2		6	18	21	44
Apoprotein	A,B,C,E		A,B,C,E	B,E	B	A,C

Figure 1   Plasma lipoproteins. FC = free cholesterol; PL = phospholipid; PT = protein; TG = triglycerides; EC = esterified cholesterol; VLDL = very low density lipoproteins; IDL = intermediate density lipoproteins; LDL = low density lipoproteins; HDL = High density lipoproteins.

shell of more soluble protein, phospholipid, and unesterified cholesterol. Their major function is the transport of lipids in the plasma for a variety of metabolic purposes (2).

Lipoproteins are traditionally subdivided into several classes based on their hydrated density (Fig. 1) (2). Chylomicrons and very low density lipoproteins (VLDL) are large (in diameter), relatively light lipoproteins that carry most of the plasma triglyceride. Low-density lipoproteins (LDL) and high-density lipoproteins (HDL) are smaller and more dense, and carry more cholesterol and protein and much less triglyceride.

B.   Apoproteins

The proteins that form part of the lipoprotein outer shell are called apolipoproteins, or apoproteins. Apoproteins also serve as the activators or inhibitors of the enzymes that catalyze lipoprotein metabolism and as ligands or recognition sites for cell surface receptors that bind circulating lipoproteins (3).

Apoproteins are named by an alphabetical nomenclature (Table 1) (4). Like lipids, they are found in more than one lipoprotein species and may exchange between lipoproteins. For example, Apoprotein B-100 is found in LDL, IDL, and VLDL.

C. Lipid Transport

Lipoprotein metabolism may be thought of as a process by which large, triglyceride-rich lipoproteins formed in the liver and intestine are converted to smaller, cholesterol-rich lipoproteins.

1.   Chylomicrons and Very Low Density Lipoproteins

Lipid transport begins in the intestine and the liver. Both the intestine and the liver produce large amounts of triglyceride that must be transported for storage in adipose tissue sites. In the intestine, triglyceride accumulates in enterocytes as a result of dietary fat ingestion. In the liver, the triglyceride is synthesized from circulating carbohydrates and free fatty acids.

Intestinal triglycerides are incorporated into lipoproteins called chylomicrons. Chylomicrons are not transported in the portal circulation but are taken up by intestinal lymphatics and enter the bloodstream via the thoracic duct. The counterparts of chylomicrons in the liver are VLDL. Both of these lipoproteins find their way into the peripheral circulation. In adipose tissue and skeletal muscle, both chylomicrons and VLDL are acted upon by lipoprotein lipase (LPL), an enzyme found on the surface of endothelial cells. Apoprotein C-II (apo-C-II), present on both chylomicrons and VLDL, acts as a cofactor to enhance the activity of this enzyme. As a result of this lipolytic reaction, 70% to 80% of the core triglyceride is converted to free fatty acids, glycerol, and monoglyceride, all of which traverse the cell membrane, are resynthesized into triglyceride, and stored.

As these large triglyceride-carrying lipoprotein particles lose their core triglyceride (but not, for the most part, their core cholesterol), they diminish in size. The redundant constituents of the outer shell (i.e., apoproteins, phospholipid, and free cholesterol) break away and join the HDL fraction. Shell re-forms around the smaller cholesterol-enriched core. The resulting smaller lipoproteins are referred to as remnants.

2.   Remnants

Chylomicron remnants are removed from circulation by the liver by binding to cell surface receptor proteins, called remnant receptors, apo-E receptors, or lipoprotein-related protein (LRP). VLDL remnants are taken up by both remnant receptors and LDL receptors. The latter recognizes the apo-B-100 on

Table 1 Characteristics of the Major Apoproteins

Apolipo-protein	Molecular weight	Lipoproteins	Metabolic functions
apo-A-1	28,016	HDL, chylomicrons	Structural component of HDL; LCAT activator
apo-A-11	17,414	HDL, chylomicrons	Unknown
apo-A-IV	46,465	HDL, chylomicrons	Unknown: possibly facilitates transfer of other apolipo-proteins between HDL and chylomicrons
apo-B-48	264,000	Chylomicrons	Necessary for assembly and secretion of chylomicrons from the small intestine
apo-B-100	514,000	VLDL, IDL, LDL	Necessary for assembly and secretion of VLDL from the liver; structural protein of VLDL, IDL, LDL; ligand for LDL receptor
apo-C-I	6630	All major lipoproteins	
apo-C-II	8900	All major lipoproteins	Activator of lipoprotein lipase
apo-C-III	800	All major lipoproteins	Inhibitor of lipoprotein lipase; may inhibit hepatic uptake of chylomicron and VLDL remnants
apo-E	34,145	All major lipoproteins	Ligand for binding of several lipoproteins to the LDL re-ceptor, and possibly to a sep-arate hepatic apo-E receptor

HDL = High-density lipoprotein; LCAT = lecithin-cholestorol acyltransterase; VLDL = very low-density lipoprotein; IDL = intermediate-density lipoprotein; LDL = low-density lipoprotein.

the surface of VLDL remnants. Chylomicron remnants, in contrast, contain another form of apo-B, apo-B-48 (Table 1) (2), which does not appear to play any role in receptor interactions and is not recognized by the LDL receptor. They attach to remnant receptors, probably by virtue of Apo-E on their surface.

When chylomicron remnants are taken up by the liver, they deliver their cholesterol to that organ. As a result of the process of chylomicron metabolism, dietary triglyceride is stored mainly in adipose tissue, while dietary cholesterol is stored in the liver.

Very low density lipoprotein remnants may, however, depending on their size, be metabolized differently. Catabolism of large VLDL by LPL results in remnants that are removed from the circulation by the liver. Catabolism of smaller VLDL, however, leads to remnants that are smaller, called intermediate-density lipoproteins (IDL). IDL may be acted on in the liver by another noncirculating lipolytic enzyme, hepatic triglyceride lipase (HTGL). IDL is then converted to LDL, the major carrier of cholesterol in the plasma.

3. LDL

Low density lipoprotein is a smaller lipoprotein than chylomicrons or VLDL, with a single apo-B-100 molecule on its surface. It carries about 75% of the circulating cholesterol but relatively little triglyceride (Table 1). Most human cells contain LDL cell surface receptors, and LDL is thought to be the main external source of cholesterol for cells. About 60% of circulating LDL is removed by the liver, the rest by peripheral tissues. Once bound to the LDL surface receptor, the LDL-receptor complex is internalized, and the cholesterol is either stored or used to make cell membranes, bile salts, or gonadal hormones, depending on the tissue involved. As intracellular cholesterol accumulates, it also inhibits cellular cholesterol synthesis as well as the synthesis of LDL receptors.

Only the liver has the ability to convert cholesterol to bile salts and excrete them. Other cells must rely on the presence of HDL to rid themselves of excess cholesterol.

4. HDL

High density lipoprotein is the smallest, densest lipoprotein with the lowest amount of triglyceride. Some nascent forms of HDL are not spherical but rather disk-shaped. These may be thought of as a lipoprotein shell lacking a lipid core. HDL may be synthesized de novo in both the liver and intestine. Some HDL components come directly from the excess surface material produced as chylomicrons, and VLDL are converted to remnants.

It is possible that cholesterol-poor HDL binds to a specific cell surface receptor, picks up free cholesterol from the cell membrane, and adds it to its own surface. In the plasma, in the presence of a protein called apoprotein D (apo-D), the free cholesterol in the lipoprotein surface is esterified by accepting a fatty acid molecule from circulating lecithin and interfacing with an enzyme called lecithin cholesterol acetyl transferase (LCAT).

Apoprotein A-I (apo-A-I) on the surface of HDL acts as a cofactor for LCAT. The cholesterol ester formed is then transferred into the HDL core and transported to the liver for excretion or passed onto other lipoproteins by combining with a circulating protein called cholesterol ester transfer protein

(CETP). In this way, excess cholesterol is eventually transported to the liver, the only organ from which it can be excreted. The cholesterol-rich HDL that actually delivers cholesterol to the liver also has on its surface apo-E, which can be recognized by both LDL and remnant receptors and may thus be an efficient mechanism for allowing HDL uptake by the liver (2).

D. Lipoproteins and Atherogenesis

At least three lipoprotein species, oxidized LDL, IDL, and chylomicron remnants, can be shown in vitro to convert scavenger cells to foam cells—that is, cells laden with cholesterol ester in their cytoplasm (2). Clinical states in which these three lipoproteins accumulate are associated with an increased risk of clinical atherosclerosis. Whether small VLDL may also be directly atherogenic is an unsettled question. The mechanisms by which the process of atherosclerosis proceeds are discussed elsewhere in this book.

HDL can be shown in vitro to clear cholesterol from foam cells. Presumably, by the process of reverse cholesterol transport, it accumulates and transports cholesterol ester to the liver, where it can be metabolized (3). It is reasonable to hypothesize that diet, exercise, weight control, and drug interventions that lead to lower LDL, IDL, and chylomicron levels and to higher HDL levels will lower the risk of clinical atherosclerosis.

E. Lipids as Coronary Risk Factors

A risk factor is a characteristic of an individual or a population that predicts the chances of the development of coronary atherosclerosis. For almost 50 years circulating levels of blood cholesterol have been recognized as powerful predictors of coronary risk (5). This has been true in comparisons of diverse populations around the world as well as within individual populations. Risk factors are usually defined by their ability to predict relative risk of coronary disease, that is, to predict the risk in a group of individuals with the characteristic compared to those without. Cholesterol and other circulating lipids, however, are also strong predictors of absolute risk. That is, they predict the absolute number of coronary events in a population. In the elderly, where the ability of lipid fractions to predict relative risk is diminished, the power to predict absolute risk is actually increased because more events occur as individuals age (6).

Observational epidemiologic studies demonstrate that cholesterol levels are a factor in the prognosis of patients with established coronary heart disease (CHD). In the Framingham Study, for example, women with cholesterol levels higher than 275 mg/dl (7.0 mmol/L) had a ninefold greater risk of recurrent myocardial infarction (MI) than women with levels < 200 mg/dl (5.2 mmol/L).

At the higher of these same levels, men have a fourfold increase in risk in recurrent events and both sexes have a doubled risk of coronary death (7).

In a 10-year follow-up of men with and without documented CHD, the Lipid Research Clinic Prevalence studies showed that both LDL cholesterol (LDL-C) and HDL cholesterol (HDL-C) levels were strong predictors of risk. In both groups, the relative risk of death from coronary disease was proportional to increased LDL-C and decreased HDL-C levels. The absolute risk of coronary death, while still proportional to LDL-C and HDL-C levels, was greater in those with established CHD. Men with LDL-C levels > 160 mg/dl (4.1 mmol/L) had five times the risk of coronary death as those without documented disease but with the same LDL-C levels (8).

1. The "Normal" Cholesterol Level

In both animal and population experiments it has been observed that atherogenesis and the development of extracellular subendothelial cholesterol pools do not proceed in the presence of circulating cholesterol levels < 160 mg/dl (4.1 mmol/L) (5,9). A "normal" circulating total cholesterol, i.e., one below which vascular disease is unlikely, is something < 160 mg/dl (4.1 mmol/L) regardless of the mean cholesterol level in a particular population. This means populations whose average cholesterol is much higher than that are likely to have much greater risk of coronary risk than the populations in which mean cholesterol is at or below that number. Other risk factors, like diabetes, cigarette smoking, and hypertension, while important in the promotion of atherogenesis, are not in themselves sufficient for the development of atherosclerosis if cholesterol levels are < 160 mg/dl (4.1 mmol/L). Thus, populations in Japan and China with high per-capita cigarette consumption, high average mean blood pressures, and comparable rates of diabetes have levels of coronary atherosclerosis one-quarter to one-fifth of those found in western populations (10).

An elevated circulating cholesterol level (in this context, > 160 mg/dl [4.1 mmol/L]), then, is a sine qua non for the development of atherosclerosis. In that sense, circulating cholesterol is the most important risk factor in the development of atherosclerosis. While diabetes, high blood pressure, or smoking alone increases the rate of coronary disease, the effect of these risk factors is greatly multiplied when cholesterol levels are also elevated (11). The implication for public health programs is that the goal of lowering rates of atherosclerosis is best served by mass dietary change to lower the average level of blood cholesterol. This is not to say that intervention on other risk factors is not important in coronary prevention. Nor is it to ignore the fact that prevention of other diseases may also be favorably affected by lowering noncholesterol coronary risk factors. For example, cessation of tobacco smok-

Table 2 Association of Hyperlipidemia and CHD Risk

| Sex and age (yr) | Relative risk | | |
	Total cholesterol	LDL-C	HDL-C
Women			
< 65	2.44	3.27	2.13
≥ 65	1.12	1.13	1.75
Men			
< 65	1.73	1.92	2.31
≥ 65	1.32	1.51	1.09

ing is likely to lower levels of not only atherosclerosis, but also chronic lung disease and lung cancer. It does mean, however, that no public health or medical program whose goal is to lower rates of atherosclerosis is likely to be fully successful without a major emphasis on cholesterol reduction.

It has become clear over the last several decades that total cholesterol, however, while a convenient and important measurement, is not as refined a predictor of risk as other circulating lipid fractions.

2. LDL-C

About 30 years ago, measures of LDL-C, that is, an estimate of the levels of LDL estimated by the cholesterol content of the fraction, were proposed as more precise measures of risk of coronary disease. This concept has taken hold more firmly in the U.S. than in other parts of the world.

There is no question that LDL-C is a major CHD risk factor. Measurements of LDL-C are more precise estimates of risk than total cholesterol, particularly in population subgroups, i.e., women, where HDL-C may carry large fractions of the total cholesterol. LDL-C is a strong predictor of risk in both men and women. However, its power to predict relative risk diminishes, in both sexes, with age (Table 2) (12). On the other hand, the power of both total cholesterol and LDL cholesterol to predict *absolute* risk in older men actually increases with age. (This finding has not been tested in older women.) In other words, the risk attributable to total or LDL-C actually increases with age.

In general, LDL-C accounts for about 75% of the total circulating cholesterol. This varies, however, from one individual to another, from one sex to the other, and even among various ethnic groups. African-Americans, for example, have on average the same total cholesterol as Caucasians, but higher HDL-C and lower LDL-C (13).

The usefulness of LDL-C is limited by the difficulties in measuring it. It can be reasonably estimated by the Friedewald formula, which estimates LDL-C by the following: LDL-C = total cholesterol minus (HDL-C + TG/5) (14). Above a triglyceride of about 400 mg/dl (4.5 mmol/L), however, this formula loses validity. The only other way to measure LDL-C is by ultra-centrifugation, a technique that is expensive, laborious, and not easily adapted to routine clinical practice.

The methods by which LDL-C is directly measured, moreover, eliminate IDL and other remnant lipoprotein particles, which themselves have a high cholesterol content and have been implicated in the atherogenic process. It has been proposed that a more rational measure of risk might be "non-HDL" cholesterol, that is, total cholesterol minus HDL-C (15,16). This would provide a better estimate not only of LDL-C but also of other cholesterol-rich atherogenic lipoproteins that are circulating. Unfortunately, in the past 30 years most of the epidemiologic and clinical data that have accumulated have emphasized either total cholesterol or LDL-C, so that substitution with non HDL-C would be fraught with translational difficulties.

LDL-C forms the basis of the intervention guidelines promulgated by the U.S. National Cholesterol Education Program (NCEP) (17). It figures less prominently in the European Atherosclerosis Society guidelines, where total cholesterol is used (18). As a predictor of CHD risk, total cholesterol is a reasonable surrogate for LDL-C levels, although it is a better substitute for LDL-C levels in men than in women. This may, in part, result simply from the fact that most coronary disease in women occurs over the age of 65, when LDL-C is, in both sexes, less predictive of relative risk (12). There are, in addition, good physiologic reasons to believe that LDL-C may be less dangerous in women than in men. It has been demonstrated, for example, that estrogen inhibits the uptake of LDL by the arterial wall (19).

Even allowing for these variations, however, it is clear that in every population in which it has been studied, there is a linear relationship between circulating LDL-C levels and coronary risk, and that both LDL-C and total cholesterol predict the degree of coronary risk.

3. HDL-C

High-density lipoprotein represents that fraction of the circulating cholesterol that is inversely associated with coronary disease risk. There is a substantial body of evidence that supports the notion that this protection is, in fact, due to HDL's function as a promoter of cholesterol efflux from cells, including those in the arterial wall. Other mechanisms, including HDL's antioxidant properties and its inverse relationship with circulating levels of atherogenic proteins, have also been proposed as explanations for the inverse relationship between circulating levels of HDL and atherosclerotic risk (20).

HDL-C levels are raised by estrogen. It is widely believed that the relative protection, particularly in premenopausal years, that women enjoy against atherosclerosis, is at least partially related to their higher circulating levels of HDL-C. Interestingly, however, HDL-C levels do not decline much in postmenopausal women, and the increasing risk of coronary disease in older women is related to the higher levels of LDL-C that are associated with aging of women in Western populations (21).

As a CHD risk factor, HDL-C is somewhat more complicated than LDL-C. In interpopulation studies, HDL-C levels are not as consistently predictive of coronary disease. Thus, in Asian populations, where dietary cholesterol and saturated-fat intake are low, and where LDL-C levels are low, HDL-C levels are, by Western standards, also low (22). This is also true of Caucasian vegetarian populations (23). This is related to the fact that dietary cholesterol and saturated fat raise both LDL and HDL cholesterol content (24). Because estimates of HDL-C, like those of LDL-C, are based on lipoprotein cholesterol content, low levels of HDL in populations with low intake of animal fat should not be surprising. Nevertheless, as is true of other coronary risk factors, low levels of HDL can be tolerated without the development of atherosclerosis when LDL-C levels are also low. It is perhaps best to think of HDL in the same way that other risk factors are regarded. It is a powerful predictor when LDL-C or total cholesterol levels are above the threshold necessary to develop atherogenesis. Like total cholesterol and LDL-C, HDL-C loses some of its power to predict relative risk of coronary disease as populations age (12). Even so, in studies of older populations, both HDL-C and total cholesterol to HDL-C ratios continue to predict both relative and absolute risk of coronary disease (25).

4. Triglyceride

Debate about whether or not triglyceride should be regarded as an independent risk factor has continued for 25 years. With few exceptions, triglycerides predict little or no additional risk when controlled for total LDL or HDL-C levels (26). The relevance of such statistical analyses can be questioned, however, since triglyceride carried mostly in the VLDL fraction is intimately related metabolically to circulating LDL and HDL.

In fact, it is that intimate interrelationship that may ultimately define the value of triglyceride as a predictor of risk. When triglyceride levels are high, HDL-C levels are low. The precise pathophysiologic mechanisms of this relationship have not been fully clarified. They may relate to several factors, including lower production of HDL particles and higher catabolic rates of triglyceride-laden HDL (27).

High triglyceride levels are also associated with formation of triglyceride-laden LDL particles. These smaller, denser LDL particles are thought to be more atherogenic (28). Thus, high triglycerides may not themselves be directly involved in atherogenesis but may be markers for lipoprotein states, including low HDL, high levels of triglyceride-laden atherogenic LDL, and high levels of triglyceride-laden remnant particles, all of which are atherogenic. Considering these relationships, the fact that triglyceride levels are not statistically independent predictors of coronary risk (and probably not *directly* involved in atherogenesis) becomes largely irrelevant. What is important is that the triglyceride levels are strong markers of metabolic changes in other lipoproteins that produce atherogenesis.

The consequences of very high levels of triglyceride (> 1000 mg/dl [11.4 mmol/L]), in particular, acute pancreatitis, occur too rarely to be accounted for in most population studies. The very large chylomicron particles that carry triglycerides at these levels, however, do not appear to be atherogenic.

Finally, high triglyceride levels are often markers of other conditions, including diabetes, hyperinsulinemia, and high levels of interabdominal fat, all of which may, either through the effects on circulating lipoproteins or through other independent effects, be predictors of and causally related to the acceleration of atherogenesis (29).

5. Apoproteins

In recent years, the ability to measure the protein components of lipoproteins, the so-called apoproteins, has led to suggestions that these circulating factors, which may be more precisely measured than the cholesterol content of lipoproteins, should be considered primary predictors of coronary risk (30). Apoprotein B (apo-B) levels, for example, which are better correlated with "non-HDL" cholesterol than with LDL-C, are reflective not only of LDL levels but also levels of other apo-B-containing remnants that may be atherogenic and, as such, may be better predictors of risk. While many studies have examined apoprotein B, apoprotein A-1, and apoprotein A-2 as predictors of risk, few have convincingly demonstrated that apoproteins are significantly better predictors than lipoprotein cholesterol levels (30,31). The lack of standardization of apoprotein measurements as well as the lack of widespread availability make them interesting items for continued research but impractical as substitutes for currently available cholesterol and triglyceride measurements.

6. Lipoprotein(a)

Lipoprotein(a) (Lp[a]) is an odd circulating complex composed of an LDL molecule joined by a disulfide bond to a complex peptide that is 80% identical to plasminogen. It has been clearly demonstrated as a strong predictor of coronary risk. This is true in both men and women and in populations around the world. Reproducible measurement of Lp(a), however, remains problematic. It is at this point unclear whether it offers any advantages over more traditional lipoprotein fractions. Its role in clinical practice is as yet unclear (32,33).

7. Ratios

It has been proposed that a better estimate of coronary risk than individual cholesterol subfractions would be ratios, either total cholesterol to HDL-C or LDL-C to HDL-C. In a sense, this is an alternative method for measuring non-HDL-C and represents an attempt to correct total cholesterol for HDL-C. It has been suggested, for example, that the total cholesterol-to-HDL ratio would be a better predictor of risk, able to select more accurately those at risk than the LDL-C levels recommended by the NCEP (34). Use of such ratios, moreover, would enable clinicians to avoid treatment of patients with high total cholesterol whose HDL-C levels were also high. As a single number, it is probably true that ratios are more useful information than LDL-C or HDL-C alone. Like non-HDL-C, however, they suffer from the lack of a strong epidemiologic and clinical trial data base. At this point, there is no general agreement as to how these ratios might best be used. Neither U.S. nor European guidelines emphasize them.

8. Intergroup Differences in Lipids as Atherosclerotic Risk Factors

Total cholesterol is a predictor of coronary risk in all populations in which it has been studied. It is a more powerful predictor in western than in non-western populations. This may relate to other factors not reflected in total cholesterol levels, including dietary levels of antioxidants and fiber, levels of physical activity and body weight, and genetic differences (35). It should be noted, however, that when Asian populations like the Japanese move and adopt western eating habits, their cholesterol levels rise, as do their coronary risk levels (36). It has already been noted that cholesterol and its subfractions are poorer predictors of relative risk of CHD in older women than in men. Triglycerides, on the other hand, appear to be stronger predictors of risk in women than in men, for reasons that are not clear (37).

Circulating lipids, then, are powerful predictors of CHD risk. When the pathogenesis of atherosclerosis is considered, they are indispensable determinants of the atherosclerotic process. Public health estimates that purport to measure coronary risk in a given population, or even in individual patients, are meaningless without measurements of cholesterol, triglyceride, and their lipoprotein subfractions. It is likely that in the future measures other than those currently used may be adopted as better predictors of coronary risk. These may include apoprotein measurements, lipoprotein ratios, or measurements of newer lipoprotein fractions like Lp(a) or various genetic markers of risk. These refinements, however, will not diminish the central importance of lipids in predicting atherosclerotic risk in individuals and in populations.

III. CLINICAL TRIALS OF LIPID LOWERING

The power of circulating lipids to predict coronary risk does not necessarily mean that changes in such risk factors produce changes in atherosclerotic risk. In fact, recommendations to intervene on a given risk factor as a means of reducing risk are usually not widely endorsed until there is clinical trial evidence that such intervention produces benefit.

The earliest trials of cholesterol lowering were done in patients with established coronary disease (38). For purposes of completeness rather than chronologic consistency, however, trials of primary prevention will first be briefly reviewed.

A. Primary Prevention Trials

A number of "primary" prevention studies, some quite large, in patients without coronary disease but with elevated cholesterol levels have been completed. Because event rates are much lower in those without clinically established disease (and presumably with less advanced atherosclerosis), the number of subjects required in these studies was much larger. Cholesterol lowering was only in the 5% to 15% range. The major studies, including the World Health Organization study using clofibrate (39), the Lipid Research Clinics Primary Prevention Trial utilizing cholestyramine (40), and the Helsinki Heart Study using gemfibrozil (41), were carried on for 5 or more years. Meta-analyses of these primary prevention trials demonstrated definite declines in coronary mortality but no decline in total mortality, since coronary mortality was offset by increases in noncardiovascular mortality (Fig. 2) (42). This last observation was particularly true in the World Health Organization study, which, as the largest of the primary prevention trials, heavily influenced all meta-analyses in which it was included. These noncardiovascular mortal events were from cancer and from nonillness causes, including suicides, homicides, or accidents. No single form of cancer could be demonstrated to be associated with cholesterol treatment. Nonillness death was only significant if suicides, homicides, and accidental deaths were added together. The validity of adding all forms of cancer or all forms of noncardiovascular, noncancer deaths, of course, is highly questionable.

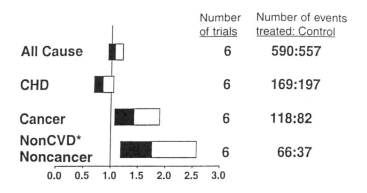

Figure 2   Meta-analysis of primary prevention trials. *Accidents, violence, trauma, suicide.

Nevertheless, meta-analyses including these studies produced concern that cholesterol lowering might itself promote noncardiovascular mortality. The means of cholesterol lowering in these studies ranged from diet through cholesterol-lowering drugs to hormones like dextrothyroxin and estrogen (in men). When analyzed in meta-analysis by treatment modality, it was clear that the excess mortality apparent in these studies was limited to studies in which other fibrates or hormones were used and was completely unrelated to the degree of cholesterol lowering (43,44).

The West of Scotland Coronary Prevention Study (WOSCPS) put to rest many of the concerns about primary prevention. In this study, middle-aged men (no women were included) without a prior history of myocardial infarction (MI) were included. This, of course, does not mean that those men included in the study were without coronary disease. In fact, it is likely that most middle-aged men in Western populations have some coronary atherosclerosis. What it does signify is the likelihood that their coronary disease, on the average, was at an earlier stage of development than those with clinical coronary disease. The average cholesterol of participants was 272 mg/dl (7.0 mmol/L); LDL cholesterol was 192 mg/dl (4.9 mmol/L).

Cholesterol in WOSCSP was lowered with pravastatin, 40 mg/day. Cholesterol fell by 20%; LDL by 26%. There was a 31% decrease in the incidence of first MI, whether fatal or nonfatal, the major endpoint of the study. Of great importance was a 21% lowering in total mortality, the first evidence that total mortality could be favorably affected in those without clinical coronary disease. There was no indication of an increase in noncardiovascular mortality, in the form of either cancer or traumatic death. The benefit of cholesterol lowering was not limited to those with other risk factors but was equivalent in those with or without other coronary risk factors. Those > 55 years of age had essentially the same benefit as those < 55 years of age. Thus, it was clearly demonstrated in this group of middle-aged men without clinical coronary disease that cholesterol lowering not only lowers coronary event rates but lowers coronary and total mortality rates as well. As a result of all these primary prevention trials, it is apparent that cholesterol lowering, at the very least, can significantly lower the likelihood of the first coronary event.

B. Secondary Prevention Trials

1. Early Trials

Many of the earliest trials of cholesterol lowering in those with established coronary disease (secondary prevention) were small and not of sufficient size to detect a significant benefit. Cholesterol lowering achieved in virtually all of these studies was in the 5% to 15% range, far from what is achievable today with the newer cholesterol-lowering drugs. Few studies measured cholesterol subfractions such as LDL or HDL cholesterol. Most did not report triglyceride levels. There is neither time nor space to review each of these studies individually. Meta-analyses of these early secondary prevention trials, however, have been done (45,46) (Fig. 3). These indicate that cholesterol reduction did indeed produce a reduction in coronary events, a borderline reduction in coronary death and total mortality, and no increase in noncardiovascular mortality. That is, the benefit on coronary morbidity and mortality was not counterbalanced by potential adverse effects leading to increased noncardiovascular events. Thus, even from these early studies, it was clear that intervention on cholesterol was important. Because meta-analysis was not

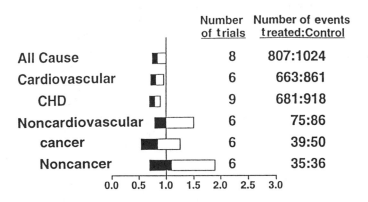

Figure 3 Meta-analysis of secondary prevention trials.

available, however, and because many of the individual studies were small and inconclusive, the message until recently was lost.

2. Trials of Vascular Endpoints

Failure to define clearly the benefits of cholesterol lowering in these studies led to attempts to examine more directly the effects on the coronary anatomy. A number of "regression" studies, some utilizing older cholesterol-lowering drugs (47–49) and, more recently, utilizing HMG-CoA reductase-inhibiting drugs (statins), which have the capacity to induce twice the cholesterol lowering achieved in older studies, have now been reported. Impressive examples of regression can be demonstrated in these studies. Overall, however, there is only slight regression in most of these studies. There are two effects that have predominated. First, the progression of atherosclerosis is slowed or halted by cholesterol lowering (50). Second, meta-analyses indicate a decline in events by about one-third (51). Since we now realize that the most active lesions are not necessarily the most occlusive ones (52), the apparent dichotomy between only modest changes in coronary anatomy and dramatic changes in events can be readily explained. Stabilization of active lesions by cholesterol lowering, even when they are not highly occlusive, while failing to alter the angiographic appearance of lesions, decreases the likelihood that they will produce the spasm, clot, and internal hemorrhage that lead to acute occlusion. Studies of LDL-cholesterol lowering on carotid wall thickening, moreover, have demonstrated similar results, i.e., small but favorable vascular changes associated with declines in coronary events.

A recent angiographic study of cholesterol lowering in 1351 men who had undergone coronary bypass surgery reaffirmed the value of aggressive LDL-C lowering. In this study, average beginning LDL-C was 156 mg/dl (4.0 mmol/L). Subjects were randomly assigned either aggressive or moderate LDL-C lowering with lovastatin, combined in some cases with cholestyramine. They were followed for approximately 4.5 years. In the aggressive group, which received on average 75 mg lovastatin per day, LDL-C levels reached a mean of 93 mg/dl (2.4 mmol/L). In contrast, the moderate group achieved an average LDL-C of 136 mg/dl (3.5 mmol/L), receiving only 4 mg of lovastatin daily. General progression of disease, luminal narrowing, and the appearance of new lesions were all more pronounced in the moderate group. After 2.5 years, repeat CABG was 39% less frequent; angioplasty was 29% less frequent, and all events were 18% less frequent in the aggressive group (53).

None of these angiographic studies were large enough to demonstrate effects on mortality. This issue, however, has been addressed in the Scandinavian Simvastatin Survival Study (4S) (54), a secondary prevention study using simvastatin in doses up to 40 mg/day to achieve total cholesterol levels between 120 and 200 mg/dl (3.0 to 5.1 mmol/L). Four thousand four hundred forty-four (4444) patients were included, of whom 81% were men. Average initial cholesterol levels of subjects were between 220 and 300 mg/dl (5.7 to 7.7 mmol/L); total and LDL cholesterol were lowered 25% and 35%, respectively. Over a 5-year period, the rate of first heart attacks fell by 37%, coronary mortality by 42%, and total mortality by 30%. The 4S demonstrated clearly for the first time that total mortality in patients with CHD could be dramatically lowered by cholesterol lowering. There was no increase in cancer or noncardiovascular, noncancer deaths in this study, and no indication that cholesterol lowering with simvastatin produced any increase in noncardiovascular mortality.

Individuals > 65 years of age in the 4S had the same rate of decline in coronary events as those < 65 years of age (55). Women in the study had the same decline in event rates as men. The small number of deaths in women, however, precluded any conclusions about effects on total mortality. An interesting sidelight was that stroke rates as well as heart attack rates were lowered by about one-third in this study, implying that cholesterol lowering could favorably affect atherosclerotic events in cerebral as well as coronary arteries.

The results of the 4S are, of course, dramatic in that they demonstrate beyond doubt that vigorous attention to cholesterol lowering in those with established coronary disease is an important means of preventing the next coronary event. Aggressive treatment of those with coronary disease is strongly recommended both in the U.S. and European cholesterol policy guidelines (17,18).

A more recent study of clinical endpoints, the Cholesterol Recurrent Events (CARE) study (56), examined the effect of LDL-C lowering in those with CHD whose cholesterol was close to the average in the United States. (It is important to repeat that "average" is not equivelent to "normal" in this context.) In this study, 3500 men and 576 women with documented CHD and average total cholesterol of 209 mg/dl (3.8 mmol/L) were treated for 5 years with pravastatin 20 to 40 mg/day. At the study's conclusion, fatal and nonfatal MI were reduced 24% overall and a surprising 45% in women. Bypass surgery, angioplasty, and stroke were reduced 26%, 22%, and 28%, respectively. Benefit was not apparent if initial LDL was < 125 mg/dl (3.2 mmol/L). Fatal or nonfatal MI declined 24% in those with initial LDL-C between 125 and 150 mg/dl (3.2 to 3.9 mmol/L), and 37% in those with initial LDL > 150 mg/dl (3.9 mmol/L). Thus, even in CHD patients with average cholesterol level, LDL-C lowering was shown to be of significant benefit.

Taken together (Fig. 4) (56), the 4S, WOSCSP, and CARE studies answer many of the important controversies that have surrounded the issue

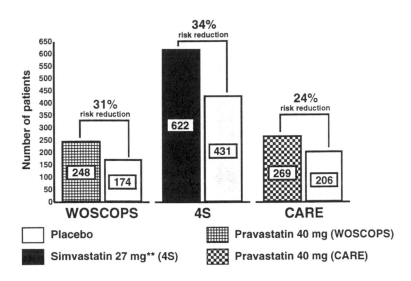

Figure 4   Coronary events in three major trials. Major coronary events were defined as coronary death or nonfatal MI. [**]Average dose in 4S.

of cholesterol lowering. It is reasonable to ask, then, if there are others that remain to be addressed.

C.   Cholesterol Lowering in the Elderly

While older individuals in both the 4S and WOSCPS seemed to have the same benefit as younger individuals, no study has ever been directed exclusively at those over the age of 65. Because the greatest burden of atherosclerosis, particularly in women, is in this age group, it is not unreasonable to ask whether cholesterol lowering has the same benefits in an age group where there are competing mortalities, higher rates of noncardiovascular illness, and the lower probability of increasing lifespan. These considerations must be coupled with the fact that cholesterol fractions seem to have less power to predict relative (although not absolute) risk in older individuals (12).

   No study has specifically addressed cholesterol lowering in older individuals, although one trial, the Antihypertensive and Lipid-Lowering Treatment to Prevent Heart Attack Trial (ALLHAT), currently in the field in the United States, is designed to address this issue by recruiting men and women > 65 years old (57).

D. Cholesterol Lowering in Women

Because women make up two-thirds of the population > 65 years of age in Western countries, a corollary to the first question is the issue of cholesterol lowering in women. What studies exist indicate that the benefits of cholesterol lowering in women are equivalent to or better than those in men (51,52,56,58). The small numbers of women included in most clinical trials, however, preclude definitive conclusions about the effects on mortality. Moreover, there has been no study in which women have been the primary targets of intervention.

Because of the poor predictability of lipoproteins as predictors of relative risk in coronary disease in older women (in whom the bulk of their coronary disease occurs), cholesterol lowering can be approached with less confidence in women than in men. Nevertheless, the process of atherogenesis appears to be identical in men and women, and incomplete results from clinical trials, as noted, appear to indicate that the benefits are the same.

E. Relative Benefits of LDL Lowering Versus Triglyceride Lowering or HDL Increasing

Virtually all studies that have been done have targeted total or LDL cholesterol as the variable to be changed. A number of studies, however, have used fibric acid derivatives, whose primary effect is to lower triglyceride and raise HDL. Many of these studies were done many years ago before triglycerides or HDLs were routinely measured and, as a result, did not report such measurements. On the other hand, in the Helsinki Primary Prevention Study (41), in which gemfibrozil was the drug used, benefit seemed to be greatest in those with the highest triglycerides and lowest HDLs. A study recruiting patients with high triglycerides and/or low HDLs as a primary inclusion criterion has not, however, been performed. Moreover, the means by which HDL might be reproducibly and significantly increased have not yet been identified, so the hypothesis is not easily tested. The Veterans Affairs High-density Lipoprotein Intervention Cholesterol Trial (HIT), designed to measure the effect of HDL raising with gemfribozil, is currently in the field (59). While there is a general agreement that, based on current information, triglyceride lowering and HDL increasing are important corollary goals, the same quality of clinical trial data does not support these conclusions as is available for LDL lowering.

1. Lipoprotein(a)

No clinical trial has yet addressed specifically the hypothesis that lowering lipoprotein(a) is of direct benefit. Some evidence exists, however, from regression studies that when LDL is lowered, the power of Lp(a) to affect

Table 3 AHA Guide to Comprehensive Risk Reduction for Patients with Coronary and Other Vascular Disease

Risk Intervention	Recommendations
Smoking: **Goal** **complete cessation**	Strongly encourage patient and family to stop smoking. Provide counseling, nicotine replacement, and formal cessation programs as appropriate.
Lipid Management: **Primary goal** LDL <100 mg/dL **Secondary goals** HDL >35 mg/dL; TG <200 mg/dL	Start AHA Step II Diet in all patients: ≤30% fat, <7% saturated fat, <200 mg/d cholesterol. Assess fasting lipid profile. In post-MI patients, lipid profile may take 4 to 6 weeks to stabilize. Add drug therapy according to the following guide:

	LDL <100 mg/dL	LDL 100 to 130 mg/dL	LDL >130 mg/dL	HDL <35 mg/dL
	No drug therapy	Consider adding drug therapy to diet, as follows:	Add drug therapy to diet, as follows:	Emphasize weight management and physical activity. Advise smoking cessation. If needed to achieve LDL goals, consider niacin, statin, fibrate.

Suggested drug therapy

TG <200 mg/dL	TG 200 to 400 mg/dL	TG >400 mg/dL
Statin Resin Niacin	Statin Niacin	Consider combined drug therapy (niacin, fibrate, statin)

If LDL goal not achieved, consider combination therapy.

Risk Intervention	Recommendations
Physical activity: **Minimum goal** 30 minutes 3 to 4 times per week	Assess risk, preferably with exercise test, to guide prescription. Encourage minimum of 30 to 60 minutes of moderate-intensity activity 3 or 4 times weekly (walking, jogging, cycling, or other aerobic activity) supplemented by an increase in daily lifestyle activities (eg, walking breaks at work, using stairs, gardening, household work). Maximum benefit 5 to 6 hours a week. Advise medically supervised programs for moderate- to high-risk patients.
Weight management:	Start intensive diet and appropriate physical intervention, as outlined above, in patients >120% of ideal weight for height. Particularly emphasize need for weight loss in patients with hypertension, elevated triglycerides, or elevated glucose levels.
Antiplatelet agents/ anticoagulants:	Start aspirin 80 to 325 mg/d if not contraindicated. Manage warfarin to international normalized ratio=2 to 3.5 post-MI patients not able to take aspirin.
ACE inhibitors post-MI:	Start early post-MI in stable high-risk patients (anterior MI, previous MI, Killip class II [S₃ gallop, rales, radiographic CHF]). Continue indefinitely for all with LV dysfunction (ejection fraction ≤40%) or symptoms of failure. Use as needed to manage blood pressure or symptoms in all other patients.
Beta-blockers:	Start in high-risk post-MI patients (arrhythmia, LV dysfunction, inducible ischemia) at 5 to 28 days. Continue 6 months minimum. Observe usual contraindications. Use as needed to manage angina, rhythm, or blood pressure in all other patients.
Estrogens:	Consider estrogen replacement in all postmenopausal women. Individualize recommendation consistent with other health risks.
Blood pressure control: **Goal** ≤140/90 mm Hg	Initiate lifestyle modification—weight control, physical activity, alcohol moderation, and moderate sodium restriction —in all patients with blood pressure >140 mm Hg systolic or 90 mm Hg diastolic. Add blood pressure medication, individualized to other patient requirements and characteristics (ie, age, race, need for drugs with specific benefits) if blood pressure is not less than 140 mm Hg systolic or 90 mm Hg diastolic in 3 months or if *initial* blood pressure is >160 mm Hg systolic or 100 mm Hg diastolic.

ACE indicates angiotensin-converting enzyme; MI, myocardial infarction; TG, triglycerides; and LV, left ventricular.

subsequent coronary disease progression is greatly diminished (60). The effect of gonadal hormones on Lp(a) is discussed in Chapter 7.

In summary, lowering of total and LDL cholesterol, then, has been shown in white, middle-aged men to lower risk of coronary morbidity and coronary and total mortality. It is likely, but not absolutely demonstrated, that these benefits accrue also to women and the elderly. It is not clear whether triglyceride lowering and/or HDL increasing have the same benefit. Clinical trials, of course, are expensive and tedious to carry out. It is reasonable to ask how many more trials are required before general recommendations to lower cholesterol by diet, or if necessary, by drugs, can be universally applied. For the foreseeable future, the answer to that question will remain a matter of individual judgment.

F. Approach to the Patient With Atherosclerosis

Treatment of CHD was once viewed as two-pronged: Drugs such as nitroglycerine, nitrates, and calcium channel blockers were prescribed to relieve ischemic symptoms and procedures, such as CABG and percutaneous transluminal coronary angioplasty (PTCA) was performed to reconstruct the coronary vasculature. Recently, the American Heart Association (AHA) and the American College of Cardiology (ACC) (61) jointly endorsed risk factor reduction—particularly in relation to lipid-lowering—as a means of significantly reducing the risk of recurrent events in patients with documented CHD (Table 3) (61).

Unlike CABG, whose effects on recurrent coronary events are limited to patients with left main or multivessel CHD, and angioplasty, which has not been shown to prevent recurrent events, lipid lowering promises to benefit many patients, with a broad range of LDL-C levels, cost-effectively.

This should not be taken to imply that angioplasty or CABG be abandoned. In a patient with angina or other symptoms of CHD, acute reduction of stenosis may be vitally important for symptom relief. In selected cases, such as those with significant occlusion of the left main coronary artery or multivessel coronary disease, CABG may be life-saving (62).

Seventy percent of myocardial infarctions, however, occur in coronary arteries that are < 50% occluded (52). This is because the degree of occlusion does not correspond to the activity of the plaque and its propensity for fissuring, rupture, clot, or spasm. Thus, angioplasty or CABG, which may not even be directed at the most dangerous or active lesions, cannot be considered as definitive treatment in patients with CHD. Such anatomic interventions should be combined with cholesterol lowering and other risk factor interventions (61) to enhance the long-term prognosis. As demonstrated in the 4S and post-CABG studies, vigorous cholesterol lowering reduces the need for anatomical intervention.

The AHA-ACC document (61) recommends other medical interventions, including aspirin therapy (63) and beta-adrenergic blockade (64) in the first year after MI. These are discussed in greater detail in other sections of this book (65,66). Cholesterol lowering is not a substitute for these interventions. In fact, in meta-analyses of cholesterol-lowering studies, conducted before the availability of statins, the same reduction in coronary events was evident with cholesterol lowering, beta-blockade, and aspirin therapy (45). More recent trials with cholesterol lowering, such as the 4S, have produced almost twice the benefits of those obtained from beta-blockade or aspirin (54). Because there is every reason to believe that these medical interventions may be at least partially additive, the use of one should not preclude the use of any or all of the others.

IV. GUIDELINES FOR SECONDARY PREVENTION OF CORONARY EVENTS

The AHA-ACC guidelines for modifying cholesterol levels in individuals with documented CHD indicate that the goal of therapy is to lower LDL-C levels to 100 mg/dl (2.5 mmol/L) (2) or below, a goal supported by the result of both CARE and post-CABG. The guidelines also recommend that a statin be the initial therapy in patients with TG levels < 400 mg/dl (4.5 mmol/L).

Four statins are available in the U.S. market; lovastatin, pravastatin, simvastatin, and fluvastatin. Their effects on lipid and lipoprotein levels are summarized in Table 4 (67). At appropriate doses, there is little difference in

Table 4 Lipid-Lowering Properties of HMG-COA Reductase Inhibitors at Recommended Daily Dose Range

Drug daily dosing regimen	(mg/day)	Change from baseline (%)			
		TC	LDL-C	HCL-C	TG
Lovastatin	10–80	16–34	↓ 21–42	↑ 2–12	↓ 10–27
Pravastatin	10–40	12.9–27.0	↓ 17.5–35.3	↑ 4.1–7.8	↓ 10.6–24.5
Simvastatin	5–40	17–32.5	↓ 23.9–40	↑ 4.8–20.6	↓ 0.9–46.2
Fluvastatin	10–40	14.6–19.5	↓ 18.9–26.1	↑ 2.5–7.8	↓ 2.7–10.6
Atorvastatin(68)	10–20	27–36	↓ 27–29	↑ 7–8	↓ 27–30

HMG-COA = hydromethylglutanyl coenzyme A; TC = total cholesterol, LDL-C = low-density lipoprotein cholesterol; HDL-C = high-density lipoprotein cholesterol; TG = triglycerides effect among lovastatin, pravastatin, or simvastatin, although the latter two require only once-a-day dosage, while lovastatin is most effective taken twice a day. At equivalent doses, fluvastatin is less potent and atorvastatin more potent. The ability of either fluvastatin or atorvastatin to protect against CHD had not been established.

All of these drugs have few adverse effects. There is a 1% incidence of liver function abnormalities and a < 0.05% incidence of skeletal myopathy. The latter may be aggravated if these drugs are used with fibric acid derivatives, niacin, cyclosporine, or erythromycin. This has particular relevance in patients requiring combination drug therapy and in patients requiring these drugs after cardiac transplantation. Table 5 summarizes the effects of these drugs compared with those of other lipid-lowering agents (69). The statins' efficacy in LDL-C lowering and infrequent side effects make them attractive choices for patients with established CHD, in whom cholesterol lowering may be life-saving.

It is unlikely that diet alone will enable many patients to decrease their high LDL-C levels to < 130 mg/dl (3.2 mmol/L). Given the early benefits of cholesterol lowering in patients with CHD and the substantial risk of recurrent, often fatal events, it is inappropriate to wait several months before beginning drug therapy. If LDL-C levels are > 100 mg/dl (2.5 mmol/L) at the time of the patient's 4 to 6 week follow-up after MI, the patient should be considered a candidate for drug intervention (61).

A. Combination Drug Therapy

The target level of 100 mg/dl (2.5 mmol/L) or below may be difficult to attain, even with the use of a statin. Consequently, therapy with a statin combined with another drug may be required in some patients (70). The best combination is one of a statin with a bile acid sequestrant, since the sequestrant adds little toxicity. Moreover, the LDL-C lowering required may not necessitate the full sequestrant dosage. Many patients will thus be able to achieve an LDL-C level < 100 mg/dl (2.5 mmol/L) with a statin plus 4 to 8 g/day of cholestyramine.

Combining a statin with niacin may also enhance LDL-C lowering, although it increases the risk of drug-induced myopathy. Because patients taking the combination may have a risk of myopathy as high as 3%, they must be instructed to report any muscle pain and immediately stop taking drugs until the source of the pain is identified and creatine kinase (CK) levels are determined. Unfortunately, regular monitoring of CK levels is of no value; CK levels do not begin to rise until the patient experiences pain.

Patients with low HDL-C, high TG, and high LDL-C levels may benefit from the combination of a statin, with either niacin or gemfibrozil. When a statin is used with gemfibrozil, however, the risk of myopathy has been

Table 5 Comparison of Lipid-Lowering Drugs

Drug	Change in lipid fraction (%)			Effect on lowering CAD risk	Adverse effects	Toxicity
	LDL-C	TG	HDL-C			
Bile acid sequestrant (cholestyramine, colestipol)	↓ 15–30	0 or ↑[a]	↑ 3–5	Yes	Constipation, bloating, belching, nausea	None
Nicotinic acid	↓ 15–25	↓ 20–50	↑ 15–30	Yes	Flushing, pruritis	Hepatotoxicity, hyperuricemia, hyperglycemia[b]
Statins[c]	↓ 20–40	↓ 10–25	↑ 15–10	Yes	Rare	Myopathy, hepatotoxicity
Gemfibrozil	↓ 0–15	↓ 20–50	↑ 10–15	Yes	Rare	Hepatotoxicity, myopathy, perhaps gallstones

LDL-C = low-density lipoprotein cholesterol: TG = triglyceride, HDL-C = high-density lipoprotein cholesterol; CAD coronary artery disease.
[a] May increase in patients with initial high TG levels.
[b] More prevalent when dose exceeds 3 g/day.
[c] HMG-CoA reductase inhibitors: lovastatin, provastatin, simvastatin, fluvastatin.

reported to be as high as 5% (70). Again, close patient monitoring is required. This combination should only be used in patients responsible enough to report early warning symptoms. A new statin, atorvastatin, lowers both LDL-C and triglyceride more effectively and may obviate the need for combination therapy in many patients (71).

B. Triple-Drug Therapy

Occasionally, lowering LDL-C levels to < 100 mg/dl (2.5 mmol/L) may require the use of three drugs (for example, the combination of a statin, niacin, and a bile acid sequestrant). Patients requiring this intensive therapy should be referred to individuals or centers with extensive experience in lipid disorders. If this is not possible, careful monitoring for signs of liver dysfunction and myopathy must be incorporated into patient management. It should also be remembered that benefits on CHD are directly related to the degree of cholesterol lowering accomplished (43), so that even if maximal LDL C lowering is not possible, there is still benefit.

V. SUMMARY

Cholesterol and related lipoprotein fractions predict recurrent events in patients with CHD. Lowering of LDL-C improves coronary anatomy and reduces recurrent events in patients with established CHD. Recent clinical studies conclusively demonstrate that statin therapy reduces coronary morbidity and mortality as well as total mortality.

While a number of cholesterol-modifying drugs, including bile acid sequestrants, niacin, and statins, are effective in LDL-C lowering and have been shown to prevent coronary events, statins have the advantages of a low side-effects profile and high compliance rate. For this reason, the AHA and ACC jointly recommend them as the drugs of choice for most patients.

Still, available evidence indicates that cholesterol lowering is underused in patients with established CHD (72,73), perhaps because of confusion over the degree of benefit they provide in patients with and without established CHD. Given the conclusive evidence of the benefits of cholesterol lowering in patients with established disease, withholding cholesterol-lowering medication in such patients is irrational and even dangerous. It is imperative that monitoring of cholesterol levels be incorporated into the management of patients with established CHD and that treatment be prompt and effective.

REFERENCES

1. Roberts WC. Preventing and arresting coronary atherosclerosis. Am. Heart J. 1995; 130:580–600.
2. Ginsberg HN. Lipoprotein metabolism and its relationship to atherosclerosis. In: Hunninghake, DB, ed. Lipid Disorders. Philadelphia: W.B. Saunders, 1994:1–20.
3. Leroy A, Dallongeville J, Fruchart JC. Apolipoprotein A-1–containing lipoproteins and atherosclerosis. Curr Opin Lipidol 1995; 6:281–285.
4. LaRosa, JC. Lipoproteins: Their role in atherosclerosis and its prevention. Needham Heights, MA. Damon Corporation, 1988, 1990. 19 pp.
5. LaRosa JC, Hunninghake D, Bush D, et al. The cholesterol facts: a summary of the evidence relating dietary fats, serum cholesterol and coronary heart disease. Circulation 1990; 81:1721–1733.
6. Rubin SM, Sidney S, Black DM, et al. High blood cholesterol in elderly men and the excess risk for coronary heart disease. Ann Intern Med 1990; 113:916–920.
7. Wong ND, Wilson PWF, Kannel WB. Serum cholesterol as a prognostic factor after myocardial infarction: the Framingham Study. Ann Intern Med 1991; 115:687–693.
8. Pekkanen J, Linn S, Heiss G, et al. Ten-year mortality from cardiovascular disease in relation to cholesterol level among men with and without preexisting cardiovascular disease. N Engl J Med 1990; 322:1700–1707.
9. St. Clair RSW. Atherosclerosis regression in animal models: current concepts of cellular and biochemical mechanisms. Prog Cardiovasc Dis 1983; 26:109–132.
10. Roberts WC. Atherosclerosis risk factors: Are there ten or is there only one? Am J Cardiol 1989; 64:552.
11. Kannel WB. Metabolic risk factors for coronary heart disease in women: perspective from the Framingham Study. Am Heart J 1987; 114:413–419.
12. Manolio TA, Pearson TA, Wenger NK, et al. Cholesterol and heart disease in older persons and women: review of an NHLBI workshop. Ann Epidemiol 1992; 2:161–176.
13. Brown SA, Hutchinson R, Morrisett J, et al. Plasma lipid, lipoprotein cholesterol, and apoprotein distributions in selected US communities. Arterioscler Thromb 1993; 13:1139–1158.
14. Friedewald WT, Levy RI, Fredrickson DS. Estimation of the concentration of low-density lipoprotein cholesterol in plasma, without use of the preparative ultracentrifuge. Clin Chem 1972; 18:499–502.
15. Sniderman AD. Apolipoprotein B and apolipoprotein AI as predictors of coronary artery disease. Can J Cardiol 1988; 4:14A–30A.
16. Vega GL, Grundy SM. Does measurement of apolipoprotein B have a place in cholesterol management? Arteriosclerosis 1990; 10:668–671.
17. Summary of the second report of the National Cholesterol Education Program (NCEP) Expert Panel on detection, evaluation, and treatment of high blood cholesterol in adults (Adult Treatment Panel II). JAMA 1993; 269:3015–3023.
18. EAS Task Force for Prevention of Coronary Heart Disease. Prevention of coronary disease: scientific background and new clinical guidelines. Nutr Metab Cardiovasc Dis 1992; 2:113–156.

19. Wagner JD, Clarkson TB, St. Clair RW. Estrogen and progesterone replacement therapy reduces low density lipoprotein accumulation in the coronary arteries of surgically postmenopausal cynomolgus monkeys. J Clin Invest 1991; 88:1995–2002.
20. Barter PJ, Rye KA. High density lipoproteins and coronary heart disease. Atherosclerosis 1996; 121:1–12.
21. Kannel WB. Nutrition and the occurrence and prevention of cardiovascular disease in the elderly. Nutr Rev 1984; 46:68–78.
22. Zhang W, Evans AE, Cambien F.et al. Distribution of lipid variables in subjects in Belfast, Northern Ireland and Taiyuan, P R China. Atherosclerosis 1993; 102:175–180.
23. Masarei JR, Rouse IL, Lynch WJ, et al. Vegetarian diets, lipids and cardiovascular risk. Aust NZ J Med 1984; 14:400–404.
24. Schaefer EJ, Lichtenstein AH, Lamon-Fava S, et al. Efficacy of a national cholesterol education program step 2 diet in normolipidemics and hypercholesterolemic middle-aged and elderly men and women. Arterioscler Thromb Vasc Biol 1995; 15:1079–1085.
25. Corti M C, Guralnik JM, Salivo ME. HDL cholesterol predicts coronary heart disease mortality in older persons. JAMA 1995; 274:539–544.
26. Gordon DJ. Role of circulating high-density lipoprotein and triglycerides in coronary artery disease: risk and prevention. Endocrinol Metabol Clin North Am, 1990; 19:299–309.
27. Sprecher DL, Feigelson HS, Laskarzewski PM. The low HDL cholesterol/high triglyceride trait. Arterioscler Thromb 1993; 13:495–504.
28. Austin MA. Small, dense low-density lipoprotein as a risk factor for coronary heart disease. Int J Clin Lab Res 1994; 24:187–192.
29. Reaven G. Syndrome X: 6 years later. J Intern Med 1994; 236(736 suppl):13–22.
30. Stampfer MJ, Sacks FM, Salvini S, et al. A prospective study of cholesterol, apolipoproteins and the risk of myocardial infarction. N Engl J Med 1991; 325:373–381.
31. Mahley RW, Innerarity TL, Rall SC Jr, et al. Plasma lipoproteins: apolipoprotein structure and function. J Lipid Res 1984; 25:1277–1294.
32. Liu A, Lawn RM. Lipoprotein(a) and atherogenesis. Trends Cardiovasc Med 1994; 4:4044.
33. Bartens W, Wanner C. Lipoprotein(a): new insights into an atherogenic lipoprotein. Clin Invest 1994; 72:558–567.
34. Grover SA, Coupal L, Hu X-P. Identifying adults at increased risk of coronary disease. JAMA 1995; 274:801–806.
35. Law MR, Wald NJ. An ecological study of serum cholesterol and ischaemic heart disease between 1950 and 1990. Eur J Clin Nutr 1994; 48:305–325.
36. Robertson TL, Kato H, Rhjoads GG, et al. Epidemiologic studies of coronary heart disease and stroke in Japanese men living in Japan, Hawaii and California. Incidence of myocardial infarction and death from coronary heart disease. Am J Cardiol 1977; 39:239–243.
37. Castelli WP. The triglyceride issue: a view from Framingham. Am Heart J 1986; 112:432–437.

38. LaRosa JC. Unresolved issues in early trials of cholesterol lowering. Am J Cardiol 1995; 76:5C–9C.
39. Report of the Committee of Principal Investigators. World Health Organization Cooperative Trial on primary prevention of ischemic heart disease using clofibrate to lower serum cholesterol: mortality follow-up. Lancet 1980; 2:379–385.
40. Lipid Research Clinics Coronary Primary Prevention Trial Results. I. Reduction in incidence of coronary heart disease. JAMA 1984; 251:351–364.
41. Frick MH, Elo O, Haapa K, et al. Helsinki Heart Study: primary-prevention trial with gemfibrozil in middle-aged men with dyslipidemia: safety of treatment, changes in risk factors and incidence of coronary heart disease. N Engl J Med 1987; 317:1237–1245.
42. Muldoon MF, Manuck SB, Matthews KA. Lowering cholesterol concentrations and mortality: a quantitative review of primary prevention trials. Br Med J 1990; 301:309–314.
43. Gould AL, Russouw JE, Santanello NC, et al. Cholesterol reduction yields clinical benefit. A new look at old data. Circulation 1995; 91:2274–2282.
44. Holme I. Cholesterol reduction and its impact on coronary artery disease and total mortality. Am J Cardiol 1995; 76:10C-17C.
45. Rossouw JE, Lewis B, Rifkind BM. The value of lowering cholesterol after myocardial infarction. N Engl J Med 1990; 323:1112–1119.
46. Holme I. Relation of coronary heart disease incidence and total mortality to plasma cholesterol reduction in randomised trials: use of meta-analysis. Br Heart J 1993; 69:S42–S47.
47. Blankenhorn DH, Nessim SA, Johnson RL, et al. Beneficial effects of combined colestipol-niacin therapy on coronary atherosclerosis and coronary venous bypass grafts. JAMA 1987; 257:3233–3240.
48. Kane JP, Malloy MJ, Ports TA, et al. Regression of coronary atherosclerosis during treatment of familial hypercholesterolemia with combined drug regimens. JAMA 1990; 264:3007–3012.
49. Brown G, Albers JJ, Fisher LD, et al. Regression of coronary artery disease as a result of intensive lipid-lowering therapy in men with high levels of apolipoprotein B. N Engl J Med 1990; 323:1289–1298.
50. Brown BG, Zhao X-Q, Sacco DE, et al. Arteriographic view of treatment to achieve regression of coronary atherosclerosis and to prevent plaque disruption and clinical cardiovascular events. Br Heart J 1993; 69:S48–S53.
51. Byington RP, Jukema JW, Salonen JT, et al. Reduction in cardiovascular events during pravastatin therapy. Pooled analysis of clinical events of the Pravastatin Atherosclerosis Intervention Program. Circulation 1995; 92:2419–2425.
52. Bogaty P, Brecker SJ, White SE, et al. Comparison of coronary angiographic findings in acute and chronic first presentation of ischemic heart disease. Circulation 1993; 87:1938–1946.
53. Post Coronary Artery Bypass Graft Trial Investigators. The effect of aggressive lowering of low-density lipoprotein cholesterol levels and low-dose anticoagulation on obstructive changes in saphenous-vein coronary-artery bypass grafts. N Engl J Med 1997; 336:153–162.

54. Scandinavian Simvastatin Survival Study Group. Randomised trial of cholesterol lowering in 4444 patients with coronary heart disease: the Scandinavian Simvastatin Survival Study (4S). Lancet 1994; 344:1383–1389.

55. Pedersen TR, Kjekshus J, Pyorala K, et al. Effect of simvastatin on survival and coronary morbidity in coronary heart disease patients 65 or older. Circulation 1995; 92(suppl 1):I-672. Abstract.

56. Sacks FM, Pfeffer MA, Moye LA, et al. The effect of pravastatin on coronary events after myocardial infarction in patients with average cholesterol levels. N Engl J Med 1996; 335:1001–1009.

57. Davis BR, Cutler JA, Gordon DJ, et al. Rationale and design for the Antihypertensive and Lipid Lowering Treatment to Prevent Heart Attack Trial (ALLHAT). Am J Hypertens 1996; 9:342–360.

58. LaRosa JC. Dyslipoproteinemia in women and the elderly. Med Clin North Am, 1994; 78:163–180.

59. Rubins HB, Robins SJ, Iwane MK, et al. Rationale and design of the Department of Veterans Affairs High-density Lipoprotein Cholesterol Intervention Trial (HIT) for secondary prevention of coronary artery disease in men with low-density lipoprotein cholesterol and desirable low-density lipoprotein cholesterol. Am J Cardiol 1993; 71:45–52.

60. Maher VMG, Brown BG, Marcovina SM, et al. Effects of lowering elevated LDL cholesterol on the cardiovascular risk of lipoprotein(a). JAMA 1995; 274: 1771–1774.

61. Smith SC Jr, Blair SN, Criqui MH, et al. Preventing heart attack and death in patients with coronary disease. Circulation 1995; 92:2–4.

62. Yusuf S, Zucker D, Peduzzi P, et al. Effect of coronary artery bypass graft surgery on survival: overview of 10–year results from randomised trials by the coronary Artery Bypass Graft Surgery Trialists Collaboration. Lancet 1994; 344:563–570.

63. Antiplatelet trialists' collaboration. Secondary prevention of vascular disease by prolonged antiplatelet treatment. Br Med J 1988; 296:320–331.

64. Yusuf S, Peto R, Lewis J, et al. Beta blockade during and after myocardial infarction: an overview of randomized trials. Prog Cardiovasc Dis 1985; 27:335–371.

65. Elliott WJ, Black HR. High blood pressure and atherosclerosis. In: LaRosa JC, ed. Medical Management of Atherogenesis, New York: Marcel Dekker, 1997.

66. Pitt B. Adjunctive non-lipid lowering strategies for the therapy of atherogenesis. In: LaRosa JC, ed. Medical Management of Atherosclerosis. New York: Marcel Dekker, 1997.

67. Hsu I, Spinler SA, Johnson NE. Comparative evaluation of the safety and efficacy of HMG-CoA reductase inhibitor monotherapy in the treatment of primary hypercholesterolemia. Ann Pharmacother 1995; 29:743–759.

68. Alaupovic P, Heinonen T, Shurzinske L, et al. Effect of a new HMG-CoA reductase inhibitor, atorvastatin, on lipids, apolipoproteins and lipoprotein particles in patients with elevated serum cholesterol and triglyceride levels. Atherosclerosis 1997; 133:123–133.

69. Hunninghake DM. Drug treatment of dyslipoproteinemia. Endocrinol Metab Clin North Am 1990; 19:345–360.

70. Blum CB. Comparison of properties of four inhibitors of 3–hydroxy-3–methyl-glutaryl oenzyme A reductase. Am J Cardiol 1994; 732:3D-11D.
71. Nawrocki JW, Weiss SR, Davidson MH, et al. Reduction of LDL cholesterol by 25% to 60% in patients with primary hypercholesterolemia by atorvastatin, a new HMG–CoA reductase inhibitor. Arterioscler Thromb Vasc Biol 1995; 15:678–682.
72. Clinical Quality Improvement Network (CQIN) Investigators. Low incidence of assessment and modification of risks in acute care patients at high risk for cardiovascular events, particularly among females and the elderly. Am J Cardiol 1995; 76:570–73.
73. Shepherd J, Pratt M. Prevention of coronary heart disease in clinical practice: a commentary on current treatment patterns in six European countries in relation to published recommendations. Cardiology 1996; 87:1–5.

2

Role of Antioxidants in Prevention of Coronary Artery Disease

Joseph L. Witztum

University of California, San Diego, La Jolla, California

I. INTRODUCTION

There is now a large body of evidence, including both primary and secondary intervention trials, that support the contention that plasma cholesterol levels are directly related to the expression of coronary artery disease (CAD). As reviewed elsewhere in this book, when plasma cholesterol levels are lowered, morbidity and mortality from CAD decrease, and with effective therapies, total mortality decreases as well. However, at any given plasma concentration of low-density lipoprotein (LDL), there remains a great diversity in the extent of atherosclerosis present and in the expression of clinical disease. For example, in the Physicians Health Study, nearly two-thirds of those who developed a clinical event had an initial plasma cholesterol level < 240 mg/dl (1). Atherosclerosis is indeed a complex disease that develops over many decades. Undoubtedly, different factors play key roles at different stages in the evolution of the atherosclerotic process. For example, pathogenic factors involved in the initiation of the lesion may be different from those involved in plaque rupture, which give rise to unstable angina or acute myocardial infarction.

This review will focus on just one of the potential processes that go "beyond cholesterol," but it is clear that many other mechanisms are involved as well. This chapter will focus on the oxidation hypothesis of atherosclerosis, which states that the oxidative modification of LDL (or other lipoproteins) is important, if not obligatory, in the pathogenesis of the atherosclerotic lesion (2–4). Not only has this hypothesis been of great heuristic value in studying the mechanisms by which atherogenesis occurs, but if the hypothesis is correct, the important corollary follows that inhibiting oxidation of LDL will decrease or prevent atherosclerosis and clinical sequelae. The possibility that an augmented intake of antioxidant vitamins or compounds could lead to a significant reduction in CAD has provoked widespread interest among scientists and the lay public as well. This review will attempt to summarize the theoretical basis of the oxidation hypothesis and what we know about the use of antioxidants in relationship to CAD.

II.   WHAT IS OXIDIZED LDL?

The fatty streak is the earliest lesion of the atherogenic process, which in turn gives rise to the transitional and the more complicated fibrous plaques, which can rupture and give rise to thrombosis, myocardial infarction, and death (5–7). The macrophage was recognized to be the predominant cell type within the artery wall that took up LDL and became the typical "foam cell" of the fatty streak. It was originally thought that this might occur via the LDL receptor pathway. However, experimental evidence indicated that incubation of macrophages with native LDL did not lead to foam cell formation, presumably because uptake via the LDL receptor pathway leads to feedback downregulation of these receptors, preventing excess cholesterol accumulation. Furthermore, human subjects with homozygous familial hypercholesterolemia, who completely lack LDL receptors, or WHHL rabbits also lacking LDL receptors, nevertheless experience greatly accelerated atherosclerotic formation. Thus, alternative pathways had to exist to allow for macrophage cholesterol accumulation. Goldstein and Brown were the first to suggest a solution to this problem. They postulated that the primary function of macrophages is to scavenge damaged material and that macrophages took up damaged or modified LDL by novel pathways. They demonstrated that LDL chemically modified by acetylation was rapidly taken up by a different receptor, which they termed the acetyl LDL or scavenger receptor (8). Although no evidence was presented that acetylation of LDL occurred to any extent in vivo, studies in La Jolla and elsewhere subsequently demonstrated that analogous modifications of LDL did occur in vivo. It was shown that preincubation of LDL with endothelial cells resulted in a modification of LDL that led to its being recognized by the macrophage acetyl LDL receptor (9), and that the modification that occurred was the oxidation of the LDL (10).

Incubations of LDL with smooth muscle cells or macrophages also produced a similar oxidized LDL (11,12). The extensive oxidation of the lipids of LDL led to a series of changes that created novel ligands leading to rapid uptake by way of the acetyl LDL receptor of macrophages. Indeed, there appears to be a whole family of different scavenger receptors on macrophages whose function is to remove modified lipoproteins, and presumably other modified structures as well (3,4).

Why is there such an elaborate system of receptors on macrophages to clear modified lipoproteins? The answer may be that oxidized LDL, as well as a large number of oxidatively modified products generated from the modified LDL, are pro-inflammatory and cytotoxic. The chemical events that occur when LDL undergoes oxidation are indeed complex, in part dependent on the method used to initiate the oxidation of LDL, and have been reviewed in detail elsewhere (5). It does not appear that oxidation of LDL occurs to any significant extent in the circulation, as there are extensive antioxidant defenses in plasma. However, once the LDL enters into the intimal space of the artery, oxidation appears to occur in microdomains presumably protected from soluble antioxidants. The exact mechanisms by which oxidation of LDL occurs in vivo are not known but probably are complex, involve multiple mechanisms, and are mediated by the cells of the artery wall, including macrophages, endothelial cells, and smooth muscle cells. In some cases, reactive oxygen species released by cells may initiate oxidation (13); in some cases products of lipoxygenase reactions could be involved (14); and in others oxidation involving myeloperoxidase and H_2O_2 released by macrophages may also occur (15).

Oxidation of the LDL presumably begins when a reactive radical abstracts a hydrogen atom from a carbon atom in a polyunsaturated fatty acid (PUFA) on a phospholipid of the LDL particle. In turn, this reacts with oxygen, leading to formation of oxygen-containing radicals, which can then initiate oxidation in neighboring fatty acids and propagate lipid peroxidation. Oxidation can spread throughout the LDL particle, leading to modifications of the surface phospholipids, the fatty acids in the cholesterol esters and triglycerides, and the cholesterol moieties themselves. Many of these oxidized and modified lipid products may be hydrophilic, can leave the LDL particle, and have a variety of effects on the artery wall, as noted below. In addition, breakdown products of the PUFA occur, leading to formation of highly reactive aldehydes, ketones, and other products. Some of these can form covalent adducts with the protein moiety of LDL, apo-B, forming new epitopes that are believed to form the new ligands by which scavenger receptors on macrophages recognize oxidized LDL (2,3).

As described above, the original impetus for studying oxidized LDL was the observation that oxidation of LDL converted it into a form that had accelerated uptake in macrophages leading to foam cell development. However, it is now apparent that products of oxidized LDL can affect the atherogenic process in many ways. Fogelman and colleagues have demonstrated that during the earliest stages of the oxidation of LDL, products are released which have profound pro-inflammatory effects on the artery wall (16). They have termed this early form of oxidized LDL minimally modified LDL (MM-LDL), to distinguish it from more heavily modified forms of oxidized LDL.

MM-LDL is not yet sufficiently modified to be recognized by scavenger receptors. Thus, it may have a more prolonged residence time within the intima, releasing products that have pro-inflammatory properties. Products of various stages of oxidized LDL can affect gene expression in cells of the artery wall both through specific pathways and through generalized shifts in intracellular redox potential. For example, modified phospholipids of MM-LDL appear to have platelet-activating-factor-like activities (17). Some products of MM-LDL can cause arterial cells to express monocyte chemoattractant protein (MCP-1) and monocyte colony-stimulating factor (M-CSF). In turn, these proteins can lead to the attraction of monocytes and their immigration into the artery wall, where their differentiation into macrophages is accelerated.

Still other products of MM-LDL or oxidized LDL may promote endothelial adhesion molecules, which should further promote mononuclear cell immigration (16). Some products of oxidized LDL can interfere with EDRF activity either directly by altering endothelial function, or indirectly by reacting with nitric oxide, leading to inhibition of normal vasodilatory activity and even paradoxical vasoconstriction (18). Other products of MM-LDL or oxidized LDL may activate macrophages to release interleukin-1 (Il-1), which in turn may initiate smooth muscle cell proliferation. Similarly, a variety of other cytokines and growth factors may be influenced by various products. Yet other products of oxidized LDL can be cytotoxic (12).

Thus, it seems reasonable that the macrophage uptake of oxidized LDL, in one sense, may actually be protective, removing the source of the many pro-inflammatory and cytotoxic molecules. However, in the face of hypercholesterolemia and/or unchecked pro-oxidant processes, the net effect of either event would be to generate both excess MM-LDL and oxidized LDL, resulting in the inflammatory state and marked accumulation of cholesterol and modified lipid molecules within macrophages. In turn, it is likely that many of these products, such as oxidized sterols, are cytotoxic to the macrophages as well, leading to their death via necrosis and/or apoptosis, which contributes to the formation of the acellular "gruel" typical of the advanced and complicated plaque. This insoluble lipid (ceroid) probably represents the products of lipid peroxidation and their conjugation to proteins, and is found in both fatty streaks and, to a much greater degree, advanced atherosclerotic plaques. Undoubtedly this is more difficult to "reverse" than free cholesterol. If this general scheme is correct, it suggests that by the time LDL becomes so extensively modified that it is recognized by macrophage scavenger receptors, it may already have adversely affected the artery wall. This formulation implies that preventing oxidation of LDL in the first place will be of therapeutic importance, not only because it will prevent foam cell formation, but because it will prevent the pro-inflammatory component of the atherosclerotic process.

III. INHIBITING LDL OXIDATION

As noted above, it is believed that LDL becomes oxidized in the artery wall, where it is exposed to a variety of pro-oxidant stresses. Thus, the direct provision of lipophilic antioxidants to the LDL particle itself should theoretically prove an effective strategy (19). The most abundant natural antioxidant in LDL is vitamin E. Supplementation of the diet with vitamin E can increase the vitamin E content of LDL and lead to enhanced protection of LDL when tested in in vitro oxidation assays. However, the maximum degree of supplementation (about 1000 to 1200 mg/day) leads to only a 2.5–fold increase in vitamin E content, which is sufficient to prolong the lag phase of susceptibility to lipid peroxidation by only 50% (20). As noted below, it is not yet clear if this degree of protection is sufficient to protect LDL under the pro-oxidant conditions that exist in vivo, and, in particular, it does not appear protective in several animal models with severe hypercholesterolemia.

Beta-carotene is the next most common antioxidant in LDL and theoretically should provide enhanced antioxidant protection, but neither our laboratory (20) nor others have been able to show this effect, even when LDL beta-carotene levels were raised more than 20-fold. By contrast, the administration of probucol, a synthetic lipophilic antioxidant, in sufficient amounts to achieve a probucol content in LDL of 2 to 4 µg/mg LDL protein, can lead to near total protection of the LDL against oxidative stress for as long as 16 hours in the in vitro assays (21). Vitamin C, which is a water-soluble antioxidant, should probably be administered with vitamin E, since it provides significant protection to LDL by maintaining vitamin E in the LDL particle in its reduced, antioxidant state (e.g. each time vitamin E acts as an antioxidant, it is oxidized in turn, requiring vitamin C to convert it back to the reduced vitamin E capable of antioxidant protection).

Finally, as noted above, it is the oxidation of the PUFA in LDL that begins the process of oxidation of LDL. Reduction of the PUFA content of LDL by dietary substitution with mono-unsaturated fatty acid, primarily oleic acid, is an effective means to inhibit the susceptibility of LDL to oxidation (22) and could be part of the explanation for the alleged protective effect of the so-called Mediterranean diet.

IV. EVIDENCE THAT OXIDATION OF LDL IS IMPORTANT IN ATHEROGENESIS

There is now an extensive series of experiments to support the hypothesis that oxidation of lipoproteins does occur in vivo and is quantitatively important, certainly in animal models of atherosclerosis. This evidence has been summarized and detailed elsewhere (2–4) but can be summarized in brief as follows:

1. Immunocytochemical studies using antibodies directed against epitopes of oxidized LDL demonstrate the presence of such epitopes in atherosclerotic lesions of experimental animal models as well as in man.
2. LDL extracted from atherosclerotic tissue of rabbits and humans has all of the physical, immunologic, and biological properties observed with LDL oxidized in vitro.
3. Oxidized lipids, including oxidized sterols as well as products of the lipoxygenase pathway, are found in atherosclerotic tissue, but not in normal aortic tissues.
4. Although oxidized LDL per se is not found in the plasma, a small fraction of circulating LDL particle displays chemical indices of early stages of oxidation and oxidation-specific epitopes can be demonstrated in some LDL particles by immunochemical techniques.
5. Oxidized LDL is immunogenic, and autoantibodies to a variety of epitopes of oxidized LDL can be found in sera of experimental animal models with atherosclerosis, as well as in humans. In studies of mice, such autoantibody titers are related to the presence of atherosclerosis, and in humans preliminary data suggest that the titers are related to the presence and/or the rate of progression of disease.
6. Autoantibodies to oxidized LDL epitopes are found in atherosclerotic lesions of rabbits and man and are present in lesions as part of immune complexes with oxidized LDL.
7. Most importantly, and most convincingly, treatment of hypercholesterolemic rabbits, mice, and nonhuman primates with a variety of antioxidants leads to inhibition of the progression of atherosclerosis, independent of any effects on plasma lipoprotein levels.

In most of these studies in experimental animals, the inhibition of atherosclerosis varied from 40 to 80%. However, these studies were carried out with potent antioxidants such as probucol, which conferred maximal protection to LDL, much greater than that achieved with a natural antioxidant such as vitamin E (as will be discussed in greater detail below). A number of major questions remain unanswered about the mechanisms by which antioxidants inhibit atherosclerosis. For example, do they achieve this protective effect by protection of the LDL, by altering the redox potential within cells of the artery (such as endothelial cells), or both? In addition, could the antioxidants affect atherogenesis by some nonantioxidant properties? Evidence that strongly supports the idea that antioxidant mechanisms are related to their protective effect is that the compounds that conferred the most potent antioxidant protection to LDL, e.g., probucol, almost universally inhibit the progression of atherosclerosis, while those compounds that are much weaker, such as vitamin E, have often failed to inhibit atherosclerosis in experimental animal models. Furthermore, in a recent study of nonhuman primates by Sasahara et al. (23), there was a significant correlation between the extent of antioxidant protection of plasma LDL and the extent of inhibition of athero-sclerosis. However, not all studies in animals have shown a positive benefit of antioxidant therapy. For example, in the study of Freubis et al. (24), probucol and a probucol analog were given to LDL receptor-negative rabbits, which have marked hypercholesterolemia even on a chow diet. Probucol provided very potent protection to the LDL from oxidation, prolonging the lag time for conjugated diene formation (an index of the extent of antioxidant protection) by as much as eightfold, whereas the probucol analog prolonged the lag time only fourfold. While probucol provided the expected degree of protection against atherosclerosis, the probucol analog did not.

This experiment and others conducted by our group in La Jolla suggest that under some circumstances the degree of protection observed in the cir-culating LDL may not necessarily be a reflection of a compound's anti-atherogenic potential. In addition, these experiments raise the very important possibility that for any given level of pro-oxidant stress there is a given level of antioxidant protection required. Thus, mild degrees of antioxidant pro-tection, as might be conferred by usual doses of vitamin E consumed by human populations (see below), may not be sufficient under certain cir-cumstances. Further support for this hypothesis can be found in the elegant studies of Parker et al. (25), who looked at the ability of probucol and vitamin E to protect against atherosclerosis in a cholesterol-fed hamster model. Under conditions of marked hypercholesterolemia, none of the agents tested were effective, whereas in the presence of only a mild degree of hypercholester-olemia, both were effective. Further studies are needed to test this "threshold hypothesis" as it has obvious clinical relevance to studies in humans. For example, it may well imply that the degree of antioxidant protection need-ed for a hypercholesterolemic individual who smokes would be signifi-cantly greater than that needed for a nonsmoking, normocholesterolemic in-dividual.

It should be noted that antioxidants may protect against atherosclerosis by means other than direct protection of LDL from oxidation. For example, in the presence of hypercholesterolemia, or as a result of some other factor leading to an altered redox state, endothelial cells may be activated, leading to increased expression of adhesion molecules, such as VCAM-1, which can bind monocytes and T-cells, and antioxidants may abrogate this. Similarly, antioxidants may restore the normal endothelial-dependent relaxing activity of endothelial cells (26) and/or directly inhibit the ability of cells to initiate oxidation of LDL (27).

V. RELATIONSHIP OF THE OXIDATION HYPOTHESIS TO HUMAN POPULATIONS

There are now many epidemiologic studies that suggest an inverse relationship between dietary intake and/or serum levels of antioxidants and CAD (28). For example, Gey demonstrated a strong inverse relationship between intake of vitamin C and vitamin E and rates of CAD in a cross-sectional study of European countries (29). Two large, prospective cohort studies in the United States which studied female nurses or male health professionals found that those who had the highest self-reported intake of vitamin E (> 100 mg/day) had up to a 30% to 50% reduction in CAD events (30,31). In another study, the 10-year follow-up of the First National Health and Nutrition Survey, vitamin C intake was inversely related to CAD and overall mortality, but this study was not controlled for vitamin E intake (32).

Epidemiologic studies are important and suggestive of relationships, but they do not demonstrate cause and effect and they do not substitute for prospective intervention trials. Unfortunately, we do not have any such prospective trials, with the exceptions noted below, which were designed to test the hypothesis that antioxidant intervention will inhibit manifestations of CAD. However, a number of trials have been completed that were aimed at assessing the effects of antioxidant therapy on other endpoints, chiefly prevention of cancer. In a clinical trial in Linxian, China, intervention with low doses of beta-carotene, vitamin E, and selenium produced a 10% lowering of cerebral vascular disease (33). However, in the Finnish ATB study, in which 30,000 male smokers were given 20 mg/day of beta-carotene or 50 mg/day of vitamin E, or both, vitamin E had no apparent effect on mortality, while total mortality was 8% higher among those who received beta-carotene (34). In a large double-blind trial in the United States, the CARET study, the effects of combined daily supplementation of 30 mg of synthetic beta-carotene and 25,000 units of vitamin E (or placebo) on incidents of cancer and cardiovascular disease in 18,000 smokers were studied. In the supplemented group, the relative risk of death from cardiovascular disease was actually 26% higher than in those in the placebo group (35). Finally, we now have results of the randomized, double-blind Physicians Health Study of over 22,000 male physicians 40 to 84 years of age in the United States who received either 50 mg beta-carotene q.o.d. or placebo for a follow-up period of 12 years. No significant difference in the number of men who suffered a stroke or myocardial infarction was observed. However, there was no indication of an adverse effect, as the overall incidence of death was unchanged (36).

A rather different result was recently reported from the Cambridge Heart Antioxidant Study (CHAOS). In this study, vitamin E supplementation of 400 or 800 IU per day or placebo was given to 2002 men with angiographic evidence of coronary atherosclerosis. After a median follow-up of only 510 days, it was reported that vitamin E supplementation significantly reduced the risk of the primary endpoint of nonfatal myocardial infarction and cardiovascular death by 47%, and produced an overall 77% decrease in the risk of nonfatal myocardial infarction. Divergence in clinical outcomes was observed after only 200 days of vitamin E therapy. Total mortality from cardiovascular disease was slightly but not significantly greater in the vitamin E-supplemented group (37). The results of the CHAOS study are most dramatic and unexpected, and must be confirmed by other studies to ensure that some unknown confounding variable was not present. Nevertheless, to date it is the first intervention trial with vitamin E to show a reduction in clinically significant coronary events.

In the absence of any definitive data, what is the individual physician to do with his or her patients while awaiting results of ongoing trials? Although the oxidation hypothesis of atherosclerosis remains alive and well, it is important to remember that it remains a hypothesis and that its importance, especially for atherosclerosis in humans, remains to be proven. Strong epidemiologic evidence suggests that there is indeed an inverse relationship between the intake of antioxidant vitamins and CAD, but whether this is a cause-and-effect association remains to be proven. People who take large amounts of antioxidant supplements are more likely to eat healthier diets, exercise more, refrain from smoking, and have a healthier lifestyle in general. Carefully controlled trials of primary and secondary prevention are urgently needed, and some studies with natural antioxidants are under way. While use of natural antioxidants may prove to be sufficient for individuals in a primary prevention trial, as suggested above, if there is indeed a threshold level of antioxidant protection that must be achieved for any given pro-oxidant setting, for some individuals it may be necessary to use more powerful antioxidants such as probucol or its equivalent. It is important for pharmaccutical companies to develop such compounds and for assays to be developed that can reflect in vivo states of oxidation of LDL and indeed of lipid pro-oxidation in general.

We are at an early phase in the testing of the oxidation hypothesis. It is not yet possible to make specific recommendations to the general public. Certainly we can recommend diets low in saturated fat and cholesterol and enriched in fruits and vegetables which will contain abundant natural antioxidants. Should we recommend to the public that they augment their intake of antioxidant vitamins? Unfortunately, at the present time we do not have an answer. In the absence of definitive data, what then is the individual physician, faced with a high-risk patient, to advise? Should the patient be encouraged to take vitamin E together with vitamin C? This is a decision that must be discussed between the individual patient and physician, with the full recognition that definitive information is not yet available. However, if a decision has been made to provide antioxidant protection, it would seem prudent to take at least 400 to 800 mg of vitamin E per day and to supplement this with vitamin C 500 to 1000 mg in divided doses. While ingestion of saturated fat should be limited, it would seem prudent to use mono-unsaturated fats in preference to PUFA, as both would effectively lower plasma cholesterol, but the mono-unsaturated is less susceptible to oxidation, as described above. Most importantly, the physician must convey to the patient that use of antioxidant vitamins should never replace attention in dealing with standard risk factors for CAD prevention.

REFERENCES

1. Young FE, Nightingale SL, Temple RA. The preliminary report of the findings of the aspirin component of the ongoing Physicians' Health Study. The FDA perspective on aspirin for the primary prevention of myocardial infarction. JAMA 1988; 259:3158–3160.
2. Steinberg D, Parthasarathy S, Carew TE, Khoo JC, Witztum JL. Beyond cholesterol. Modifications of low-density lipoprotein that increase its atherogenicity. N Engl J Med 1989; 320:915–924.
3. Witztum JL. The oxidation hypothesis of atherosclerosis. Lancet 1994; 344:793–795.
4. Steinberg D. Oxidative modification of LDL and atherogenesis. The 1995 Lewis A. Conner Memorial Lecture. Circulation 1997; 95:1062–1071.
5. Witztum JL, Steinberg D. Role of oxidized low density lipoprotein in atherogenesis. J Clin Invest 1991; 88:1785–1792.
6. Ross R. The pathogenesis of atherosclerosis: a perspective for the 1990s. Nature 1993; 362:801–809.
7. Libby P. Molecular bases of the acute coronary syndromes. Circulation 1995; 91:2844–2850.
8. Goldstein JL, Ho YK, Basu SK, Brown MS. Binding site on macrophages that mediates uptake and degradation of acetylated low density lipoprotein, producing massive cholesterol deposition. Proc Natl Acad Sci USA 1979; 76:333–337.
9. Henriksen T, Mahoney EM, Steinberg D. Enhanced macrophage degradation of low density lipoprotein previously incubated with cultured endothelial cells: recognition by receptors for acetylated low density lipoproteins. Proc Natl Acad Sci USA 1981; 78:6499–6503.
10. Steinbrecher UP, Parthasarathy S, Leake DS, Witztum JL, Steinberg D. Modification of low density lipoprotein by endothelial cells involves lipid peroxidation and degradation of low density lipoprotein phospholipids. Proc Natl Acad Sci USA 1984; 81:3883–3887.
11. Heinecke JW, Rosen H, Chait A. Iron and copper promote modification of low density lipoprotein by human arterial smooth muscle cells in culture. J Clin Invest 1984; 74:1890–1894.

12. Chisolm GM. Oxidized lipoproteins and leukocyte-endothelial interactions: growing evidence for multiple mechanisms. Lab Invest 1993; 68:369–371. Editorials.
13. Chisolm GM, Ma G, Irwin KC, et al. 7 Beta-hydroperoxycholest-5–en-3 beta-ol, a component of human atherosclerotic lesions, is the primary cytotoxin of oxidized human low density lipoprotein. Proc Natl Acad Sci USA 1994; 91:11452–11456.
14. Yla-Herttuala S, Rosenfeld ME, Parthasarathy S, et al. Colocalization of 15–lipoxygenase mRNA and protein with epitopes of oxidized low density lipoprotein in macrophage-rich areas of atherosclerotic lesions. Proc Natl Acad Sci USA 1990; 87:6959–6963.
15. Hazen SL, Hsu FF, Duffin K, Heinecke JW. Molecular chlorine generated by the myeloperoxidase-hydrogen peroxide-chloride system of phagocytes converts low density lipoprotein cholesterol into a family of chlorinated sterols. J Biol Chem 1996; 271:23080–23088.
16. Berliner JA, Navab M, Fogelman AM, et al. Atherosclerosis: basic mechanisms. Oxidation, inflammation, and genetics. Circulation 1995; 91:2488–2496.
17. Navab M, Berliner JA, Watson AD, et al. The Yin and Yang of oxidation in the development of the fatty streak. A review based on the 1994 George Lyman Duff Memorial lecture. Arterioscler Thromb Vasc Biol 1996; 16:831–842.
18. Keancy JF, Vita JA. Atherosclerosis, oxidative stress, and antioxidant protection in endothelium-derived relaxing factor action. Prog Cardiovasc Dis 1995; 38:129–154.
19. Esterbauer H, Ramos P. Chemistry and pathophysiology of oxidation of LDL. Rev Physiol Biochem Pharmacol 1996; 127:31–64.
20. Reaven PD, Khouw A, Beltz WF, Parthasarathy S, Witztum JL. Effect of dietary antioxidant combinations in humans. Protection of LDL by vitamin E but not by beta-carotene. Arterioscler Thromb 1993; 13:590–600.
21. Reaven PD, Parthasarathy S, Beltz WF, Witztum JL. Effect of probucol dosage on plasma lipid and lipoprotein levels and on protection of low density lipoprotein against *in vitro* oxidation in humans. Arterioscler Thromb 1992; 12:318–324.
22. Reaven PD, Witztum JL. Oxidized LDL in atherogenesis: role of dietary modification. In: McCormack D, ed. Annual Review of Nutrition. Palo Alto: Annual Reviews Inc. 1996:51–71.
23. Sasahara M, Raines EW, Chait A, et al. Inhibition of hypercholesterolemia-induced atherosclerosis in the nonhumanprimate by probucol. I. Is the extent of atherosclerosis related to resistance of LDL to oxidation? J Clin Invest 1994; 94:155–164.
24. Fruebis J, Steinberg D, Dresel HA, Carew TE. A comparison of the antiatherogenic effects of probucol and of a structural analogue of probucol in low density lipoprotein receptor-deficient rabbits. J Clin Invest 1994; 94:392–398.
25. Parker RA, Sabrah T, Cap M, Gill BT. Relation of vascular oxidative stress, alpha-tocopherol, and hypercholesterolemia to early atherosclerosis in hamsters. Arterioscler Thromb Vasc Biol 1995; 15:349–358.
26. Keaney JF, Guo Y, Cunningham D, Shwaery GT, Xu A, Vita JA. Vascular incorporation of alpha-tocopherol prevents endothelial dysfunction due to oxidized LDL by inhibiting protein kinase C stimulation. J Clin Invest 1996; 98:386–394.

27. Devaraj S, Li D, Jialal I. The effects of alpha tocopherol supplementation on monocyte function. Decreased lipid oxidation, interleukin 1 beta secretion, and monocyte adhesion to endothelium. J Clin Invest 1996; 98:756–763.

28. Jha P, Flather M, Lonn E, Farkouh M, Yusuf S. The antioxidant vitamins and cardiovascular disease. A critical review of epidemiologic and clinical trial data. Ann Intern Med 1995; 123:860–872.

29. Gey KF. The antioxidant hypothesis of cardiovascular disease: epidemiology and mechanisms. Biochem Soc Trans 1990; 18:1041–1045.

30. Stampfer MJ, Hennekens CH, Manson JE, Colditz GA, Rosner B, Willett WC. Vitamin E consumption and the risk of coronary disease in women. N Engl J Med 1993; 328:1444–1449.

31. Rimm EB, Stampfer MJ, Ascherio A, Giovannucci E, Colditz GA, Willett WC. Vitamin E consumption and the risk of coronary heart disease in men. N Engl J Med 1993; 328:1450–1456.

32. Enstrom JE, Kanim LE, Klein MA. Vitamin C intake and mortality among a sample of the United States population. Epidemiology 1992; 3:194–202.

33. Blot WJ, Li JY, Taylor PR, et al. Nutrition interventions trials in Linxian, China: supplementation with specific vitamin/mineral combination, cancer incidence, and disease-specific mortality in the general population. J Natl Cancer Inst 1993; 85:1483–1492.

34. Heinonen OP, Albanes D. The effect of vitamin E and beta carotene on the incidence of lung cancer and other cancers in male smokers. N Engl J Med 1994; 330:1029–1035.

35. Omenn GS, Goodman GE, Thornquist MD, et al. Effects of a combination of beta carotene and vitamin A on lung cancer and cardiovascular disease. N Engl J Med 1996; 334:1150–1155.

36. Hennekens CH, Buring JE, Manson JE, et al. Lack of effect of long-term supplementation with beta carotene on the incidence of malignant neoplasms and cardiovascular disease. N Engl J Med 1996; 334:1145–1149.

37. Stephens NG, Parsons A, Schofield PM, et al. Randomised controlled trial of vitamin E in patients with coronary disease: Cambridge Heart Antioxidant Study (CHAOS). The Lancet 1996; 347:781–785.

3
High Blood Pressure and Atherogenesis

William J. Elliott and Henry R. Black
Rush University, Chicago, Illinois

I. INTRODUCTION

It is difficult for most physicians to make the distinction between the common pathophysiological process of atherogenesis (which occurs in the arteries of very young subjects in Western societies) and the atherosclerotic diseases commonly seen by physicians in older individuals, who typically have more than just a single risk factor for myocardial infarction, stroke, or renal disease. Clearly, hypertension increases the risk for both processes, but how it does so, and which confounding variables are important, highlight some of the differences between hypertension as a risk factor for atherogenesis, and how blood pressure (BP) control can limit the adverse clinical sequelae of atherosclerosis.

Theories about how hypertension increases the rate of atherogenesis fall into four general categories: a) barotrauma to the arterial intima; b) endothelial dysfunction within the lining of the hypertensive arterioles; c) hyperstimulation of the adrenergic nervous system; or d) an underlying endocrine abnormality (e.g., elevated circulating levels of insulin). Advocates of the "damaged artery" hypothesis point to a biophysical alteration of the shear stress induced on arterial walls as the starting point for a broad cascade of adverse effects, eventually leading to microtrauma to the endothelial lining, which attempts to heal and leads to intimal hyperplasia, smooth muscle proliferation, and calcium deposition and "fatty streak" formation, followed by accumulation of connective tissue in the area of barotrauma. Devotees of endothelial dysfunction (which is commonly seen in hypertension) suggest that this could lead to lipid deposition in the vascular wall, proliferation of smooth muscle cells, and a higher propensity for platelet-vessel wall adhesion. Those who favor "adrenergic stimulation" as a pathophysiological origin for hypertension can easily explain altered lipolysis rates and enhanced very low density lipoprotein (VLDL) synthesis in animal models. Proponents of an endocrinological origin of hypertension (e.g., hyperinsulinemia) use this as a very convenient way to explain the effects of dyslipidemia at the microcirculatory level, which could alter local lipoprotein metabolism and disposition at the arterial wall.

What is abundantly clear, however, is that elevated blood pressure greatly increases the risk of atherosclerosis, especially in the presence of dyslipidemia. Experimental studies have demonstrated that without dyslipidemia, hypertensive animals and man generally develop fibrin-containing plaques but little atheromata; populations of humans with hypertension without dyslipidemia have a higher risk of stroke than myocardial infarction. Perhaps the best demonstration of the enhancing effect of blood pressure on atherogenesis in the presence of dyslipidemia is a comparison of the pulmonary and coronary arteries in Western peoples: there is seldom any atherosclerosis in the low-pressure pulmonary arteries, whereas the originally high-pressure coronaries are typically loaded with atherosclerotic plaque, which still is the No. 1 killer in the U.S. and most other industrialized nations.

In this chapter, then, we will try to highlight some of the links between hypertension and atherogenesis, and focus on the data from clinical trials in humans which have attempted to limit atherosclerosis by giving antihypertensive drugs. Although this chapter, by design, focuses on blood pressure, most astute clinicians would agree that managing *all* important risk factors (especially hypertension, smoking, and dyslipidemia) is likely to lead to the best result for an individual patient.

II. HYPERTENSION AND ATHEROGENESIS

A. Hypertension as a Contributor to the Atherogenic Process

Clinical and experimental hypertension and atherogenesis are highly interrelated. An overwhelming body of evidence indicates that when both are present, hypertension most commonly precedes the atherogenic process, although extensive atherosclerosis in the renal arterial bed can be the cause of elevated blood pressure in patients with renovascular hypertension. Although it is beyond the scope of this chapter to review all of the data which support the view that hypertension is one of the most important risk factors for the development of atherosclerosis in humans (and perhaps the most important risk factor for the development of the clinically recognized sequelae of coronary heart disease and stroke), some of the salient points will be summarized.

There is abundant evidence from laboratory studies of rats, dogs, monkeys, and other animals which demonstrates that atherogenesis appears after various interventions which increase systemic blood pressure—e.g., clipping a renal artery (1), feeding salt to DOC-treated animals (2), or banding the aorta (3). Two great advantages of these studies (compared to observational and epidemiological studies in humans) are that they can be interrupted at will (leading to measurements of the extent, grade, and location of atheromata), and the endpoints can be quantitated by histological and pathological techniques (4). Whole-animal experiments have now been interpreted on a cellular and molecular level, and the events that contribute to the atherosclerotic lesion (which are often exacerbated by hypertension) have been described (5–7).

The epidemiological studies supporting the conclusion that hypertension is a major risk factor for atherosclerosis are numerous, wide-ranging, and definitive. Hypertension and clinical events resulting from atherosclerotic lesions (e.g., coronary heart disease death, myocardial infarction, stroke) are highly correlated in large populations: both tend to occur more frequently in older individuals, and the prevalence of both problems across countries, peoples, or populations is also tightly correlated (8,9). Studies of young individuals—free-living children (10), deceased children (11), or adolescents (12,13), or young soldiers (14)—have shown that aortic atherosclerosis begins early in life, and is more extensive and more advanced in those who had higher blood pressures earlier during life.

Data have now been collected from many population-based observational studies in several countries which clearly indicate that hypertension is a major definitive antecedent which increases the risk of myocardial infarction, stroke, and cardiovascular death, all of which are common clinical sequelae of atherosclerosis (15). The most important American study of this type is the Framingham Heart Study, begun in the late 1940s, which has been able to demonstrate an independent, direct, and significant association between elevated levels of both systolic and diastolic blood pressure (separately) and stroke and coronary heart disease. The associations became apparent even after a short number of years of observation (16), and have remained strong during the more than 40 years of follow-up (17). While other risk factors (e.g., dyslipidemia, obesity, diabetes, and hyperuricemia) tend to "cluster" and to be found more among hypertensive individuals (18), the adverse effect of hypertension alone to increase the risk of clinical sequelae of atherosclerosis is clearly and distinctly independent of each of these other factors (19).

B.   Atherosclerosis as a Contributor to Elevated Blood Pressure

In addition to the overwhelming evidence linking hypertension as a risk factor which temporally precedes atherosclerosis and its clinical sequelae, there is now renewed appreciation of the fact that renal artery atherosclerosis can cause hypertension. Although the vast majority of hypertensives have no other definable reason for their elevated blood pressure (thus being called "essential" or "primary" hypertension), the prevalence of atherosclerotic renovascular hypertension appears to be rising, especially in the elderly population. This may be due to an increased number of elderly hypertensives and improvements in our ability both to better detect it and to intervene both to reduce blood pressure and to avoid the ischemic nephropathy which results.

1.   Renal Artery Disease/Renovascular Hypertension

When atherosclerosis or another process causes a major diminution in the caliber of a renal artery, blood pressure increases, as shown by the classic experiments of Goldblatt (20). Atherosclerosis is the most common cause of renovascular hypertension among older individuals, especially cigarette smokers with known obstructive atherosclerotic disease in another vascular bed. The "vicious cycle" of renal arterial atherosclerosis increasing blood pressure, which then accelerates atherosclerosis in this and other vascular beds, has been shown in case control (21) and other studies of patients with renovascular hypertension (22), who have more abnormalities in other arteries than matched controls with essential hypertension (23). This occurs even in cases of fibromuscular hyperplasia, in which aortic and carotid atherosclerosis is uncommon, due to the early age of the affected patients (21). Although some have attributed this phenomenon directly to an activation of the renin-angiotensin-aldosterone system (24,25), some (26,27) but not all prospective studies have demonstrated an increased risk of future sequelae of atherosclerosis in patients with elevated plasma renin activity (28,29).

2.   Associated Risk Factors

As noted above, hypertension is most commonly found in patients in whom cardiovascular risk factors "cluster" (18). Thus, in an older population of cigarette smokers with dyslipidemia, obesity, diabetes, and other traditional cardiac risk factors, it would be surprising to find many who did not also have at least "high normal" blood pressures. Many such patients would have some of the cellular and biological markers which are possibly related pathophysiologically to both the development of atherosclerosis, hypertension, and occlusive vascular disease. Some of these markers are listed in Table 1.

Table 1 Cellular and Biological Markers Common to Hypertension and Atherogenesis

---

Peripheral insulin resistance (and resultant hyperinsulinemia)
Endothelial dysfunction
Impaired nitric oxide synthesis
Abnormal endothelin synthesis, metabolism, and response
Enhanced endothelial permeability to plasma proteins and other components
Abnormal response to angiotensin II
Abnormal platelet function
Abnormal migration and proliferation of smooth muscle cells
Heightened free radical synthesis
Diminished ability to metabolize and remove reactive oxygen species

---

Although some have suggested that the simultaneous occurrence of these in many patients is merely a result of "lifestyle defects" common in western societies, two intriguing hypotheses have been advanced that might link many of these biological markers and their clinical sequelae pathophysiologically. Hyperinsulinemia and peripheral insulin resistance (30), and/or oxidative stress in and around arterial walls (31) are the two leading mechanisms that might explain why hypertension and factors that increase the risk of atherosclerosis are seen so commonly together; the evidence for each has been recently reviewed in detail (30–32).

III. SUMMARY OF EVIDENCE

A. Laboratory and Animal Studies

Although the foregoing epidemiological information linking hypertension and atherogenesis is compelling, perhaps the most convincing way to prove the hypothesis is to show that lowering blood pressure prevents either the progression of atherosclerosis or the clinical sequelae that result from it. The advantage of laboratory and animal studies is that direct inspection of the arterial walls can be done, with quantitation of the atherosclerotic lesions, and that appropriate controls can be carried simultaneously in which the only difference between them and the experimental animals is that the controls do not have blood pressure-lowering procedures or drugs administered to them.

There are now numerous studies of animal models of atherosclerosis which prove that blood pressure lowering limits the atherosclerotic process; some have tied these results directly to specific drugs or classes of drugs. Calcium antagonists and angiotensin-converting enzyme (ACE) inhibitors have been the most extensively studied recently; some older data about β-adrenergic blocking agents and at least two relatively positive studies of α_1-adrenoceptor blocking agents have been reported (33).

1. Intact Hypercholesterolemic Animals

There are several classes of antihypertensive drugs which have been shown to reduce the extent or severity of the arterial surface covered by atherosclerotic plaque. These experiments are typically done in animals fed a cholesterol-laden diet, or in animals rendered hypothyroid by pharmacological means.

Nifedipine was the first antihypertensive agent to demonstrate a reduction in aortic plaque in cholesterol-fed rabbits (34), and subsequent follow-up studies done with different classes of drugs, different agents within the same class, different durations of treatment, different routes of administration, and different doses have generally (but not always) shown similar results (35). More than 25 such studies have now been reported, and most of the results have been positive: the great majority of the treated animals have less severe or less extensive atherosclerotic plaquing than control animals.

The longest list of agents showing the antiatherogenic properties belongs to the dihydropyridine calcium antagonist class (and includes nifedipine, nicardipine, lacidipine, nisoldipine, isradipine, nivaldipine). The doses of dihydropyridine calcium antagonists used in these animal experiments have in general been quite high, resulting in much higher plasma concentrations than can be achieved safely in humans (36). The most notable exception has been isradipine, which has shown an antiatherogenic effect, even when given at doses which result in tissue and plasma levels comparable to those seen in humans (37,38). Direct comparisons of several dihydropyridines have generally shown that all of these drugs are reasonably effective, albeit at suprapharmacological doses (compared to humans). Because the antiatherogenic effect occurs even in normotensive animals, the specific drug therapy is thought to be the inhibitor of atherogenesis rather than the BP-lowering effect of the drug.

Nondihydropyridine calcium antagonists have similar effects on atherogenesis in animal studies, although again the effective doses are far higher than the usual doses used in humans (39). It appears that all calcium antagonists so far studied can inhibit the stimulatory effects of epidermal growth factor on intracellular calcium concentrations and DNA synthesis in cultured rat aortic smooth muscle cells. They also have been reported to stimulate prostacyclin production and weakly inhibit 12–hydroxyeicosatetrenoic acid-induced vascular smooth muscle cell migration, thus preventing both platelet aggregation and arterial intimal thickening (40,41). Some investigators have been able to demonstrate one or two of the changes listed above in treated animals, which occurred simultaneously with inhibited atherogenesis, which lends credence to the postulated pathophysiological mechanism.

The other class of antihypertensive agents that has been carefully and thoroughly studied in animals is the ACE inhibitors (42,43). Probably the most closely related animal model to human atherosclerosis is the cynomolgus monkey, which can be fed sufficient cholesterol so it develops aortic atheromata. In one of the better studies of this animal model, captopril (25 or 50 mg/kg/day, a suprapharmacological dose) reduced the severity and extent of atherosclerotic lesions in all arteries studied; in many arteries, there was a dose-response relationship (44). Several possible mechanisms for these effects have been postulated (45).

Antiatherogenic effects of β-adrenergic blocking agents have been reported in 16 of 19 studies done in five different animal species (46). Although there are multiple possible mechanisms (47), β-blockers have greater effects on atherogenesis than hydralazine, which actually lowers blood pressures more, suggesting that the antiatherogenic effects of β-blockade are independent of blood pressure reduction (48).

Although animal and human studies have consistently shown that α_1-adrenergic blocking agents reduce blood pressure and favorably alter the lipid profile, few data about atherogenesis have been developed using these agents (49).

2.   Genetically Hypercholesterolemic Animals

Another type of experimental model of atherosclerosis is the Watanabe hyperlipidemic rabbit, which at a very young age develops aortic and other arterial atheromata which resemble those seen in humans. This strain of rabbits is thought to be a reasonable model for human familial hypercholesterolemia, as it lacks a low-density lipoprotein (LDL) receptor. Two ACE inhibitors, captopril and trandolapril, are remarkable for their ability to limit atherogenesis in this model (50,51), although other compounds have shown similar effects in related animal models (52). Some of these studies have also demonstrated important physiological correlates (e.g., changes in parameters listed in Table 1) which occur simultaneously. Several studies have also been done in Watanabe rabbits using the same doses and routes of administration of propranolol (53) or calcium antagonists which have been found to inhibit atherogenesis in diet-induced hypercholesterolemic animals but have demonstrated no significant effects in these rabbits (54–56). Although the exact reason for this is still debated (35), the simplest explanation may be that some calcium antagonists may have preventive effects on the formation of new plaques but little therapeutic effect on established atherosclerotic lesions. This view is consistent with the results of some of the human studies, to be discussed below.

3. Iatrogenically-Damaged Arteries

A third type of animal experiment that may be particularly relevant to human atherosclerosis involves administering any one of several antihypertensive agents immediately before and then continuously after arterial intimal disruption by balloon catheters, cuffs, allografting, or other instruments designed to denude the vascular endothelium (as might happen in humans undergoing angioplasty, for example).

In rats or rabbits, several calcium antagonists (nilvadipine [57], isradipine [58], and amlodipine [59]), several ACE inhibitors (perindopril [60,61], cilazapril [62,63], lisinopril [64], and quinapril [65]) and at least one α_1-adrenoceptor blocker (prazosin [66]) and one angiotensin II receptor antagonist (losartan [67]) have been shown to reduce several aspects of atherogenesis, including thickening of the intima-media stratum and subsequent proliferation of endothelium. Typically the antihypertensive agent must be given before, during, and after the endothelial injury to be effective. Even then, the damage is less than in control animals, but more extensive than in uninjured arteries. The results of similar experiments, often using the same doses of the same drugs, in either pigs or baboons, have not confirmed the previous work in rats or rabbits (68).

Despite their generally positive conclusions, there are a number of limitations to even the very well done animal studies, especially when attempts are made to extrapolate the results to humans. Pathologists can recognize histological differences between experimental plaques raised by iatrogenically and even pharmacologically manipulated animals and those that occur commonly in humans. The atherogenic response to stimuli in animals appears to be even more highly variable in animals (across strains, species, and individual animals from the same litter) than in humans. Some animal models (e.g., the Watanabe heritable hyperlipidemic rabbit) appear to be much more resistant to drug interventions than most humans. As noted above, the doses of antihypertensive drugs used in animal studies have in general been much higher than achievable in humans. And lastly, the drugs appear to have their greatest effects in animals that begin to receive the drugs at a very early age, even before atherosclerosis is found in untreated control animals. This last point has important implications for human therapy, in that optimal inhibition of atherogenesis may be achievable only in humans who receive effective agents from a very early age.

B. Human Studies Using Surrogate Endpoints

In contrast to the overwhelming number of studies in laboratory animals indicating that blood pressure lowering and certain antihypertensive drugs can be generally quite effective at limiting the progression and extent of atherogenesis, the clinical studies designed to reach similar conclusions in humans have been disappointing. This appears to be particularly true of studies that use "surrogate endpoints" (e.g., narrowing of arterial lumina or biological markers of the atherosclerotic process) as distinguished from "clinical endpoints" (e.g., cardiovascular death, acute myocardial infarction, or atherosclerotic cerebrovascular disease events like acute stroke). It is essentially impossible to reproduce in humans the types of experiments that were successful in dyslipidemic animals (e.g., direct pathological examination of arteries for atherosclerotic plaque, using Oil Red O, Sudan Red, or other sensitive methodologies).

There have been, nonetheless, several clinical trials designed that have as one of the endpoint measurements a direct attempt to measure atherosclerosis and atherogenesis. These have attempted to build on the generally positive experience of the animal studies, but they have not been as successful.

1. Atherogenesis in a Native, Diseased Coronary Bed

One of the more ambitious prospective, randomized, controlled trials to grow out of the laboratory work with nifedipine was INTACT (International Nifedipine Trial on Antiatherosclerotic Therapy) (69). The investigators had been impressed with the efficacy of nifedipine in reducing atherogenesis in animals, and wished to extend this observation to humans with mild coronary artery disease. Thus, patients from multiple centers with catheterization-documented coronary lesions were randomly allocated to a high dose of short-acting nifedipine (20 mg q.i.d.) or placebo, in a double-blind fashion, and an elective follow-up cardiac catheterization was performed 36 months later in 348 patients. The interval change between the two cardiac catheterizations was evaluated blindly by a set of independent angiographers and a computerized image processing program; similar conclusions were reached after both methods of analysis. The results indicated that, although there were no significant between-group differences on progression of already existing coronary stenoses, there was an effect on de novo atherogenesis. There was only a nonsignificant trend in favor of nifedipine in the percentage of patients with new lesions (40% vs. 49%; $P = .129$), but the number of new lesions per patient was reported to be statistically significantly reduced in the nifedipine-treated group (0.59 vs. 0.82; $P = .034$). The latter analysis is considered less appropriate by some, since the power calculation should depend on the number of patients enrolled, not on the outcome, and because the randomization was performed for each patient rather than for each unaffected artery (36).

These results and their interpretation have been criticized on a number of grounds, perhaps most important of which was a difference in mortality, which was higher in the nifedipine group, although not quite statistically significantly so (70). Justifiable concern has also been expressed about the formulation of nifedipine used, which may have had acute, short-lived, untoward effects on blood pressure, heart rate, and/or coronary blood flow (71). The experiment may have been unrealistically ambitious, because most of the laboratory experiments began with very young animals without any atherosclerosis, and because INTACT studied older humans in which atherosclerosis was judged to be absent in a given arterial segment (despite its presence in a nearby arterial segment), based on a two-dimensional lumenogram.

There have also been several analyses of other cardiac catheterization data (some collected retrospectively, some unrandomized) to support this methodology as being able to quantitate atherogenesis and to establish the antihypertensive agent as being effective in preventing coronary stenoses. Loaldi et al. reported that, after 2 years, short-acting nifedipine significantly reduced the progression of existing coronary lesions and development of new stenoses, compared to either propranolol or isosorbide dinitrate, in only 36 to 39 patients per group (72). A randomized study of short-acting nicardipine vs. placebo for 2 years enrolled 383 patients with catheterization-documented coronary disease; repeat catheterization in 335 showed similar protection against de novo atherogenesis ($P = 0.038$ in the most favorable subgroup analysis), but little effect on existing stenoses (73). In this study, a trend (although $P = 0.21$, and far from statistically significant) was again seen in the numbers of patients with severe adverse events (death, MI, or unstable angina), with the higher risk in patients given the calcium antagonist. Immediate-release verapamil was initially reported to slow progression, increase regression, and reduce the number of new coronary stenoses in a small, retrospective series (74), but this promising conclusion was not verified in a subsequent prospective randomized trial in 159 patients recatheterized after 3 years (75).

In progress is a study of ACE inhibitor therapy (SCAT), that will compare enalapril (± simvastatin) with placebo in 468 patients with documented coronary disease and moderate hypercholesterolemia; computerized quantitative coronary angiography is planned 5 years following initial catheterization.

2.   Other Studies of Atherogenesis in the Coronary Bed

Another excellent candidate for prophylactic antiatherogenesis treatment is the autologously transplanted heart. Perhaps due to the high-dose immunosuppressive therapy in a typically hypertensive host, most heart transplant recipients develop accelerated atherosclerosis, especially in the transplanted coronary bed, which sometimes necessitates a second transplant or an aorto-coronary bypass procedure in the heart which previously had not had significant coronary stenoses. Probably the best-quality data from a properly designed, randomized, blinded, prospective, controlled clinical trial demonstrating the efficacy of antihypertensive drug therapy in these patients has been obtained by the Stanford heart transplant group using short-acting diltiazem (30 to 90 mg t.i.d.) (76). Although the study was, by design, unblinded and a randomized consecutive series without placebo control, patients catheterized 2 years after initiation of treatment with that preparation of diltiazem showed no increase in coronary arterial diameter, which was highly statistically significantly different from the decrease seen in the control (untreated) patients. The number of patients who developed stenoses > 50% were small, but higher in the control than diltiazem-treated group (7 vs. 2); all five episodes of cardiovascular death or retransplantation occurred in control patients. Further follow-up in this cohort, and results of other randomized trials will be of great interest to cardiac transplantation centers.

Some similar data have been obtained at Johns Hopkins using short-acting nifedipine (20 mg t.i.d.) in patients undergoing venous aortocoronary bypass grafting. In a preliminary analysis of 144 patients, there was a statistically significant reduction in formation of new atherosclerotic lesions in the transplanted veins at 1 year, with 67% of the grafts free of lesions in the nifedipine-treated group, vs. only 52% in the placebo-treated grafts (77). Another study randomizing patients to either verapamil or placebo after coronary artery bypass grafting in Frankfurt has been plagued by a high dropout and crossover rate, and final results are not yet available (78). The PREVENT (Prospective Randomized Evaluation of the Vascular Effects of Norvasc Trial) plans to subject 720 patients with mild coronary artery disease to a repeat catheterization after 3 years of treatment with either amlodipine or placebo; a subgroup of these patients will have additional carotid ultrasonic evaluations. HOPE (Heart Outcomes Prevention Evaluation) is a 3-year study in 9541 coronary artery disease patients, using a factorial design (ramipril and/or vitamin E), but the endpoints will be clinical events rather than an evaluation for atherosclerosis (79). A "large, simple" 5-year study of trandolapril is expected to enroll 14,000 patients with documented coronary heart disease and follow them until death or acute myocardial infarction. Similar (but smaller) studies using other ACE inhibitors (enalapril, captopril) have also been planned.

There has been a great deal of interest in studying the effects of antihypertensive agents in patients undergoing coronary angioplasty, based on encouraging results in animals subjected to iatrogenic instrumentation of an artery (typically a carotid, where the contralateral side can be studied as a control). Perhaps because the drug can be administered in this setting immediately prior to the endothelial injury, there is a close parallel in humans to the animal experiments.

Unfortunately, the results of administering antihypertensive agents to patients undergoing angioplasty have not been very successful. Probably the earliest disappointment was with nifedipine (80), although subsequent studies with diltiazem (81) fosinopril (82), and cilazapril (83) (in what may have been the best study design of this type, despite its short 6-month duration [84]) showed no significant difference between the groups who received antihypertensive drug or placebo. A very similar trial of higher dose cilazapril in Canada and the U.S. should be published shortly (85). There is a preliminary report claiming improvement with high doses of verapamil in angioplasty patients with stable angina, although the benefit was not seen in unstable angina patients (86).

Quinapril is being compared with placebo in the 3–year randomized, double-blind, prospective study named QUIET (Quinapril Ischemic Event Trial) in 1700 patients with normal LV function and a recent coronary angioplasty. The planned comparison of a prospectively identified nearby minimally diseased coronary artery in the very same patients will presumably allow assessment of the efficacy of ACE inhibitors in limiting plaque deposition in already established lesions, as well as de novo atherogenesis (87). QUIET will follow the smaller Trial on Reversing Endothelial Dysfunction (TREND) study of 129 patients, which showed a beneficial effect of quinapril over placebo in endothelium-dependent vasoconstriction (in response to acetylcholine) 6 months after the initial cardiac catheterization which demonstrated obstructive coronary disease (88). The population studied was, by design, normotensive with intact left ventricular function (situations for which ACE inhibitors typically have little salutary effect), and because the changes in endothelial function were achieved despite no alteration in lipid levels.

3. Atherogenesis in the Carotid Bed

Probably the most interesting clinical trial of antihypertensive drug therapy with a primary atherosclerosis endpoint was MIDAS (Multicenter Isradipine Diuretic Atherosclerosis Study), the final results of which have recently been published (89). Hypertensive patients with carotid stenoses by ultrasound were randomized to either isradipine (2.5 or 5 mg b.i.d.) or hydrochlorothiazide (HCTZ) (12.5 or 25 mg b.i.d.), and serial measurements of carotid intimal-medial wall thickness were made every 6 months during a 3-year follow-up period. Despite an initial difference in wall thickness after just 6 months ($P < .02$), subsequent measurements did not sustain the difference, and the comparison over the entire 3-year interval did not achieve statistical significance (90). The biggest confounder may have been the 3.5 mm Hg lower average systolic blood pressure achieved in the HCTZ group, which maintained statistical significance across the duration of the trial. Part of the design was that both groups were to receive enalapril if blood pressure was not adequately controlled with the initially assigned drug therapy; eventually about 25% of the isradipine patients and 28% of the HCTZ patients required this. Furthermore, there were 18% in the isradipine group and 20% in the HCTZ group who ended up not taking the medication to which they were initially assigned, which confounds the results of the intention-to-treat analysis. The data were reanalyzed and the wall thickness measurements reread, due to some possible technical problems with across-reader variability, but this extra work changed the conclusions only slightly. Great concern had already been raised, even prior to publication, because of the higher number of severe adverse events in the group originally assigned to take isradipine (25 vs. 14, $P = .07$; mostly due to a difference in hospitalization for presumed angina pectoris and "rule out MI," for which $P = .03$) (91). Despite the not quite significant difference in major vascular endpoints, the *a priori* statistical power of a 3-year study in 883 patients with hypertension and carotid atherosclerosis to detect a significant difference in serious cardiovascular event rates must have been small, and appropriate concern has been voiced about overgeneralizing or misinterpreting these limited data (89,92,93).

Studies similar in some ways to MIDAS have begun with verapamil, lacidipine, fosinopril, and doxazosin. In the Italian Verapamil in Hypertension Atherosclerosis Study, 1450 patients have been randomized to verapamil or chlorthalidone, 450 of whom had quantitative Doppler-ultrasound evaluations of their carotid arteries (94). Results after 3 years in both the main trial and the carotid atherosclerosis substudy should be presented shortly. Doxazosin is being studied in hypertensive patients with carotid atherosclerosis in the Netherlands (95). A 5-year randomized comparison of lacidipine or atenolol in 3708 hypertensive patients (ELSA: European Lacidipine Study of Athero-sclerosis), stratified by severity of plaquing or thickening of carotid wall thickness, will compare not only the progression of carotid disease by ultra-sound, but also clinical events and blood pressures, using ambulatory monitors (96). PART will compare ramipril with placebo treatment for 4 years in 600 patients with documented atherosclerosis, using B-mode ultrasound measure-ments of carotid intimal thickness as a primary endpoint. Using a similar end-point, two doses of ramipril are being compared (± vitamin E) in 732 patients at high risk for cardiovascular disease in a 4-year study (SECURE). PHYLLIS (Plaque Hypertension Lipid Lowering Italian Study) is a 3-year factorial design clinical trial of pravastatin and/or fosinopril in 800 hypertensive and dyslipidemic patients with at least one uncomplicated carotid stenosis by ultrasound (97).

C. Human Studies Using Clinical Endpoints

If one accepts the premise that, in Western societies, most myocardial infarc-tions and cerebrovascular accidents are related to atherosclerosis, the true test of whether hypertension is related to atherosclerosis (and the process of how it develops—atherogenesis) is whether or not therapies that lower blood pressure lead, in clinical trials against placebo, to lower rates of the atherosclerotic clinical sequelae. Such clinical trials began with the first Department of Veterans' Affairs Study, and continue even today.

It now seems clear (at least in the aggregate, based on meta-analyses, if not from individual studies themselves) that the blood pressure-lowering drugs that have been tested in long-term clinical trials are effective in reducing both myocardial infarction and stroke rates better than placebo (98). While some have argued that the reduction in myocardial infarction rates has been somewhat less impressive than epidemiology-based expectations, more recent meta-analyses and different groupings of studies have suggested that studies that used as first-line therapy either low-dose diuretics or beta-blockers have nearly achieved the goal reduction in MI rates, whereas older studies, which used high-dose diuretics, were not as successful (99).

These important results from double-blind, randomized, placebo-controlled, multicenter clinical trials convinced the Fifth U.S. Joint National Committee on Detection, Evaluation and Treatment of High Blood Pressure that diuretics and beta-blockers should be "preferred" for patients with hypertension in whom they are not contraindicated, ineffective, or not tolerated, or when there was no specific reason to start treatment with a drug from another class. Variants of the recommendation to use antihypertensive drug therapy to reduce the clinical sequelae of elevated blood pressure have been given also in Australia, Canada, Great Britain, New Zealand, and the World Health Organization/International Society of Hypertension. A more ringing endorsement of routinely using antihypertensive drug therapy to avoid atherosclerotic clinical events (in patients for whom a trial of lifestyle modification has been insufficient) is difficult to imagine.

The dichotomy about which drug therapy ought to be used initially for hypertension (JNC V recommendation vs. data from clinical practice) is a troubling one. Since 1994 (the year after publication of JNC V's recommendations), America's physicians are prescribing calcium antagonists or ACE inhibitors as the two most common choices for antihypertensive drug therapy. Some have suggested this is potentially dangerous (70,71), unwise (91), unscientific, and wasteful of scarce national health resources (100).

Data from clinical trials in heart failure and post-MI patients have proven the efficacy of some ACE inhibitors in reducing cardiovascular death and/or recurrent myocardial infarction rates. Somewhat less encouraging data are available about calcium antagonists in these diseases.

There have now been launched a number of clinical trials (see Table 2) that will eventually provide the answer to the question of whether the newer drugs (ACE inhibitors, calcium antagonists, α_1-adrenoceptor blockers, or angiotensin II receptor antagonists) reduce rates of cardiovascular death, acute

Table 2 Some Long-Term Clinical Trials of Newer Drugs for Hypertension

Acronym (name)	New drug(s)	Comparator	Patients	Comments
ALLHAT (Antihypertensive and Lipid Lowering Prevention of Heart Attack Trial)	Amlodipine, doxazosin, lisinopril	Chlorthalidone	40,000 in > 500 centers	NIH-funded, 5-year follow-up planned
CAPPP (Captopril Primary Preventive Project)	Captopril	Diuretic or beta-blocker	10,800 at 275 centers	Sweden and Finland
CONVINCE (Controlled-Onset Verapamil Investigation of Cardiovascular Endpoints)	COER-verapamil	HCTZ or atenolol	15,000 in > 300 North American and European centers	5-year follow-up planned
HOT (Hypertension Optimal Treatment)	Felodipine	None	18,000 patients in > 18 countries	Randomized to 1 of 3 BP goals
INSIGHT (International Nifedipine GITS Study Intervention as a Goal in Hypertension Treatment)	Nifedipine GITS	HCTZ + amiloride	6600 patients in 9 European countries	3-year minimum follow-up planned
LIFE (Losartan Intervention for Endpoint Reduction)	Losartan	Atenolol	9224 patients in > 300 centers	EKG-LVH only; 5-year follow-up planned
NORDIL (Nordic Diltiazem Study)	Diltiazem	Diuretic or beta-blocker	12,000 patients in 480 centers	Sweden and Norway, 5-year follow-up planned
STOP-Hypertension 2 (Swedish Trial in Old Patients with Hypertension 2)	ACE inhibitor or calcium antagonist	Diuretic or beta-blocker	6600 patients in 300 centers	Sweden, 2-year follow-up planned

myocardial infarction, or stroke. With rare exception, however, these trials are not placebo-controlled, but instead are "equivalence" trials against a representative of the diuretic or beta-blocker classes that have been used in previous trials against placebo. The much larger number of patients, the extended length of the trials, and the greater expense of these trials have now been justified to the appropriate funding agencies, and results in many of these are expected around the turn of the millennium. Until then, however, there is nearly universal agreement that hypertension is a major contributor to the atherogenic process and should be controlled with whatever therapy is effective in a given patient over the long term.

REFERENCES

1. McGill HC, Carey KD, McMahan CA, et al. Effects of two forms of hypertension on atherosclerosis in the hyperlipidemic baboon. Arteriosclerosis 1983; 5:481–493.
2. Lichtenstein AH, Brecher P, Chobanian AV. Effects of deoxycorticosterone-salt hypertension on cell ploidy in the rat aorta. Hypertension 1986; 8(suppl II):1150–1154.
3. Haudenschild CC, Prescott MF, Chobanian AV. Effects of hypertension and its reversal on aortic intima lesions of the rat. Hypertension 1980; 2:33–44.
4. Chobanian AV. Vascular effects of systemic hypertension. Am J Cardiol 1992; 69:3E–7E.
5. Ross R. The pathogenesis of atherosclerosis: An update. N Engl J Med 1986; 314:488–500.
6. Chobanian AV. Effects of hypertension on arterial gene expression and atherosclerosis. Adv Exp Med Biol 1991; 308:45–53.
7. Ross R. Cell biology of atherosclerosis. Annu Rev Physiol 1995; 57:791–804.
8. McGill HC, Arias-Stella J, Carbonell LM, et al. General findings of the international atherosclerosis project. Lab Invest 1968; 18:498–502.
9. Doyle AE. A review of the short-term benefits of antihypertensive treatment with emphasis on stroke. Am J Hypertens 1993; 6 (3 Pt 2):6S–8S.
10. Berenson GS, Srinivasan SR, Webber LS, et al. Cardiovascular Risk in Early Life: The Bogolusa Heart Study: Current Concepts. Chicago: Upjohn, 1991.
11. Zeek P. Juvenile arteriosclerosis. Arch Pathol 1930; 10:417–446.
12. Relationship of atherosclerosis in young men to serum lipoprotein cholesterol concentrations and smoking. A preliminary report from the Pathobiological Determinants of Atherosclerosis in Youth (PDAY) Research Group. JAMA 1990; 264:3018–3024.
13. McGill HC Jr, Strong JP, Tracy RE, McMahan CA, Oalmann MC. Relation of a post-mortem renal index of hypertension to atherosclerosis in youth. The Pathobiological Determinants of Atherosclerosis in Youth (PDAY) Research Group. Arterioscler Throm Vasc Biol 1995; 15:2222–2228.
14. Enos WF, Holmes RH, Boyer J. Coronary disease among United States soldiers killed in action in Korea: preliminary report. JAMA 1953; 152:1090–1093.

15. Keys A, Aravanis C, Blackburn HW, et al. Epidemiological studies related to coronary heart disease: characteristics of men aged 40–59 in seven countries. Acta Med Scand Suppl 1966; 460:1–392.
16. Kannel WB. Contribution of the Framingham Study to preventive cardiology. J Am Coll Cardiol 1990; 15:206–211.
17. Kannel WB. Hypertension as a risk factor for cardiac events—epidemiologic results of long-term studies. J Cardiovasc Pharmacol 1993; 21(suppl 2):S27–S37.
18. Williams RR, Hunt SC, Hopkins PN, et al. Familial dyslipidemic hypertension. Evidence from 58 Utah families for a syndrome present in approximately 12% of patients with essential hypertension. JAMA 1988; 259:3579–3586.
19. MacMahon S, Peto R, Cutler J, et al. Blood pressure, stroke, and coronary heart disease. Part 1. Prolonged differences in blood pressure: prospective observational studies corrected for the regression dilution bias. Lancet 1990; 335:765–774.
20. Goldblatt H, Lynch J, Hanzal RF, Summerville WW. Studies on experimental hypertension. I. The production of persistent elevation of systolic blood pressure by means of renal ischemia. J Exp Med 1934; 59:347–378.
21. Rossi GP, Rossi A, Zanin L, et al. Excess prevalence of extracranial carotid artery lesions in renovascular hypertension. Am J Hyperten 1992; 5:8–15.
22. Chiesura-Corona M, Feltrin GP, Sevastano S, et al. Excess prevalence of supra-aortic artery lesions in renovascular hypertension: an angiographic study. Cardiovasc Intervent Radiol 1994; 17:264–270.
23. Davis BA, Crook HE, Vestal RE, Oates JA. Prevalence of renovascular hypertension in patients with grade III or IV hypertensive retinopathy. N Engl J Med 1979; 301:1273–1276.
24. Rossi GP, Pavan E, Pessina AC. Role of genetic, humoral, and endothelial factors in hypertension-induced atherosclerosis. J Cardiovasc Pharmacol 1994; 23(suppl 5):S75–S84.
25. Rossi G, Rossi A, Sacchetto A, Pavan E, Pessina AC. Hypertensive cerebrovascular disease and the renin-angiotensin system. Stroke 1995; 26:1700–6.
26. Brunner HR, Laragh JH, Baer L, et al. Essential hypertension: renin and aldosterone, heart attack and stroke. N Engl J Med 1972; 286:441–449.
27. Alderman MH, Madhavan S, Ooi WJ, Cohen H, Sealey JE, Laragh JH. Association of the renin-sodium profile with the risk of myocardial infarction in patients with hypertension. N Engl J Med 1991; 324:1098–1104.
28. Meade TW, Cooper JA, Peart WS. Plasma renin activity and ischemic heart disease. N Engl J Med 1993; 329:0000–0000.
29. Alderman MH, Madhavan S, Cohen H, Sealey JE, Laragh JH. Low urinary sodium is associated with greater risk of myocardial infarction among treated hypertensive men. Hypertension 1995; 25:1144–1152.
30. Sowers JR, Sowers PS, Peuler JD. Role of insulin resistance and hyperinsulinemia in development of hypertension and atherosclerosis. J Lab Clin Med 1994; 123:647–652.
31. Alexander RW. Theodore Cooper Memorial Lecture. Hypertension and the pathogenesis of atherosclerosis. Oxidative stress and the mediation of arterial inflammatory response: a new perspective. Hypertension 1995; 25:155–161.

32. Reaven GM, Lithell H, Landsberg L. Hypertension and associated metabolic abnormalities—the role of insulin resistance and the sympathoadrenal system. N Engl J Med 1996; 334:374–381.
33. Omoigui N, Dzau VJ. Differential effects of antihypertensive agents in experimental and human atherosclerosis. Am J Hypertens 1993; 6(3 Pt 2):30S–39S.
34. Henry PD, Bentley KI. Suppression of atherogenesis in cholesterol-fed rabbits treated with nifedipine. J Clin Invest 1981; 68:1366–1369.
35. Holzgreve H, Burkle B. Anti-atherosclerotic effects of calcium antagonists. J Hypertens Suppl 1993; 11:S55–S59.
36. Waters D, Lespérance J. Calcium channel blockers and coronary atherosclerosis: from the rabbit to the real world. Am Heart J 1994; 128:1309–1316.
37. Habib JB, Bosaller C, Wells S, Williams C, Morisett JD, Henry PD. Preservation of endothelium-dependent vascular relaxation in cholesterol-fed rabbits by treatment with the calcium blocker PN 200–110. Circ Res 1986; 58:305–309.
38. Handley DA, Van Valen RG, Melden MK, et al. Suppression of rat carotid lesion development by the calcium channel blocker PN 200–110. Am J Pathol 1986; 124:88–93.
39. Leonetti G, Sampieri L, Bragato R, Comerio G. Effect of verapamil on atherosclerosis. Drugs 1993; 2:75–81.
40. Ouchi Y, Orimo H. The role of calcium antagonists in the treatment of atherosclerosis and hypertension. J Cardiovasc Pharmacol 1990; 16(suppl 2):S1–S4.
41. Rafflenbeul W. Hypertension treatment and prevention of new atherosclerotic plaque formation. Drugs 1994; 48(suppl 1):11–15.
42. Riezebos J, Vleeming W, Beems RB, et al. Comparison of the antiatherogenic effects of isradipine and ramipril in cholesterol-fed rabbits. I. Effect on progression of atherosclerosis and endothelial dysfunction. J Cardiovasc Pharmacol 1994; 23:415–423.
43. Riezebos J, Vleeming W, Beems RB, et al. Comparison of the antiatherogenic effects of isradipine and ramipril in cholesterol-fed rabbits. II. Effect on regression of atherosclerosis and restoration of endothelial function. J Cardiovasc Pharmacol 1994; 23:424–431.
44. Aberg G, Ferrer P. Effects of captopril on atherosclerosis in cynomolgus monkeys. J Cardiovasc Pharmacol 1990; 15(suppl 5):S65–S75.
45. Dzau VJ. Vascular renin-angiotensin system and vascular protection. J Cardiovasc Pharmacol 1993; 22(suppl 5):S1–S9.
46. Kaplan JR, Manuck SB. Antiatherogenic effects of beta-adrenergic blocking agents: theoretical, experimental, and epidemiologic considerations. Am Heart J 1994; 128:1316–1328.
47. Bondjers G. Anti-atherosclerotic effects of beta-blockers. Eur Heart J 1994; 15(suppl C):8–15.
48. Spence JD, Perkins DG, Klein RL, Adams MR, Haust MD. Hemodynamic modifications of aortic atherosclerosis: effects of propranolol versus hydralazine in hypertensive hyperlipidemic rabbits. Atherosclerosis 1984; 50:325–333.
49. Kowala MC, Nicolosi RJ. Effect of doxazosin on plasma lipids and atherogenesis: A preliminary report. J Cardiovasc Pharmacol 1989; 13(suppl 2):S45–S49.

50. Chobanian AV, Handenscheild CC, Nickerson C, Drago R. Antiatherogenic effect of captopril in the Watanabe heritable hyperlipemic rabbit. Hypertension 1990; 15:327–331.

51. Chobanian AV, Haudenschild CC, Nickerson C, Hope S. Trandolapril inhibits atherosclerosis in the Watanabe heritable hyperlipidemic rabbit. Hypertension 1992; 20:473–477.

52. Hudson P, Holland TK, McCraw AP, Duffen J, Sim AK. Evaluation of the effect of cicletanine on genetic atherosclerosis in the rabbit. Arch Mal Coeur 1989; 82:71–77.

53. Lichtenstein AH, Drago R, Nickerson C, Prescott MF, Lee SQ, Chobanian AV. The effect of propranolol on atherogenesis in the Watanabe heritable hyperlipidemic rabbit. J Vasc Med Biol 1989; 1:248–254.

54. Watanabe N, Ishikawa Y, Okamoto R, Watanabe Y, Fukazaki H. Nifedipine suppressed atherosclerosis in cholesterol-fed rabbits but not in Watanabe heritable hyperlipidemic rabbits. Artery 1987; 14:283–294.

55. van Niekerk JLM, Hendriks TH, De Boer HHM, Van't Laar A. Does nifedipine suppress atherogenesis is WHHL rabbits? Atherosclerosis 1984; 53:91–98.

56. Tilton GD, Buja LM, Bilheimer DW, et al. Failure of slow channel calcium antagonist, verapamil, to retard atherosclerosis in the Watanabe heritable hyperlipidemic rabbit: an animal model of familial hypercholesterolemia. J Am Coll Cardiol 1985; 6:141–144.

57. Nomoto A, Hirosumi J, Sekiguchi C, et al. Antiatherogenic activity of FR 34.235 (nilvadipine), a new potent calcium-antagonist. Atherosclerosis 1987; 64:255–261.

58. Sinzinger H, Lupatelli G, Virgolini I, et al. Isradipine, a calcium entry blocker, decreases the vascular ^{125}I low density lipoprotein entry in hypercholesterolemic rabbits. J Cardiovasc Pharmacol 1991; 17:546–550.

59. Atkinson JB, Wudel JH, Hoff SJ, Stewart JR, Frist WH. Amlodipine reduces graft coronary artery disease in rat heterotopic cardiac allografts. J Heart Lung Transplant 1993; 12:1036–1043.

60. Christensen HRL, Nielsen H, Christensen KL, et al. Long-term hypotensive effects of an angiotensin-converting enzyme inhibitor in spontaneously hypertensive rats: is there a role for vascular structure? J Hypertens 1988; 6(suppl 3):S27–S31.

61. Plissonnier D, Amichot G, Duriez M, Legagneux J, Levy BI, Michel JB. Effect of converting enzyme inhibition on allograft-induced arterial wall injury and response. Hypertension 1991; 18(suppl II):II-47–II-54.

62. Powell JS, Clozel JP, Muller RKM, et al. Inhibitors of angiotensin-converting enzyme prevent myointimal proliferation after vascular injury. Science 1989; 245:186–188.

63. Hajdu MA, Heistad DD, Baumbach GL. Effects of anti-hypertensive therapy on mechanics of cerebral arterioles in rats. Hypertension 1991; 17:308–316.

64. Bell L, Madri JA. Influence of the angiotensin system on endothelial and smooth muscle cell migration. Am J Pathol 1990; 137:7–12.

65. Rakugi H, Wang DS, Dzau VJ, Pratt RE. Potential importance of tissue angiotensin-converting enzyme inhibition in preventing neointimal hyperplasia. Circulation 1994; 90:449–455.

66. O'Malley MK, McDermott EWM, Mehigan D, O'Higgins NJ. Role for prazosin in reducing the development of rabbit intimal hyperplasia after endothelial denudation. Br J Surg 1989; 76:936–938.

67. Kauffman RF, Bean JS, Zimmerman KM, Brown RF, Steinberg MI. Inhibition by DuP 753, a non-peptide angiotensin II antagonist, of neointima formation following balloon injury of rat carotid arteries. Circulation 1991; 84(suppl II):II–141. Abstract.

68. Pepine CJ. Angiotensin converting enzyme inhibition and coronary artery disease. J Hypertens Suppl 1994; 12:S65–S71.

69. Lichtlen PR, Hugenholz PG, Raffenbeul W, Hecker H, Jost S, Deckers JW. Retardation of angiographic progression of coronary artery disease by nifedipine. Lancet 1990; 335:1109–1113.

70. Furberg CD, Psaty BM, Meyer JV. Nifedipine: Dose-related increase in mortality in patients with coronary heart disease. Circulation 1995; 92:1326–11331.

71. Furberg CD, Psaty BM. Should dihydropyridines be used as first-line drugs in the treatment of hypertension? The con side. Arch Intern Med 1995; 155:2157–2161.

72. Loaldi A, Polese A, Montorsi P, et al. Comparison of nifedipine, propranolol, and isosorbide dinitrate on angiographic progression and regression of coronary arterial narrowings in angina pectoris. Am J Cardiol 1989; 64:433–439.

73. Waters D, Lespérance J, Francetich M, et al. A controlled clinical trial to assess the effect of a calcium channel blocker on the progression of coronary atherosclerosis. Circulation 1990; 82:1940–1953.

74. Kober G, Nickelsen T, Jakobs B, Kaltenbach M. The influence of long-term therapy with verapamil on the development of coronary artery stenosis. In: Rosenthal J, ed. Calcium Antagonists and Hypertension: Current Status Symposium. New York: Excerpta Medica, 1986: 97–105.

75. Kober G, Schneider W, Cieslinki G, Kaltenbach M. Can the coronary atherosclerosis process be influenced by calcium-antagonists? Drugs 1992; 44(suppl 1): 123–127.

76. Schroeder JS, Gao SZ, Alderman EL, et al. A preliminary study of diltiazem in the prevention of coronary artery disease in heart transplant patients. N Engl J Med 1993; 328:164–170.

77. Gottlieb SO, Brinker JA, Mellits ED, et al. Effect of nifedipine on the development of coronary bypass graft stenoses in high-risk patients: A randomized, double-blind, placebo-controlled trial. Circulation 1989; 80(suppl II):228. Abstract.

78. Schneider W, Kober G, Roebruck P, et al. Retardation of development and progression of coronary atherosclerosis, a new indication for calcium antagonists? Eur J Clin Pharmacol 1990; 39(suppl 1):S17–S23.

79. HOPE (Heart Outcomes Prevention Evaluation) Study. The design of a large, simple randomized trial of an angiotensin-converting enzyme inhibitor (ramipril) and vitamin E in patients at high risk of cardiovascular events. The HOPE Study Investigators. Can J Cardiol 1996; 12:127–137.

80. Marcus AJ. Aspirin: an antithrombotic medication. N Engl J Med 1983; 309: 1515–1517.

81. Corios T, David PR, Val PG. Failure of diltiazem to prevent restenosis after percutaneous transluminal coronary angioplasty. Am Heart J 1985; 109:926–931.

82. Desmet W, Vrolix M, De Scheerder I, Van Lierde J, Willems JL, Piessens J. Angiotensin-converting enzyme inhibition with fosinopril sodium in the prevention of restenosis after coronary angioplasty. Circulation 1994; 89:385–392.

83. Faxon DP. Angiotensin converting enzyme inhibition and restenosis: the final results of the Mercator trial. Circulation 1992; 86(suppl I):I–53. Abstract.

84. Multicenter European Research Trial with Cilazapril after Angioplasty to Prevent Transluminal Coronary Obstruction and Restenosis (MERCATOR) Study Group. Does the new angiotensin converting enzyme inhibitor cilazapril prevent restenosis after percutaneous transluminal coronary angioplasty? Results of the MERCATOR study: a multicenter, randomized, double-blind placebo-controlled trial. Circulation 1992; 86(suppl I):100–110.

85. Faxon DP. Angiotensin converting enzyme inhibition and restenosis: The final results of the MERCATOR Trial. Circulation 1992; 86(suppl I):I-53. Abstract.

86. Hoberg E, Kübler W. Effects of calcium-antagonist treatment on late restenosis after PTCA. Thrombos Res 1992; 65(suppl I):63. Abstract.

87. Texter M, Lees RS, Pitt B, Dinsmore RE, Uprichard ACG. The Quinapril Ischemic Event Trial (QUIET): design and methods: evaluation of chron- ic ACE inhibitor therapy after coronary artery intervention. Cardiovasc Drugs Ther 1993; 7:273–282.

88. Mancini GBJ, Henry GC, Macaya C, et al. Angiotensin-converting enzyme inhibition with quinapril improves endothelial vasomotor dysfunction in patients with coronary artery disease: The TREND (Trial on Reversing Endothelial Dysfunction) Study. Circulation 1996; 94:258–265.

89. Borhani NO, Mercuri M, Borhani PA, et al. Final outcome results of the Multicenter Isradipine Diuretic Atherosclerosis Study (MIDAS). JAMA 1996; 276:785–791.

90. McClellan K. Unexpected results from MIDAS in atherosclerosis. Inpharma 1994; 932:4.

91. Furberg CD, Psaty BM. Calcium antagonists: not appropriate as first line antihypertensive agents. Am J Hypertens 1996; 9:122–124.

92. Brogden RN, Sorkin EM. Isradipine. An update of its pharmacodynamic and pharmacokinetic properties and therapeutic efficacy in the treatment of mild to moderate hypertension. Drugs 1995; 49:618–649.

93. Chobanian AV. Calcium channel blockers: lessons learned from MIDAS and other clinical trials. JAMA 1996; 276:829–830.

94. Zanchetti A, Magnani B, Dal Palù C. Atherosclerosis and calcium-antagonists: The VHAS study. J Human Hypertens 1992; 6(suppl 2):1–8.

95. Barth JD, De Heide L, Van Swijndrecht A. Doxazosin atherosclerosis progression study in hypertension in the Netherlands. Symposium on the Atherosclerotic Process in Hypertensive Patients. Toledo, Spain, 1992. Abstract.

96. Bond G, Dal Palù C, Hansson L, et al. The ELSA trial: protocol of a randomized trial to explore the differential effect of antihypertensive drugs on atherosclerosis in hypertension. J Cardiovasc Pharmacol 1994; 23(suppl 5):S85–S87.

97. Borghi C, Bacchelli S, Ambrosioni E. The use of zofenopril and fosinopril in acute myocardial infarction and carotid artery disease. Am J Hypertens 1994; 7(9 Pt 2):96S-101S.
98. Collins R, Peto R, MacMahon S, et al. Blood pressure, stroke, and coronary heart disease. Part 2. Short-term reductions in blood pressure: Overview of randomised drug trials in their epidemiological context. Lancet 1990; 335:827–838.
99. Psaty BM, Smith NL, Siscovick DS, et al. Health outcomes associated with antihypertensive therapies used as first-line agents: a systematic review and meta-analysis. JAMA 1997; 277:739–745.
100. Manolio TA, Cutler JA, Furberg CD, Psaty BM, Whelton PK, Applegate WB. Trends in pharmacologic management of hypertension in the United States. Arch Intern Med 1995; 155:829–837.

4
Smoking and Atherogenesis

Thomas E. Kottke, Antonio Cabrera,[*] and Miriam A. Marquez[†]
Mayo Clinic and Foundation, Rochester, Minnesota

I. INTRODUCTION

Although the first scientific data that tobacco causes disease were case control studies on tobacco and the risk of lung cancer (1,2), atherosclerotic diseases are the dominant manifestation of smoking in the United States and Europe. After 40 years of follow-up of the British doctors' smoking study, Doll et al. (3) found that between 1971 and 1991, half of deaths were from vascular causes, 25% were from neoplasms, and 12% were from nonneoplastic respiratory diseases. In this cohort, the only cardiovascular diseases that did not show a dose-response relationship between the amount smoked and risk of death were venous thrombosis and rheumatic heart disease. The data suggest that half of all regular cigarette smokers will eventually die from their habit (3).

Epidemiological (4–8) evidence has also been presented to demonstrate that environmental tobacco smoke (ETS) raises the risk of atherosclerotic disease for nonsmokers. The epidemiological evidence is bolstered by observations that urinary levels of cotinine, a nicotine metabolite, parallel exposure to environmental tobacco smoke in the home and work site (9). Experimental data also demonstrate that exposure to environmental tobacco smoke 6 hours a day for a period of only 6 weeks increases myocardial infarction size in rats (10).

Current affiliations:
[*] Hospital de la Candelaria, Santa Cruz de Tenerife, Canary Islands, Spain
[†] University of Puerto Rico, San Juan, Puerto Rico

Although the first data to be presented on the hazards of environmental tobacco smoke were also on the relationship between tobacco smoke and lung cancer (11), Glantz and Parmley have demonstrated that the majority of the burden from environmental tobacco smoke in the United States is due to atherosclerotic diseases. It is accepted that ETS causes 35,000 to 40,000 premature deaths each year from cardiovascular disease in the United States (6,12). This is nearly 10% of all deaths attributable to tobacco.

Even though there are data to support the hypothesis that both active smoking and environmental tobacco smoke cause atherosclerotic disease, two critical observations do not support this conclusion. First, in Japan, where more than 80% of men smoked in the 1950s and 60% of men currently smoke, the levels of coronary heart disease are very low (13). Second, smoking does not affect total cholesterol levels in the blood (14–18).

While a hypothesis of genetically inferred susceptibility or resistance in different populations might be proposed, data from the MRFIT study do not support one. The four racial groups (blacks, Hispanics, Orientals, and whites) in this study all showed a risk of coronary heart disease death that was at least doubled in smokers of 20 to 39 cigarettes per day when compared to nonsmokers (19). It might also be proposed that smoking promotes the clinical manifestations of atherosclerosis without causing atherosclerosis. However, this in not the case in smokers in the United States and western Europe (20–23).

A plausible alternative hypothesis why tobacco smoke can be athero-genic in some populations but not in others is that an additional factor must be present if injury to the arterial endothelium, activation of platelets, and oxidative damage to the myocardium, all caused by exposure to tobacco smoke or components of tobacco, are to progress to atherosclerosis. This factor appears to be high levels of low-density lipoprotein (LDL)—a risk factor that is nearly ubiquitous in the United States, western Europe, and other parts of the world where smoking has been shown to be a risk factor for atherosclerosis. The remaining sections of this chapter review the nature and strength of the evidence that supports this hypothesis.

II. HOW TOBACCO SMOKE DAMAGES BLOOD VESSELS

A. Endothelial Desquamation and Platelet Aggregation

Both active (24) and passive smoking (25) increase endothelial desquamation and platelet activation. Temporary increases in platelet thrombus formation has been shown to occur in smokers immediately after they have smoked a cigarette (26). Smoking is also associated with an increase in the mean platelet volume, probably by consumption of older platelets and activation of mega-cariocytes to produce younger, larger platelets (27). These larger platelets are more active and may contribute to the acceleration of atherosclerosis.

To document the effects of smoking on platelets and endothelial des-quamation, Davis et al. (25) recruited 10 healthy male medical students and physicians who were nonsmokers and had them participate in two 20–min experimental periods. Five men participated in the control period first, and five men participated in the passive smoking period first. The periods were separated by 1 week, and the participants were prohibited from taking aspirin or other nonsteroidal anti-inflammatory agents beginning 10 days before the experiments. The control period consisted of sitting in a laboratory where smoking was prohibited, and the passive smoking period consisted of sitting where hospitalized patients came to smoke of their own accord. Blood was collected from an antecubital vein before and after the control and passive smoking periods to determine the platelet aggregation ratio, the endothelial cell count, the plasma nicotine concentration, and the carboxyhemoglobin level.

The mean values before and after the control period were unchanged for the platelet aggregation level (0.88 ± 0.05 vs. 0.88 ± 0.04), endothelial cell count (2.2 ± 0.8 vs. 2.3 ± 1.0), plasma nicotine concentration (0 vs. 0), and blood carboxyhemoglobin level (1.1 ± 0.6 vs. 1.2 ± 0.7). After the passive smoking period, carboxyhemoglobin levels rose from 0.9% ± 0.3% (mean ± SD) to 1.3% ± 0.6% (P = .004) and plasma nicotine levels rose from undetectable to 2.8 ± 1.2 ng/ml (P = .004). The platelet aggregation level declined from 0.87 ± 0.06 to 0.78 ± 0.07 (P = .002), and, as can be seen in Figure 1, the endothelial cell count rose significantly from 2.8 ± 0.9 to 3.7 ± 1.1 per counting chamber (P = .002). It is inferred from the decline in platelet activation in vitro that the platelets were activated by the tobacco smoke in vivo.

In another series of experiments, this same group compared the effects of tobacco and nontobacco cigarettes. They found that the tobacco cigarettes had a far greater effect on both endothelial cell counts and platelet aggregation ratios than nontobacco cigarettes (24). This observation confirmed Levine's finding that smoking a lettuce leaf cigarette did not cause the same perturba-tion of platelet aggregation as smoking a tobacco cigarette (28).

To define the mechanism by which tobacco smoke increases the propen-sity of platelets to aggregate when exposed to tobacco smoke, Burghuber et al. (29) tested the effects of active and passive smoking on platelet sensitivity to prostaglandin (PG) I_2. In the active smoking experiment, seven nonsmokers and seven moderate to heavy smokers were recruited to smoke two cigarettes within 10 min. Immediately before and 15 min after smoking the two cigarettes, blood pressure, pulse rate, and ventilatory function were measured, and blood

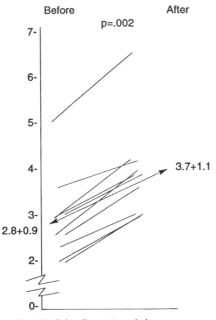

Figure 1 Exposure to environmental tobacco smoke significantly increases endothelial desquamation. From: Davis JW, Shelton L, Watanabe IS, Arnold J. Passive smoking affects endothelium and platelets. Arch Intern Med 1989; 149:386–389, with permission.

was drawn from a previously inserted plastic cannula. Platelet-rich and platelet-poor plasma were produced for each subject and then mixed to produce a platelet count of approximately $250 \times 10^3 / \mu l$. Irreversible ADP-induced platelet aggregation was measured in a Born-type aggregometer. The sensitivity index of platelets to PGI_2 was calculated by adding increasing concentrations of PGI_2 (1, 2, 3 ng/ml) 60 sec before adding the ADP.

In the passive smoking experiment, 13 smokers and nine nonsmokers were exposed to environmental tobacco smoke for 20 min at a concentration that had been calculated to be present in restaurants and night clubs. The same aggregation studies were performed for the passive smoking as for the active smoking experiment.

Prior to smoking two cigarettes, the aggregation of platelets in response to ADP was the same in smokers and nonsmokers, but the platelet sensitivity to PGI_2 was significantly lower in smokers than nonsmokers (Fig. 2). After

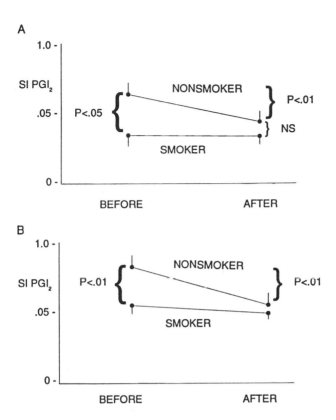

Figure 2 Both active (A) and passive (B) smoking reduces the sensitivity of non-smokers' platelets to PGI_2. The sensitivity index, SI PGI_2, is defined as the inverse of the concentration of PGI_2 necessary to inhibit ADP-induced platelet aggregation by 50%. Lower values of SI PGI_2 indicate greater platelet aggregation. Modified from Burghuber OC, Punzengruber CH, Sinzinger H, Haber P, Silberbauer K. Platelet sensitivity to prostacyclin in smokers and nonsmokers. Chest 1986; 90: 34–38, with permission.

two cigarettes were smoked, platelet sensitivity to PGI_2 did not change for the smokers but decreased significantly in the nonsmokers so that no significant differences were present between smokers and nonsmokers.

In the passive smoking experiment, a similar pattern was observed (Fig. 2). Exposure to tobacco smoke did not change the sensitivity of smokers' platelets to PGI_2 while nonsmokers' platelets became significantly less sensitive to PGI_2 after exposure to tobacco smoke.

B.   Nicotine-Induced Free Radical Formation

Although there is a clear association between tobacco smoke and atherosclerosis, the causative agent remains elusive. It has been demonstrated experi-
mentally that the carbon monoxide but not the nicotine in smoke increases
the permeability of the arterial wall to the fibrinogen (30). The level of plasma
fibrinogen is positively correlated to the adherence of circulating monocytes
on endothelial cells (31). Even though nicotine does not raise levels of fibrinogen, nicotine raises the concentration of endothelin-1, a powerful vasoconstrictor that might play a role in mechanisms of atherosclerosis in smokers
(32).

To test whether nicotine might have a direct effect on ischemic myocardium through the action of free radicals, Przyklenk isolated two segments
of the left anterior descending artery (LAD) in 34 mongrel dogs and monitored
segmental shortening and other physiologic parameters under three conditions:
nicotine administered before coronary occlusion, nicotine administered after
coronary occlusion, and saline administration (33). The dose of nicotine was
80 µg/kg dissolved in 15 ml saline.

The proportion of the left ventricle represented by the occluded LAD
bed did not differ among the three groups, there was no evidence of infarction
with LAD occlusion, and infusion of the nicotine did not cause a significant
hemodynamic response before occlusion of the LAD. All dogs experienced
dyskinesis in the LAD bed during LAD occlusion, and, as expected, the
segment remained "stunned" after reperfusion. The segments recovered to a
mean of 54%±6% of baseline at 1 hour after reflow and 50%±4% at 3 hours
after reflow. In the dogs that were given nicotine before coronary occlusion,
fractional shortening recovered to only 29%±9% and 22%±5% at one and
three hours respectively (both $P < .01$). In the animals randomized to receive
nicotine after reperfusion, segmental shortening was not different from control
group dogs at 1 hour (47%±11%; $P = $ NS) but at 3 hours after reperfusion
averaged only 7%±13% of baseline ($P < .01$).

To test the hypothesis that free radicals were causing the depressed
fractional shortening, the investigator randomized eight dogs to receive the
free radical scavenging agent *N*-2–mercaptopriopionyl glycine (MPG) plus
nicotine or MPG plus saline 45 min after reperfusion. In the experiment, area
at risk and regional myocardial blood flow were similar in the two groups,
and MPG administered 45 minutes after reperfusion had no significant beneficial effect on the contractile function of the myocardium that had been
stunned by ischemia. In contrast to a decline in segmental shortening in dogs
receiving postreflow nicotine without MPG, segmental shortening in the dogs
that received MPG plus nicotine remained constant, averaging 54%±11% and
56%±9% of baseline at 1 and 3 hours after reperfusion. The investigator

concluded that the slow, low-dose infusion of nicotine had a selective effect on the ischemic/reperfused tissue and that this effect was not secondary to unfavorable changes in hemodynamics, perfusion, or nicotine-induced necrosis. Rather, the data were interpreted as suggesting that the dysfunction caused by the infusion of nicotine could be due to free radicals acting on reversibly injured myocytes. The clinical correlation of this experiment is the observation that smokers with occlusion of their left anterior descending coronary artery have left ventricular dysfunction that is out of proportion to their coronary artery disease (34).

C. Serum Lipid Alterations

Smoking has little or no effect on total cholesterol levels (14–18). However, in these same populations, smokers have lower high-density lipoprotein (HDL) levels. This appears to be, in part, due to the effect of smoking on lecithin-cholesterol acyltransferase (LCAT) activity (35). This plasma enzyme maintains the unesterified cholesterol concentration gradient, permitting cholesterol efflux from cholesterol-laden cells to HDL where it is esterified.

McCall et al. (35) investigated the direct effects of gas-phase cigarette smoke on plasma constituents, including HDL, LDL, and LCAT, in an in vitro model. They collected blood from eight nonsmoking volunteers who did not supplement their diets with vitamins. The investigators exposed the freshly isolated human plasma to gas-phase cigarette smoking in a side-arm flask connected to a vacuum line that drew smoke from a research cigarette into the flask. Plasma samples were subjected to agarose gel electrophoresis to determine whether electrophoretic mobilities of specific lipoprotein classes were altered by smoke exposure.

The investigators found that in vitro exposure of plasma to filtered cigarette smoke dramatically inhibited LCAT activity. At 1 hour, the smoke-exposed plasma possessed less than half the activity of the air-exposed control, and by 6 hours only 22% of control activity was observed in the smoke-exposed plasma. The apo-A-I and apo-A-II components of HDL were rapidly crosslinked by exposure to cigarette smoke. The authors suggest that crosslinkage of apo AI results in its destruction in vivo, and that the reduced HDL concentrations observed in smokers are the result of increased HDL catabolism rather than reduced HDL synthesis.

Heitzer et al. (36) have shown that smoking and hypercholesterolemia act synergistically to impair endothelial function. In a study designed to examine the effect of smoking on endothelium-dependent relaxation in patients with and without hyperlipidemia, 55 subjects were examined: 15 nonsmokers with hypercholesterolemia, 15 longterm smokers, 15 smokers with hypercholesterolemia, and 10 normal subjects. Hypercholesterolemia was de-

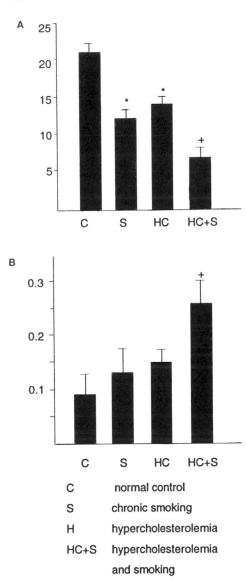

C   normal control

S   chronic smoking

H   hypercholesterolemia

HC+S   hypercholesterolemia
            and smoking

Figure 3   (A) Maximal acetylcholine-induced forearm blood flow in ml/min/100 ml of tissue in normal subjects, hypercholesterolemic subjects, long-term smokers, and patients with hypercholesterolemia who smoked (n = 8 for each group). (B) Plasma levels of autoantibody titer against oxidized LDL in the same subjects. Data are mean ± SEM. *P < .05 vs. normal subjects and patients with hypercholesterolemia and smoking; P < .05 vs. all three other groups. Modified from: Heitzer T, Yla-Herttuala S, Luoma J, et al. Cigarette smoking potentiates endothelial dysfunction of forearm resistance vessels in patients with hypercholesterolemia. Role of oxidized LDL. Circulation 1996; 93:1346–1353, with permission.

fined as an LDL greater than the 75th percentile for age and gender, and smoking was defined as > 20 pack-years of smoking. Subjects with hematological, renal, or hepatic dysfunction were excluded, and no subject had diabetes mellitus, arterial hypertension, congestive heart failure, vasculitis, Raynaud's phenomenon, or cardiac disease. Forearm blood flow (FBF) was measured, and forearm vascular resistance was calculated as the ratio of mean blood pressure to FBF. To assess endothelium-dependent vasodilatation, acetylcholine was administered in increasing dosages of 7.5, 15, 30, and 60 μg/min. To evaluate vascular smooth muscle relaxation independent of endothelial factors, each study participant received an intra-arterial infusion of sodium nitroprusside at dosages of 1, 3, and 10 μg/min. In a subset of patients, blood samples were obtained to measure autoantibodies against oxidized LDL.

In the normal subjects, stepwise-increasing dosages of acetylcholine augmented FBF from 2.9 ± 0.3 to 21.2 ± 0.8 ml/min/100 ml forearm tissue. The vasodilator response in the other three groups was significantly less (Fig. 3). There was also a difference among (a) the group with hypercholesterolemia *and* smoking in comparison to (b) the group with smoking alone and (c) the group with hypercholesterolemia alone. Alpha adrenoreceptor blockade with phentolomine did not erase these differences. There were no differences among the four groups to increasing doses of sodium nitroprusside, a non-endothelial-dependent vasodilator.

Compared to normal controls, smoking by hyperlipidemic patients was associated with a 2.5-fold increase in plasma levels of autoantibodies against oxidized LDL. Compared to subjects who only smoked or subjects who were only hyperlipidemic, smokers who were hyperlipidemic had twofold increases in autoantibodies against oxidized LDL. In a multivariate analysis that included LDL, HDL, triglycerides, LDL-to-HDL ratio, oxidized LDL, and autoantibodies against oxidized LDL, the presence of autoantibodies against oxidized LDL was the only independent factor related to endothelial dysfunction ($P < .005$).

D. Smoking and Peroxidation

Mezzetti et al. analyzed the levels of vitamins E and C and lipid peroxidation in plasma and arterial tissue of smokers and nonsmokers (37). They carried their study out in 48 male patients (24 smokers and 24 nonsmokers) who were undergoing aortocoronary bypass surgery. Patients with diabetes mellitus, systolic blood pressure > 160 mm Hg, or diastolic blood pressure > 100 mm Hg were excluded from the study. No patient had been taking lipid-lowering drugs, vitamin supplements containing E or C, or antioxidants within 30 days. The smokers had smoked at least 15 cigarettes a day for over 2 years and currently averaged 30 cigarettes per day. All were still active

Table 1   Tissue and Plasma Levels of Vitamins C and E and Levels
of Fluorescent Products of Peroxidation in Smokers and Nonsmokers

	Smokers	Nonsmokers	P
Tissue vitamin E	0.23 ± 0.03	0.41 ± 0.04	.0006
Tissue vitamin C	4.35 ± 0.30	8.58 ± 1.03	.0005
Tissue FPL[a]	1.32 ± 0.09	0.77 ± 0.07	.0005
Plasma vitamin E	28.8 ± 2.7	31.6 ± 3.0	NS
Plasma vitamin C	15.5 ± 1.6	24.5 ± 1.6	.0002
Plasma FPL	17.6 ± 1.7	9.7 ± 1.1	.0005
Vitamin E/cholesterol	5.52 ± 0.56	5.45 ± 0.39	NS

Source: Adapted from Mezzetti A, Lapenna D, Pierdomenico SD, et al. Vitamins E, C,
and lipid peroxidation in plasma and arterial tissue of smokers and nonsmokers.
Atherosclerosis 1995; 112:91–99.
[a]Fluorescent products of peroxidation

smokers. The two groups did not differ with respect to age, serum lipids, or
the prevalence of hypertension. A fasting venous blood sample was taken
from each patient before surgery, and a small segment of internal mammary
artery was harvested from each patient during surgery.

Serum levels of total cholesterol, HDL, LDL, apo-A-I and apo-B were
not significantly different between the two groups. However, coronary atherosclerotic involvement, measured by a coronary stenosis score, was significantly greater in the smokers than the nonsmokers (20.6 ± 1.3 vs. 16.6 ± 0.8;
$P < 0.02$). Tissue vitamin E and C levels were significantly lower in the
smokers than in the nonsmokers as were plasma levels of vitamin C (Table
1). Plasma levels of vitamin E were not different between the two groups.
Fluorescent products of lipid peroxidation were significantly higher in the
tissue and plasma of the smokers. The coronary stenosis score was inversely
related to tissue vitamin E levels in smokers ($r = -.57$, $P < .06$) and in
nonsmokers ($r = -.42$, $P < .05$). It was directly related to fluorescent products
of lipoperoxidation ($r = 0.59$ in smokers, $P < .005$; $r = .48$ in nonsmokers,
$P < .025$). No significant correlation between coronary score and plasma
levels of vitamins or lipid peroxidases was found.

McCall et al. (35), in the same set of in vitro experiments described
above, measured the effect of gas-phase cigarette smoke on plasma antioxidant
concentrations. Ascorbic acid was not detectable after 1 hour of exposure.
Alpha-tocopherol and urate concentrations decreased gradually after an initial
lag period of about an hour. Concentrations of alpha-tocopheral and urate
were 40% and 25%, respectively, of control values after 6 hours.

Miwa et al. (38) studied 29 patients with active variant angina who had spontaneous angina with ST-segment elevation at least twice a week, 13 patients with inactive variant angina, 32 patients with stable effort angina due to fixed stenoses, and 30 patients without coronary artery disease or angina. They obtained blood for analysis of lipids and vitamin E, and the patients with active variant angina were treated with diltiazem or nifedipine to control their angina. In six of these patients who still had variant angina on calcium channel blockers, 300 mg/day vitamin E acetate was added.

A significantly greater proportion of the patients with variant angina were smokers, but neither their total cholesterol levels nor their triglyceride levels differed from the other three groups. The HDL levels (mean and SEM = 39 mg/dl ± 3) of the patients with variant angina were significantly lower than those of the normal control group (45 mg/dl ± 3; $P < .05$). Vitamin E levels were not different between the group with active variant angina plus organic stenosis and the group with active variant angina but no stenoses. Vitamin E levels were also similar for smokers and nonsmokers with active variant angina. However, the nonsmokers in the normal control group had significantly higher levels of vitamin E than the normal control group smokers.

III. ADMINISTRATION OF ANTIOXIDANTS

Given the evidence that smoking causes atherosclerosis in part by oxidizing LDL, it is attractive to hypothesize that smokers might be protected from the harm of their habit by simultaneously taking antioxidants. However, this does not seem to be the case for all antioxidant compounds. Having earlier established that aspirin does not block the effect of smoking on endothelial cell desquamation (39), Davis et al., in a random-order, double-blind crossover study, tested the effect of a flavonoid on endothelial cell desquamation and platelet function (40). In the experiment, 24 male smokers and 22 male nonsmokers smoked two cigarettes during each of two 20–min periods separated by one week. The subjects were asked to take a flavonoid or a placebo four times before each experimental smoking period and to abstain from smoking for 12 hours before each period. The mean endothelial cell count increased and the platelet aggregation ratio decreased to a statistically significant extent in both smokers and nonsmokers and were unaffected by the flavonoid. This experiment did not test whether lipid peroxidation was modified by the flavonoid.

Reilly at al. (41) examined the production of 8-*epi*-prostaglandin (PG) $F_{2\alpha}$, a stable product of lipid peroxidation in vivo, and its modulation by aspirin and antioxidant vitamins in 18 chronic cigarette smokers and 24 nonsmokers. 8-*epi*-$PGF_{2\alpha}$ has the potential to be both an endogenous ligand for the thromboxane receptor and a marker of in vivo oxidant stress. It is a vasoconstrictor in the renal and pulmonary vasculature and a mitogen in smooth muscle cells.

All smokers and control subjects were apparently healthy and ranged in age from 20 to 47 years. No smokers or control subjects were taking any medications, including vitamins. The investigators found a dose response relationship between both urinary 8-*epi*-PGF$_{2\alpha}$ and cotinine on the one hand and amount smoked on the other. The correlation between urinary cotinine and 8-*epi*-PGF$_{2\alpha}$ in chronic smokers was 0.46 ($P = .09$).

Aspirin failed to suppress urinary 8-*epi*-PGF$_{2\alpha}$ but did suppress urinary 11-dehydro thromboxane (Tx) B$_2$. Aspirin suppressed both serum 8-*epi*-PGF$_{2\alpha}$ and serum 11-dehydro TxB$_2$. In contrast to aspirin, vitamin C, but not vitamin E suppressed urinary 8-*epi*-PGF$_{2\alpha}$ ($P < .05$). The authors concluded that the suppression of urinary 8-*epi*-PGF$_{2\alpha}$ but not serum 8-*epi*-PGF$_{2\alpha}$ suggests that the cyclooxygenase-dependent pathway may be a significant contributor to serum 8-*epi*-PGF$_{2\alpha}$ production while it is a trivial component of overall 8-*epi*-PGF$_{2\alpha}$ biosynthesis.

To test whether intra-arterial vitamin C might block the vasoconstrictive effects of smoking, Heitzer et al. (42) recruited 10 control subjects and 10 chronic smokers who had at least 20 pack-years of smoking. No participant has a history of hypercholesterolemia, arterial hypertension, diabetes mellitus, or other systemic disease predisposing them to endothelial dysfunction. No subjects were taking either antioxidants or vasoactive medications.

Forearm blood flow was measured and forearm vascular resistance was calculated while acetylcholine chloride was administered at increasing concentrations of 7.5, 15, 30 and 60 µg/min. Sodium nitroprusside was also infused at 1, 3, and 10 µg/min as a model of endothelium-independent vasodilatation. Each concentration of acetylcholine and nitroprusside was infused for 5 min and forearm blood flow was measured during the last 2 min of the infusion period. After a rest period of 40 min, 1 g vitamin C was infused intraarterially.

Increasing concentrations of acetylcholine dose-dependently increased forearm blood flow and decreased forearm vascular resistance. The vasodilator responses to acetylcholine, but not nitroprusside, were significantly attenuated in chronic smokers ($P < .05$). In control subjects, vitamin C had no effect on vasodilatory responses to either acetylcholine or nitroprusside. In contrast, vitamin C markedly improved endothelium-dependent vasodilatation ($P < .05$), but not response to nitroprusside. The investigators concluded that their findings support the hypothesis that oxygen-derived free radicals contribute to endothelial dysfunction in smokers but stop short of concluding that a daily dose of vitamin C may limit the cardiovascular consequences of smoking.

Among the patients studied by Miwa et al. (38) who took vitamin E supplements for active variant angina, vitamin E levels rose significantly and the mean number of attacks per week declined from 1.8±0.3 to 0.3±0.2 ($P <$ .05). However, there was no control group for this intervention. As discussed below, a randomized trial of vitamin E in the treatment of angina pectoris failed to demonstrate efficacy.

IV. RANDOMIZED CLINICAL TRIALS

The clinical trial experience with antioxidants in smokers has been disappointing to date. For example, the Alpha Tocopherol, Beta Carotene Cancer Prevention Study randomized 29,133 male smokers aged 50 through 69 years to 50 mg/day alpha tocopherol, 20 mg/day beta carotene, both, or placebo in a 2 × 2 design (43). An incident case of angina pectoris was defined as the first occurrence of typical angina pectoris identified in the annual administration of the World Health Organization (Rose) Chest Pain Questionnaire. During a median follow-up time of 4.7 years in 22,269 men considered free of coronary heart disease at baseline, 1983 new cases of angina pectoris were detected. Compared with men receiving placebo, the relative risk of angina pectoris incidence was 0.97 (95% confidence interval = 0.85 to 1.10) for men receiving alpha tocopherol and 1.13 (95% confidence interval = 1.00 to 1.27) for men receiving beta carotene. The authors concluded that the preventive effect of vitamin E on the incidence of angina pectoris among male smokers was small and not of public health significance. Supplementation with beta carotene had no salutary effect at all and may have had some negative effect.

After 12 years of supplementation with beta carotene in the Physicians' Health Study, there were no differences in incidence rates of malignant neoplasms, cardiovascular diseases, or death from all causes in the placebo and beta carotene groups (44). For current smokers in the beta carotene arm, relative risk compared to current smokers in the placebo arm were 1.08 (95% CI = 0.80 to 1.48) for myocardial infarction, 1.13 (0.80 to 1.16) for death from cardiovascular causes, 1.15 (0.93 to 1.43) for all important cardiovascular events, and 1.05 (0.86 to 1.29) for death from all causes.

In the Beta-Carotene and Retinol Efficacy Trial (45), 18,314 smokers, former smokers, and workers exposed to asbestos were randomized to 30 mg beta carotene per day and 25,000 IU of retinol (vitamin A) or placebo. The trial was stopped prematurely because the active treatment group had a relative risk of lung cancer of 1.28 (95% CI 1.04 to 1.57) compared with the placebo group. The relative risk of death from cardiovascular disease was 1.26 (0.99 to 1.61) and the relative risk of death from any cause was 1.17 (1.03 to 1.33) (Fig. 4). The investigators concluded that after an average of 4 years of supplementation, the treatment was of no benefit and may have had an adverse effect on the incidence of lung cancer and risk of death from

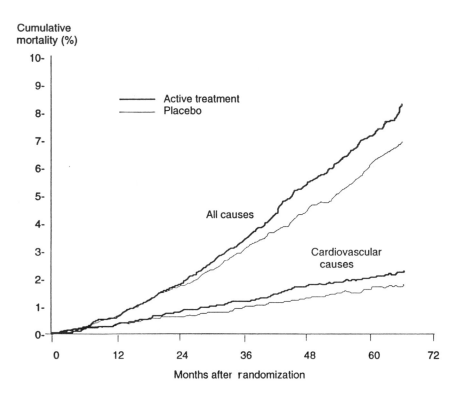

Figure 4   Kaplan-Meier curves of the cumulative incidence of death from all causes and confirmed cardiovascular causes among participants receiving active treatment and those receiving placebo. From: Omenn GS, Goodman GE, Thornquist MD, et al. Effects of a combination of beta carotene and vitamin A on lung cancer and cardiovascular disease. N Engl J Med 1996; 334(18):1150–1155, with permission.

lung cancer, cardiovascular disease, and death from any cause in smokers and workers exposed to asbestos.

V.   CLINICAL MANAGEMENT OF EXPOSURE TO TOBACCO SMOKE

A.   Active Smoking

The only effective therapy currently available to counteract the atherogenic properties of cigarette smoking is abstinence from smoking. Based on a systematic analysis of the smoking intervention trial literature, the AHCPR

Smoking Cessation Clinical Practice Guideline Panel concluded that the critical elements of smoking cessation are skills to quit, social support for quitting and remaining abstinent, and nicotine replacement (46). They outlined a five-step intervention strategy for clinicians: Ask about smoking at every visit; advise all smokers to quit; identify smokers willing to make a quit attempt; assist the smoker in quitting; and arrange follow-up (Table 2). The panel found that nicotine is the only drug with demonstrated efficacy for smoking cessation. Other substances, including clonidine or buspirone, lack evidence of efficacy.

Recognizing the importance of organizational support for the individual clinician, the panel also recommended that all institutions address six needs: implementation of a system that identifies smokers at every visit; education, resources, and feedback to promote provider intervention; dedicated staff to provide tobacco intervention treatment; hospital policies that support and provide tobacco intervention services; inclusion of tobacco intervention treatment as paid services for all subscribers; and, reimbursing fee-for-service clinicians for providing cessation intervention and including cessation intervention in salaried clinicians' scope of work (Table 3).

B. Environmental Tobacco Smoke

While adult smokers have the right to smoke in private, the health hazards and financial burden of environmental tobacco smoke gives license to eliminate tobacco smoke from public areas and from areas where children usually congregate (47). The sole exposure to tobacco smoke for many Americans is the work site. Smoke-free policies have been shown to reduce involuntary exposure to environmental tobacco smoke from > 50% to < 10% of workers (48). This type of evidence is the basis for the American Heart Association Council on Cardiopulmonary and Critical Care recommendation to eliminate environmental tobacco smoke from homes, public buildings, and workplaces (49). Samuels and Glantz (50), analyzing local efforts to make public areas smoke-free, have concluded that communities can win this battle if they work together in a cooperative effort. If, on the other hand, the community allows itself to become fragmented, tobacco industry counterefforts generally succeed.

VI. CONCLUSIONS

In populations with elevated levels of low-density lipoprotein, smoking causes atherosclerosis and the clinical manifestations of atherosclerosis in both smokers and nonsmokers exposed to environmental tobacco smoke. The mechanisms of actions include, but are probably not limited to, endothelial desquamation

Table 2 Intervention Actions and Strategies for the Primary Care Clinician Recommended by the Agency for Health Care Policy & Research Smoking Cessation Clinical Practice Guideline Panel

Action	Strategies for implementation
Step 1. Ask—systematically identify all tobacco users at every visit	
Implement and office wide system that ensures that for every patient at every clinic visit, tobacco-use status is queried and documented[a]	Expand the vital signs to include tobacco use. Data should be collected by the health care team. The action should be implemented using preprinted progress note paper that includes the expanded vital signs, a vital signs stamp, or, for computerized records, an item assessing tobacco use status. Alternatives to the vital signs stamps are to place tobacco use status stickers on all patients' charts or to indicate smoking status using computerized reminder systems.
Step 2. Advise—strongly urge all smokers to quit	
In a clear, strong and personalized manner, urge every smoker to quit	Advice should be *Clear:* " I think it is important for you to quit smoking now, and I will help you." "Cutting down while you are ill is not enough." *Strong:* "As your clinician, I need you to know that quitting smoking is the most important thing you can do to protect your current and future health." *Personalized:* Tie smoking to current health or illness and/or the social and economic costs of tobacco use, motivational level/readiness to quit, and the impact of smoking on children and others in the household. Encourage clinic staff to reinforce the cessation message and support patient's quit attempt.
Step 3. Identify smokers willing to make a quit attempt	
Ask every smoker if he or she is willing to make a quit attempt at this time.	If the patient is willing to make a quit attempt at this time, provide assistance (see step 4). If the patient prefers a more intensive treatment or the clinician believes that more intensive treatment is appropriate, refer the patient to interventions administered by a smoking cessation specialist and follow up with him or her regarding quitting (see step 5). If the patient clearly states he or she is not willing to make a quit attempt at this time, provide a motivational intervention.

Table 2   (Continued)

Step 4. Assist—aid the patient in quitting

A. Help the patient with a quit plan.

Set a quit date: Ideally the quit date should be within 2 weeks, taking patient preference into account.

Help the patient prepare for quitting: the patient must *inform* family friends, and co-workers of quitting and request understanding support.

Prepare the environment by removing cigarettes from it. Prior to quitting the patient should avoid smoking in places where he or she spends a lot of time (e.g., home, car).

Review previous quit attempts. What helped? What led to relapse?

Anticipate challenges to the planned quit attempt, particularly during the critical first few weeks.

B. Encourage nicotine replacement therapy.

Encourage the use of the nicotine patch or nicotine gum therapy for smoking cessation except in special circumstances.

C. Give key advice on successful quitting.

Abstinence: Total abstinence is essential. "Not even a single puff after the quit date."

Alcohol: drinking alcohol is highly associated with relapse. Those who should review their alcohol use and consider limiting or abstaining from alcohol use during the quit process.

Other smokers in the household: the presence of other smokers in the household, particularly a spouse, is associated with lower success rate. Patients should consider quitting with their significant others and/or developing specific plans to maintain abstinence in a household where others still smoke.

D. Provide supplementary materials.

Source: Federal agencies, including the National Cancer Institute and the Agency for Health Care Policy and Research; nonprofit agencies (American Cancer Society, American Lung Association, American Heart Association); or local or state health departments.

Selection concerns: The material must be culturally, racially, educationally, and age-appropriate for the patient.

Location: Readily available in every clinic office.

Table 2 (Continued)

Step 5. Arrange—schedule follow-up contact

Schedule follow-up contact, either in person or via telephone.

Timing: Follow-up contact should occur soon after the quit date, preferably during the first week. A second follow-up contact is recommended within the first month. Schedule further follow-up contacts as indicated.

Actions during follow-up: Congratulate success. If smoking occurred, review the circumstances and elicit recommitment to total abstinence. Remind the patient that a lapse can be used as a learning experience and is *not* a sign of failure. Identify the problems already encountered and anticipate challenges in the immediate future. Assess nicotine replacement therapy use and problems. Consider referral to a more intense or specialized program.

---

[a] Repeated assessment is not necessary in the case of the adult who has never smoked or not smoked for many years, and for whom this information is clearly documented in the medical record.

Table 3 Institutional Policies to Promote Smoking Cessation Intervention Recommended by the Agency for Health Care Policy & Research Smoking Cessation Clinical Practice Guidelines Panel[a]

Action	Strategies for Implementation
1. Implement a tobacco-user identification system in every medical setting	
Implement an officewide system that ensures that for every patient at every clinic visit, tobacco use status is queried and documented [b]	*Office system change:* Expanding the vital signs to include tobacco.
	Responsible staff: Nurse, medical assistant, receptionist, or other individual already responsible for measuring the vital signs; no additional staff requirements. Staff must be instructed regarding the frequency and importance of this activity.
	Frequency of utilization: Every visit for every patient regardless of the reason that brought the individual to the clinic[b]. In other words, whenever health care staff collect the traditional vital signs data, they also query and document tobacco use.
	System implementation steps: Preprint progress note paper or preprogram the computer record for every patient visit to include tobacco use along with the traditional vital signs. A vital sign stamp can also be effective.
2. Provide education, resources, and feedback to promote provider intervention	
Health care systems should ensure that clinicians have the knowledge and training to treat patients who smoke, that clinicians and patients have cessation resources, and that clinicians are given feedback about their cessation practices.	*Educate*: On a regular basis, offer lectures/seminars/in-service training with CME[a] and other credit for smoking cessation treatment.
	Provide resources: Have patient self-help materials and nicotine replacement starter kits readily available in every examination room.
	Provide feedback: Draw on data from chart audits, electronic medical records, and computerized patient databases to evaluate the degree to which clinicians are identifying, documenting, and treating patients who smoke and provide feedback to clinicians about their level of intervention.

Table 3 (Continued)

3. **Dedicate staff to provide tobacco intervention treatment and assess delivery of this treatment in staff performance evaluations**

Clinical sites should communicate to staff the importance of intervening with smokers and should designate 1 staff person (e.g., a nurse, medical assistant, or other clinician) to coordinate and provide tobacco dependence treatments.

Communicate to each staff member (e.g., nurses, medical assistants, and other clinicians) his or her responsibilities in the provision of smoking cessation services.

Designate a smoking cessation treatment coordinator for every clinical site.

Delineate the responsibilities of the smoking cessation coordinator, including instructing patients on the effective use of cessation treatments (e.g., nicotine, replacement therapy, telephone calls to and from prospective quitters, and scheduled follow-up visits, especially in the immediate postquit period).

4. **Promote hospital policies that support and provide tobacco intervention services**

Provide smoking cessation inpatient consultation services to all smokers admitted to a hospital.

Implement a system to identify and document the tobacco use status of all hospitalized patients who use tobacco.

Offer cessation treatment to all hospitalized patients who use tobacco.

Identify clinician(s) to provide smoking cessation inpatient consultation services for every hospital.

Reimburse providers for smoking cessation inpatient consultation services.

Expand hospital formularies to include effective smoking cessation pharmacotherapy such as the nicotine patch and nicotine gum.

Ensure compliance with JCAHO[a] regulations mandating that all sections of the hospital be entirely smoke free.

Educate all hospital staff regarding nicotine withdrawal, including effective treatments such as nicotine replacement therapy and counseling.

Table 3 (Continued)

5. **Include tobacco intervention treatments (both pharmacotherapy and counseling) identified as effective in AHCPR[a] guideline as paid services for all subscribers of health insurance packages**

Provide all insurance subscribers coverage for *effective* tobacco intervention treatments, including pharmacotherapy (nicotine replacement therapy) and counseling.

Cover: Include effective smoking cessation treatment (both pharmacotherapy and counseling) as part of the basic benefits package for all individual, group, and HMO[a] insurance packages.

Evaluate: Include the provision of smoking cessation treatment as part of "report cards" for managed care organizations and other insurers (e.g., HEDIS[a]).

Educate: Inform subscribers of the availability of covered smoking cessation services and encourage patients to use these services.

6. **Reimburse fee-for-service clinicians for provision of effective tobacco intervention treatments and include these interventions among the defined duties of salaried clinicians**

Reimburse fee-for-service clinicians for provision of effective tobacco intervention treatments; include smoking cessation treatments in the defined duties of salaried clinicians.

Include smoking cessation treatment as reimbursable activity for fee-for-service providers.

Inform fee-for-service clinicians that they will be reimbursed for using effective tobacco intervention treatments with every patient who uses tobacco.

Include tobacco intervention in the job description and performance evaluation of salaried clinicians.

[a] CME indicates continuing medical education; JCAHO is Joint Commission on Accreditation of Healthcare Organizations; HMO, health maintenance organization; HEDIS, Health Plan Employer Data and Information Set; AHCPR, Agency for Health Care Policy and Research.

[b] Repeated assessment is not necessary in the case of the adult who has never smoked or not smoked for many years, and for whom this information is clearly documented in the medical record.

of the blood vessels; platelet aggregation; free radical formation; alterations in LCAT, HDL, apo-A-I and apo-A-II; and, consumption of antioxidant compounds resulting in increased peroxidation. While these data suggest that the administration of antioxidants to smokers ought to be protective, randomized controlled trials of up to 12 years in length have failed to demonstrate any beneficial effect. In fact, at least one trial was stopped early because of higher mortality rates in the intervention arm of the trial.

The only effective intervention to reduce the health impact of tobacco smoke that is currently available is avoidance. Avoidance must include both avoidance of active smoking and avoidance of environmental tobacco smoke. A careful analysis of randomized clinical trials of smoking cessation interventions indicates that these interventions do have an effect. Efficacy is the result of training the smoker with the skills to avoid cigarettes and resist the urge to smoke, social support to become and remain a nonsmoker, and nicotine replacement. Avoidance of environmental tobacco smoke requires public policy that allows nonsmokers to attend to school, work, public events, and other activities of daily life without exposure to tobacco smoke. Ideally, smoking cessation should occur in the milieu of other lifestyle changes, which are reviewed in Chapter 5.

REFERENCES

1. Doll R, Hill AB. Smoking and carcinoma of the lung. Preliminary report. BMJ 1950; ii:739–748.
2. Wynder EL, Graham EA. Tobacco smoking as possible etiologic factor in bronchogenic carcinoma. JAMA 1950; 143:329–336.
3. Doll R, Peto R, Wheatley K, Gray R, Sutherland I. Mortality in relation to smoking: 40 years' observations on male British doctors. BMJ 1994; 309:901–911.
4. Glantz SA, Parmley WW. Passive smoking and heart disease. Mechanism and risk. JAMA 1995; 273:1047–1053.
5. Glantz SA, Parmley WW. Passive smoking and heart disease. Epidemiology, physiology, and biochemistry. Circulation 1991; 83:1–12.
6. Steenland K. Passive smoking and the risk of heart disease. JAMA 1992; 267:94–99.
7. Dobson AJ, Alexander HM, Heller RF, Lloyd DM. Passive smoking and the risk of heart attack or coronary death. Med J Aust 1991; 154:793–797.
8. Helsing KJ, Sandler DP, Comstock GW, Chee E. Heart disease mortality in nonsmokers living with smokers. Am J Epidemiol 1988; 127:915–922.
9. Matsukura S, Taminato T, Kitano N, et al. Effects of environmental tobacco smoke on urinary cotinine excretion in nonsmokers. Evidence for passive smoking. N Engl J Med 1984; 311:828–832.
10. Zhu BQ, Sun YP, Sievers RE, Glantz SA, Parmley WW, Wolfe CL. Exposure to environmental tobacco smoke increases myocardial infarct in rats. Circulation 1994; 89:1282–1290.

11. Hirayama T. Passive smoking—a new target of epidemiology. Tokai J Exp Clin Med 1985; 10:287–293.

12. Council of Scientific Affairs, American Medical Association. Environmental tobacco smoke. Health effects and prevention policies. Arch Fam Med 1994; 3:865–871.

13. Daida H, Kottke TE. The epidemiology of coronary disease. Case of five countries. Physical Med Rehab Clin North Am 1995; 6:15–35.

14. Dawber TR. The Framingham Study. The Epidemiology of Atherosclerotic Disease. Cambridge, MA; Harvard University Press, 1980; 128.

15. Sirisali K, Kanluan T, Poungvarin N, Prabhant C. Serum lipid, lipoprotein-cholesterol and apolipoproteins A-1 and B of smoking and non-smoking males. J Med Assoc Thai 1992; 75:709–713.

16. Tao S, Xiao Z, Cen R, et al. Serum lipids and their correlates in Chinese urban and rural populations of Beijing and Guangzhou. Int J Epidemiol 1992; 21:893–903.

17. Bruckert E, Jacob N, Lamaire L, Truffert J, Percheron F, de Gennes JL. Relationship between smoking status and serum lipids in a hyperlipidemic population and analysis of possible confounding factors. Clin Chem 1992; 38/39:1698–1705.

18. Casasnovas JA, Lapetra A, Puzo J, et al. Tobacco, physical exercise and lipid profile. Europ Heart J 1992; 13:440–445.

19. Kuller LH. Cigarette smoking and coronary heart disease. In: Yamamoto A, ed. Multiple risk factors in cardiovascular disease. Osaka: Churchill Livingstone Japan KK, 1994; 237–241.

20. Sackett DL, Gibson RW, Bross IDJ, Pickren JW. Relation between aortic atherosclerosis and the use of cigarettes and alcohol: an autopsy study. N Engl J Med 1968; 279:1413–1420.

21. Diez-Roux AV, Nieto FJ, Comstock GW, Howard G, Szklo M. The relationship of active and passive smoking to carotid atherosclerosis 12–14 years later. Prev Med 1995; 24:48–55.

22. Howard G, Burke GL, Szklo M, et al. Active and passive smoking are associated with increased carotid wall thickness. The Atherosclerosis Risk in Communities Study. Arch Intern Med 1994; 154:1277–1282.

23. Witteman JC, Grobbee DE, Valkenburg HA, van Hermett AM, Stijnen T, Hofman A. Cigarette smoking and the development and progression of aortic atherosclerosis. A 9–year population based follow-up study in women. Circulation 1993; 88:2156–2162.

24. Davis JW, Shelton L, Eigenberg DA, Hignite CE, Watanabe IS. Effects of tobacco and non-tobacco cigarette smoking on endothelium and platelets. Clin Pharmacol Ther 1985; 37:529–533.

25. Davis JW, Shelton L, Watanabe IS, Arnold J. Passive smoking affects endothelium and platelets. Arch Intern Med 1989; 149:386–389.

26. Roald HE, Lyberg T, Dedichen H, et al. Collagen induced thrombus formation in flowing nonanticoagulated human blood from habitual smokers and nonsmoking patients with severe peripheral atherosclerotic disease. Arterioscler Thrombo Vasc Biol 1995; 15:128–132.

27. Kario K, Matsuo T. Platelet size (mean platelet volume) and cigarette smoking. In: Yamamoto A, ed. Multiple Risk Factors in Cardiovascular Disease. Osaka: Churchill Livingstone Japan, 1994; 255–258.

28. Levine PH. An acute effect of cigarette smoking on platelet function. A possible link between smoking and arterial thrombosis. Circulation 1973; 48:619–623.

29. Burghuber OC, Punzengruber CH, Sinzinger H, Haber P, Silberbauer K. Platelet sensitivity to prostacyclin in smokers and non-smokers. Chest 1986; 90:34–38.

30. Allen DR, Browse NL, Rutt DL, Butler L, Fletcher C. The effect of cigarette smoke, nicotine, and carbon monoxide on the permeability of the arterial wall. J Vasc Surg 1988; 7:139–152.

31. Duplaa C, Couffinhal T, Labat L, et al. Monocyte adherence to endothelial cells in patients with atherosclerosis: relationships with risk factors. Eur J Clin Invest 199; 23:474–479.

32. Haak T, Jungmann E, Raab C, Usadel KH. Elevated endothelin-1 levels after cigarette smoking. Metab Clin Exp 1994; 43:267–269.

33. Przyklenk K. Nicotine exacerbates postischemic contractile dysfunction of "stunned" myocardium in the canine model. Possible role of free radicals. Circulation 1994; 89:1272–1281.

34. McKenzie WB, McCredie RM, McGilchrist CA, Wilcken DE. Smoking: a major predictor of left ventricular dysfunction after occlusion of the left anterior descending coronary artery. Br Heart J 1986; 56:496–500.

35. McCall MR, van den Berg JJ, Kuypers FA, et al. Modification of LCAT Activity and HDL structure. New links between cigarette smoke and coronary heart disease risk. Arterioscler Thrombo 1994; 14:248–253.

36. Heitzer TH, Yla-Herttuala S, Luoma J, et al. Cigarette smoking potentiates endothelial dysfunction of forearm resistance vessels in patients with hypercholesterolemia. Role of oxidized LDL. Circulation 1996; 93:1346–1353.

37. Mezzetti A, Lapenna D, Pierdomenico SD, et al. Vitamins E, C, and lipid peroxidation in plasma and arterial tissue of smokers and non-smokers. Atherosclerosis 1995; 112:91–99.

38. Miwa K, Miyagi Y, Igawa A, Nakagawa K, Inoue H. Vitamin E deficiency in variant angina. Circulation 1996; 94:14–18.

39. Davis JW, Shelton L, Eigenberg DA, Hignite CE. Lack of effect of aspirin on cigarette smoke-induced increase in circulating endothelial cells. Haemostasis 1986; 17:66–69.

40. Davis JW, Shelton L, Hartman CR, Eigemberg DA, Ruttinger HA. Smoking-induced changes in endothelium and platelets are not affected by hydroxyethylrutosides. Br J Exp Pathol 1986; 67:765–771.

41. Reilly M, Delanty N, Lawson JA, FitzGerald GA. Modulation of oxidant stress in vivo in chronic cigarette smokers. Circulation 1996; 94:19–25.

42. Heitzer T, Just H, Münzel T. Antioxidant vitamin C improves endothelial dysfunction in chronic smokers. Circulation 1996; 94:6–9.

43. Rapola JM, Virtamo J, Haukka JK, et al. Effect of vitamin E and beta carotene on the incidence of angina pectoris. A randomized, double-blind, controlled trial. JAMA. 1996; 275(9):693–698.

44. Hennekens CH, Buring JE, Manson JE, et al. Lack of direct effect of long-term supplementation with beta carotene on the incidence of malignant neoplasms and cardiovascular disease. N Engl J Med 1996; 334:1145–1149.
45. Omenn GS, Goodman GE, Thornquist MD, et al. Effects of a combination of beta carotene and vitamin A on lung cancer and cardiovascular disease. N Engl J Med 1996; 334(18):1150–1155.
46. Smoking Cessation Clinical Practice Guidelines Panel and Staff. The Agency for Health Care Policy and Research Smoking Cessation Clinical Practice Guideline. JAMA 1996; 275:1270–1280.
47. Kottke TE, Solberg LI, Brekke ML. Health plans helping smokers. HMO Pract 1995; 9:128–133.
48. Borland R, Pierce JP, Burns DM, Gilpin E, Johnson M, Bal D. Protection from environmental tobacco smoke in California. The case for a smoke-free work place. JAMA 1992; 268:749–752.
49. Taylor AE, Johnson DC, Kazemi H. Environmental tobacco smoke and cardiovascular disease. A position paper from the Council on Cardiopulmonary and Critical Care, American Heart Association. Circulation 1992; 86:699–702.
50. Samuels B, Glantz SA. The politics of local tobacco control. JAMA 1991; 266:2110–2117.

5

Lifestyle Interventions in Atherosclerosis

Neil J. Stone

Northwestern University School of Medicine, Chicago, Illinois

"Genetics load the gun, but environment pulls the trigger"—Elliot Joslin (1)

I. INTRODUCTION

Genetic predisposition determines susceptibility for atherosclerotic vascular disease (ASCVD) in our society. Environmental or "lifestyle" factors greatly affect the probability that the genetic fault(s) translate into clinical events that we recognize as coronary heart disease (CHD), peripheral vascular disease (PVD), or cerebrovascular disease. This chapter will address the major lifestyle changes of diet, exercise, tobacco, and alcohol usage and their relationship to ASCVD.

Public awareness of risk factors and diet has been increasing since the 1980s (2). Moreover, research interest has increased as well with a marked increase in the number of citations for the word lifestyle since 1966. Despite the heightened interest among the public and researchers, the ranks of the obese have continued to expand. There was a dramatic increase in overweight prevalence of about 8% between the 1976 to 1980 and 1988 to 1991 surveys with clear increases in all race/sex groups (3). During this period, for adult men and women aged 20 through 74 years, mean body weight increased 3.6 kg and the mean body mass index (BMI) increased from 25.3 to 26.3. This means that 33.4% of U.S. adults 20 years of age or older were estimated to be overweight. In contrast, the goal for the year 2000 is only 20%.

Any discussion of lifestyle changes in the 1990s must consider cost-effectiveness of any therapy recommended. In this regard, it is important to consider the role of lifestyle change in primary and secondary prevention efforts to reduce events of CHD. In primary prevention, the target is the population. Yusuf and Anand have reminded us that a shift in the mean cholesterol level of the population by 10% would prevent 30% of all CHD events (4). This is contrasted to secondary prevention where the target is the high-risk individual. Here lifetime treatment with statin therapy of those with increased risk as defined by cholesterol values in the upper 10% would prevent only about 15% to 20% of all events of CHD. This underscores the power of nutritional-hygienic approaches that were advised three decades ago by Stamler (5).

II. DIET, LIPIDS, AND CHD

The relationships between circulating lipids and coronary disease are reviewed in Chapter 2. The hallmark of the nutritional approach to prevent CHD has been to reduce dietary saturated fats, cholesterol, and excess calories leading to obesity (6). Americans have been successful in the first two cases as average values for saturated fats and dietary cholesterol have fallen according to NHANES III data (7). In this last survey, 34% of kilocalories was from total dietary fat and 12% of kilocalories was from saturated fat. This is a marked improvement from estimates of prior surveys where total dietary fat was 35% to 40% of kilocalories and saturated fat 17% (8).

Dietary cholesterol affects blood cholesterol values, but its effects are not as potent as the effects of saturated fats according to the Keys and Hegsted equations (9,10). The change with feeding, however, is variable (11). In addition, recent dietary studies suggest that consumption of one or two eggs per day in an otherwise low-saturated-fat, high-fiber diet may have only a small effect on blood cholesterol values (12,13). On the other hand, when an ethnically diverse population of normolipidemic young men was fed low and high levels of cholesterol, variation in cholesterol rather than the proportions of saturated and polyunsaturated fat had the strongest influence on LDL-C levels. Among non-Caucasians it was the only significant factor (14).

The marked variability likely has a strong genetic basis. Recent egg feeding studies suggest that those with combined hyperlipidemia may be particularly sensitive to dietary cholesterol (15). Also, those with the apo-E-4 phenotype absorb more dietary cholesterol than those with apo-E-2 phenotype (16). The apo-A-IV phenotype (17) and the XbaI site on the apo-B gene (18) may also be important genetic determinants.

Table 1 Lifestyle Effects on Lipoprotein Levels

Lipids/lipoproteins	Elevate	Lower
Cholesterol and LDL-C	Dietary cholesterol and saturated fats, excess calories	Mono- and poly-unsaturated fats, soy protein, fiber (soluble), garlic
HDL-C	Exercise, dietary fat, alcohol, weight reduction	Dietary carbohydrate, weight gain, cigarette smoking
Triglycerides	Excess calories, alcohol, acute carbohydrate feeding	Exercise, weight reduction, n-3 PUFA (fish oil)

Finally, the effect of dietary cholesterol on CHD cannot be ignored. Four studies from several decades ago showed that a high cholesterol intake was associated with an increased rate of CHD (19,20). The carefully done Western Electric study noted that dietary cholesterol was significantly associated with CHD risk and that this was independent of the serum cholesterol level.

Dietary saturated fat intake is the major dietary determinant of blood cholesterol levels (8,9). Saturated fats are solid at room temperature and appear to suppress low-density lipoprotein (LDL) receptor activity (21). Sources of saturated fatty acids include fatty cuts of meat, butterfat-rich dairy products, and vegetable fats such as coconut oil and palm kernel oil. Saturated fatty acids in the diet include lauric, myrisitic, palmitic, and stearic. In the Seven Countries study, the average population intake of lauric and myristic acid was most strongly related to the average serum cholesterol level ($r > .8$, $P < .001$) (22). Stearic acid is converted after ingestion to oleic acid and does not raise cholesterol (23). Beef products are the most common source of dietary stearic acid in the United States. Beef fat, however, contains beef tallow, which is cholesterol-raising, so only lean cuts of beef are appropriate for a cholesterol-lowering diet (24). While there is unanimous agreement that reduction in dietary saturated fats is desirable, there is considerable disagreement as to how this should be accomplished. There is a rationale for using unsaturated fatty acids, carbohydrate, or protein as replacements for saturated fats in the diet, and these will be discussed separately. See Table 1.

Mono-unsaturated fatty acids (MUFAs), when substituted for saturated fats, effectively lower LDL-C (25). The chief mono-unsaturated fatty acid is oleic acid. Common sources include canola (rapeseed) oil, olive oil, peanut oil, and avocados. Since Mediterranean countries have diets that use olive oil as the principal source of fat, an olive oil-based diet has been referred to as the "Mediterranean diet." MUFAs do not appear to lower HDL-C when added to the diet. Most importantly, LDL isolated from subjects on diets rich in MUFA is less susceptible to oxidation than that seen after subjects were on diets rich in polyunsaturated fats (26,27) This may be particularly true in those with small, dense LDL-C (28). Caution is needed, however, when advocating increased MUFAs to replace saturated fats because of the higher fat content as compared to diets that replace saturated fats with complex carbohydrates. Although the Mediterranean diet is an excellent dietary approach to a lower saturated-fat intake, grams of fat can add up, leading to unwanted weight gain.

One group that may benefit from an emphasis on more mono-unsaturated fat as canola or olive oil in the diet are diabetic patients (29). Diets that are severely restricted in fat may be supplemented with sweetened food items. These calories from simple sugars can worsen blood sugar control and increase levels of triglycerides. Avoidance of simple sugars and decreasing some of the complex carbohydrate in favor of mono-unsaturated fat can better maintain HDL-C levels.

Another form of fatty acids is the trans isomers of unsaturated fatty acids. These so-called trans fatty acids are consumed as partially hydrogenated oils in stick margarines and shortenings, milk, butter or cheese, and also in vegetable oils used for frying. The most common trans fatty acid in the American diet is elaidic acid, a trans isomer of oleic acid. They have taken the place of the tropical oils, although there is a continuing controversy as to whether this is a healthful substitute (30). Trans fatty acids raise total cholesterol and LDL-C and can lower HDL-C when ingested as more than 7% of daily energy (31). This may be mediated through an increase in cholesterol ester transfer protein (32). Furthermore they may increase lipoproteins(a), Lp(a), which is associated with an increased risk of heart disease (33). Most Americans consume much less trans fatty acid. Nonetheless, the magnitude of the hazard from trans fatty acids in the food supply remains controversial (34). An expert panel in 1995 concluded, "Data supporting a relation between trans fatty acid intake and CHD risk are equivocal compared with extensive data from studies in animals and humans linking saturated fat intake to CHD" (35).

Polyunsaturated fatty acids (PUFAs), when substituted for saturated fats, also lower blood cholesterol levels. They are divided into two groups by the position of the first double bond from the terminal end of the carbon chain. The omega 6 (n-6) fatty acids include linoleic acid, an 18-carbon fatty acid, which is an essential fatty acid for humans in that it cannot be synthesized by the body. Examples include the seed oils, namely, corn, safflower, and cottonseed oils. The n-3 PUFAs are also known as marine lipids or fish oils. They will be considered under dietary interventions to lower triglycerides.

The Keys equation stressed that to counterbalance the adverse influence of saturated fats on the cholesterol level, you needed gram-for-gram twice as much n-6 PUFA. The older literature characterized diets by the P/S ratio referring to the n-6-polyunsaturated-fat-to-saturated-fat ratio of these diets. Diets with a high polyunsaturated-to-saturated fat ratio were used in early clinical trials. In one of these, cholelithiasis, was a documented complication (36). The benefits and negative aspects or risks of PUFA continue to be investigated. Linoleic acid is needed for normal immune response, and essential fatty-acid deficiency impairs B- and T-cell-mediated responses (37). Excess linoleic acid has been associated with tumor growth in animals, an effect not verified by data from diverse human studies. Nonetheless, for safety reasons, the total PUFA intake is recommended to be < 10% of calories by NCEP guidelines.

A high-carbohydrate diet is typical of an Asian-style diet. Often the percentage of energy as carbohydrate will be on the order of 60% to 65%, allowing total fat calories to be as low as 15% to 20% of total energy. Thus, intakes of saturated fat and dietary cholesterol are very low. The usual response upon changing such a high-carbohydrate diet, however, is to increase triglyceride levels and lower HDL-C. Ullman and co-workers have demonstrated that when patients are *gradually* introduced to a high-carbohydrate, low-fat diet, significant reductions of plasma total and LDL cholesterol can occur without the carbohydrate-induced hypertriglyceridemia that occurs with immediate exposure to such a diet (38). A diet high in soy protein can lower high cholesterol values in those who are found to be hypercholesterolemic (39). Asian populations have consumed diets rich in soy protein for centuries, suggesting a lack of important toxicity per se. Thus, it is quite reasonable to choose soy-based food products within an overall balanced diet. It is not clear how the soy effect, which is rather modest when consumed in practical amounts, matches up against the effects of other cholesterol-lowering dietary changes. An exciting research question is whether the phytoestrogen content of soy protein will prove of importance to overall health in general and cardiovascular health in particular.

Fiber is an important part of a balanced diet. Soluble fiber lowers LDL-C when added to a step I NCEP diet in hypercholesterolemic subjects. Davidson and co-workers showed that a dose-dependent effect for oat products was due to β-glucan (40). Another form of soluble fiber, psyllium hydrophilic mucilloid, can lower LDL-C as much as 20% (41). In addition, even when saturated fat and dietary cholesterol are greatly reduced, very high intakes of foods rich in soluble fiber lower blood cholesterol and LDL-C and HDL-C, although to a lesser degree (42). Fiber can mitigate the hypercholesterolemic effects of dietary cholesterol as well, even among subjects characterized as hyperresponders (43). Improvements with increased fiber are not temporary.

A recent study used 20 g/day of fiber, particularly guar gum and pectin, in 59 subjects with mild to moderate increases in LDL-C (131 to 191 mg/dl) on a step I diet . After approximately 1 year, the mean percentage reductions from baseline were approximately 5% for TC, 9% for LDL-C, and 11% for the LDL/HDL ratio. Changes were apparent after 3 weeks of treatment, with the maximum reductions occurring by the 15th week of treatment (44). Thus, the addition of fiber plays an important role in the cholesterol-lowering diet.

Garlic has received considerable attention from the lay press regarding its effects on health. A recent meta-analysis did suggest that there was a small yet significant effect in those with cholesterol levels > 200 mg/dl (45). The data showed that garlic, in an amount approximating one-half to one clove per day, decreased total serum cholesterol levels by about 9%. Preliminary short-term data suggest that garlic may decrease the ex vivo susceptibility of apolipoprotein-B-containing lipoproteins to oxidation, despite lack of effect on cholesterol levels (46). It is important to view this in perspective and realize that much further information is needed before garlic can be recommended as part of a healthful diet.

The following paragraphs will deal with nutritional changes that cause improved levels of triglycerides and HDL-C. An important therapeutic aspect of such diets is their ability to promote loss of weight. The most dramatic changes in lipids are seen with the very low fat diets as espoused by Pritikin (47) and Ornish (48). The Pritikin diets have a small amount of animal protein while the Ornish approach is a < 10% total fat, vegetarian type of diet. The initial improvements in total cholesterol and LDL-C can be dramatic. Grundy has cautioned that the short-term gains seen with these diets could be due to regression to the mean effect of institutionalization if the diet was introduced in such a facility, reduction in saturated fatty acids and dietary cholesterol, regular exercise, and weight loss (49). A diet that promotes weight loss may be crucial in obtaining advantageous lipoprotein profiles. When Schaefer and colleagues compared a reduced-fat, a low-fat diet without change in energy, and a low-fat diet where decreased caloric intake was allowed to occur, only in the latter instance was the overall change in LDL-C/HDL-C ratio favorable (50). The studies from Dr. Schaefer's group seemed to indicate that when the diet is as low as 15% in fat, patient tolerability is strained. As will be pointed out later in this chapter, exercise is also an important way to increase the lowered HDL-C that occurs when fat is suddenly removed from the diet and replaced with carbohydrate.

Avoidance of sugar calories is particularly important since they promote dental caries and can add extra calories that lead to obesity. The current trend of "no-fat" foods has produced many foods that are high in calories due to corn syrup solids or sucrose. Patients need to know that these are not part of a nutritious diet.

The n-3 PUFAs are known as fish oils, although one of them, alpha linolenic acid, is actually plant-based. Common sources of alpha linolenic are tofu, soybean and canola oil, and nuts, which are an important source of n-3 PUFA for vegetarians and non-seafood eaters. Eicosapentenoic acid (EPA) and docosahexenoic acid (DHA) are long-chain n-3 PUFAs which are added together to determine the amount of fish oil in a food. Fatty fish like salmon and mackrel are good examples of n-3 fatty acids. These PUFAs have important effects on coagulation parameters. Those populations with a diet rich in marine lipids show reduced platelet aggregation and prolonged bleeding times (51). The major effect on lipids is to lower triglyceride values. This can be of clinical importance in those with severe hypertriglyceridemia for whom correction of secondary causes, diet, exercise, and gemfibrozil have proven inadequate (52). Unfortunately, in those with milder forms of hypertriglyceridemia, the beneficial fall in triglyceride is accompanied by a rise in LDL-C (53). Two carefully done trials of n-3 PUFA in diabetics demonstrated triglyceride lowering with no deterioration in glucose homeostasis (54,55). In both of these trials, the associated rise in LDL-C was seen. This clearly has to be considered when fish oil is used therapeutically. Finally, when a step II National Cholesterol Education Program (NCEP) diet is enriched with fish, there are changes in delayed hypersensitivity seen (56).

Alcohol raises triglycerides by increasing very low density lipoprotein (VLDL) synthesis (57) but, unlike high carbohydrate diets, also raises HDL-C. On the other hand, excess alcohol usage is a common cause of secondary hyperlipidemia (58). Alcohol not only exacerbates fasting hypertriglyceridemia, but also augments postprandial lipemia. Although not seen in exercise-trained subjects, delayed triglyceride clearance occurs in inactive subjects (59). In those with severe hypertriglyceridemia, alcohol usage must be prohibited or it can exacerbate triglyceride levels and lead to or aggravate a chylomicronemia syndrome. In these patients, acute pancreatitis can ensue with its high morbidity and even occasional mortality.

Transcountry data shows that alcohol consumption is negatively correlated with CHD mortality (60). This was further examined in the large MRFIT prospective experience of middle-aged men who were light to moderate drinkers. Five percent of the men abstained from alcohol during the trial, 81% consumed less than 21 alcoholic drinks per week, and 14% consumed more than 21 alcoholic drinks per week. HDL-C levels appeared to explain the inverse association between alcohol consumption and death from CHD. HDL-C may explain as much as 50% of the variance seen (61). An additional 18% of this protection is attributable to a decrease in LDL-C, but is counterbalanced by a 17% increase in risk due to increased systolic blood pressure. The residual variance is unexplained, but it is reasonable to speculate on an effect on coagulation.

In fact, some attribute the increased wine consumption as the explanation of the paradoxical situation in France where there is a high intake of saturated fat, but a low mortality from CHD (62). A possible explanation for alcohol's beneficial effects is derived from cross-sectional data showing that increased platelet aggregation, which would favor an increase in events of CHD, is inhibited significantly by alcohol at levels of intake associated with reduced risk of CHD (63). Also, alcohol usage is associated with lower fibrongen levels (64). Some have argued that red wine may be more protective against CHD than white wine, but this is not supported by epidemiologic data (65).

There seems to be general agreement that there can be no public health recommendation for use of alcohol to prevent CHD because of the known adverse effects. Excess alcohol use is clearly related to an increase risk of liver disease, accidents, and suicide (66). For the cardiac patient, this includes aggravation of hypertension, symptomatic supraventricular arrhythmias, alcoholic cardiomyopathy, and even left ventricular hypertrophy (67).

III. SPECIFIC DIETARY TRIALS AND CHD

Analysis of interventions to reduce CHD shows that drug trials have greater efficiency in cholesterol lowering and hence are more conclusive than dietary trials (68). Several diet trials, however, have increased our understanding of the potential benefit that can be seen with a cholesterol-lowering diet. Unfortunately, careful analysis of the design of these trials demonstrates the great difficulty in putting these trials together in a simple meta-analysis. For example, the Oslo trial changed smoking habits as well as diet (69), the VA trial included patients both with and without CHD (70), the Finnish trial randomized beds, not patients (71), and the Minnesota coronary survey suffered from not having enough patients on diet long enough to see an effect if one was, in fact, present (72). Informative results were gleaned from the Oslo dietary and smoking intervention trial which documented that those randomized to a modifed-fat diet and counseling to reduce smoking had a 47% less incidence of sudden death and heart attack than in the control group. This marked change is certainly greater than would be expected with cholesterol lowering alone and suggests a synergy between smoking reduction and cholesterol lowering. Interestingly, statistical analysis suggested that the cholesterol lowering played a stronger role than the smoking reductions that were seen. This study was important because the 5-year followup data documented a significant reduction in mortality which heretofore had not been seen with a trial of nonpharmacologic methods for reducing risk of CHD (73).

Three multiple risk factor intervention trials have been completed (74–76). In each case, the amount of cholesterol lowering was less than anticipated. These trials underscore the need for cholesterol lowering to exceed 10% between groups before conclusions regarding lowering risk of CHD can be made for any intervention(s).

Recent evidence supporting the role of diet in reducing atherosclerosis has come from angiographic trials. Although most of these trials have involved drug therapy, several have looked at either diet alone. The Leiden study was an uncontrolled study of the effects of a vegetarian diet in 39 men with angina pectoris who had coronary angiograms performed 2 years apart (77). The effectiveness of diet was seen in lower body weights and lower systolic blood pressure along with lower values for total cholesterol and the total cholesterol/HDL-C ratio. Disease progression was signficant in those with total/HDL-C ratios > 6.9. Those with improvement in cholesterol/HDL-C ratio had the least progression.

Blackenhorn and colleagues compared the dietary habits of the 18 men in the placebo group of the Cholesterol Lowering Atherosclerosis Study in whom new lesions of the native coronary vessels developed at follow-up angiography 2 years later to the 64 men in whom they did not (78). Subjects who did not show progression had increased their dietary protein to compensate for reduced intake of fat by substituting low-fat meats and dairy products for high-fat products. Moreover, each quartile of increased intake of total, saturated, and polyunsaturated fat was associated with increased risk of new lesion development. Although observational, the results suggested that diets low in total fat and saturated fat could be effective in reducing coronary progression.

Three studies (79–81) using change in follow-up coronary angiogams as the primary endpoint have suggested considerable benefits of varying levels of restriction of dietary fat along with regular physical exercise. LDL-C fell 37.8% in the Lifestyle Heart trial where a motivated, highly selected group (49% refused to participate after randomization) consumed a diet with < 10% of calories as fat and no cholesterol as part of an intensive lifestyle intervention involving exercise and stress reduction. The Heidelberg trial restricted fat to < 20% of calories and showed initial LDL-C declines of 25% in subjects after 3 weeks on a metabolic ward. At the end of 1 year, the decline in LDL-C had fallen to 4% (although the average over the year was 8%). The St. Thomas Atherosclerosis Trial (STARS) contrasted a diet restricted in total fat to 27% with saturated fat limited to 8% to 10% of calories with a usual care group. The therapeutic diets were high-fiber, chiefly as pectin. Although there was a drug treatment arm, the diet arm was particularly informative. The course of CAD over 3 years was measured by quantitative coronary angiography, i.e., as the per-patient change in the mean absolute width of coronary segments (Δ MAWS). The decrease in Δ MAWS which represented progression of CAD was significantly correlated with in-trial plasma total cholesterol, LDL-C, apolipoprotein-B (apo-B), and Lp(a). Of note, no significant associations were found with HDL-C, apo-A-I, vitamin E, thyroid hormones, fibrinogen, von Willebrand factor, or postload plasma glucose and insulin concentrations By multiple regression analysis, LDL-C was the best predictor of Δ MAWS, the adjusted model explaining 22% of the variance ($P = .04$). This effect of LDL suggests that the major benefit may have been dietary reduction of LDL-C.

In addition, a low-fat diet may help symptomatically through other mechanisms apart from the lipid-lowering effects. Ornish reported that patients in the experimental group of his Lifestyle Trial had a 91% reduction in frequeny of angina, 42% reduction in duration of angina, and 28% reduction in severity of angina, whereas worsening of anginal symptoms was seen in the control group. Also, in the Heidelberg trial, the number of positive ECGs in the intervention group had significantly decreased ($P < .05$) and fewer patients stopped their treadmill stress test as a result of progressive angina ($P = .06$). The sudden improvement in symptoms raises speculations regarding nonatherogenic effects of a low-fat diet. While exercise may have played an im- portant role in reducing sympathetic tone, recent work on vascular reactivity showing reversal of impairment of endothelium-dependent relaxation in hyper- cholesterolemic patients after cholesterol-lowering therapy (diet and resin) may well be the mechanism by which these favorable clinical changes arise (82).

IV. LIFESTYLE CHANGE AND HYPERTENSION

Lifestyle changes affect hypertension as well. The relationship between dietary salt and hypertension has been studied in animals and humans in great detail. The importance of salt restriction is underscored by numerous studies, including randomized trials of nonpharmacologic intervention including salt restriction in mild hypertensives (83), persons with borderline high blood pressure (84), and normals (85). While attention to weight, potassium, and alcohol are also important in deriving the benefits noted, the large body of information indicates that dietary sodium restriction by itself is crucial. Law examined 33 trials lasting 5 weeks or longer and noted that the predicted reductions in individual trials closely matched a wide range of observed reductions (86). This applied for all age groups and for people with both high and normal levels of blood pressure. His analysis suggested that for people aged 50 to 59 years, a reduction in daily sodium intake of 50 mmol, which is about 3 g salt and achievable by moderate dietary salt reduction, would, after a few weeks, lower systolic blood pressure by an average of 5 mm Hg, and by 7 mm Hg in those with high blood pressure (170 mm Hg) whereas diastolic blood pressure would be lowered by about half as much. He estimated that such a reduction in salt intake by a whole Western population would reduce the incidence of stroke by 22% and of CHD by 16%.

Recently, a meta-analysis based on 56 trials suggested that the effect of reducing dietary sodium in normotensives is so minimal as to argue against limitations on sodium intake for the general public (5,87). The authors did state that dietary sodium restriction for older hypertensives might be considered. A letter to the editor from the Nutrition Committee of the American Heart Association noted that a majority of the trials in normotensives in the meta-analysis were 2 weeks or less in duration (88). This would clearly tend to underestimate the effect of reduced salt intake on blood pressure. Almost simultaneously, an updated analysis from the Intersalt Study was published (89). The investigators of this large, multicenter observational study corrected their earlier estimates of the association of salt intake with both level of blood pressure and increase of blood pressure with age, taking into account regression dilution bias (90). They noted that the estimated association of higher dietary sodium with systolic and diastolic blood pressure was larger than that previously reported. For example, estimates of the effect of median sodium excretion by 100 mmol/day over the 30-year period from 25 years of age to 55 years of age suggested a difference of 10 to 11 mm Hg for systolic blood pressure and 6 mm Hg for diastolic blood pressure. This extrapolates to a large effect on reducing stroke risk. These results of Intersalt support population based recommendations for *reduction of high salt intake* for the prevention and control of adverse blood pressure levels.

It is important to note the phrase "high salt intake." Alderman and co-workers reported that drug-treated hypertensive men who had the lowest urinary excretion of sodium had a significant increase in cardiovascular disease and myocardial infarction after an average followup of 3.8 years. The authors suggested that because sodium and renin are inversely related, a low-sodium diet could have deleterious effects due to its stimualtion of the renin-angiotensin system. Since this was an observational study, the potential for undetected confounding must be considered before these results are generalized. The authors suggested that further data be examined before there is any attempt to establish causality.

The TOMS study put some of these data to the test for patients with stage I (mild) hypertension with DBP 90 to 99 and SBP 140 to 159 mm Hg where the goal for nutritional-hygienic intervention would be SBP < 140 and DBP < 90. All participants received advice on the need for weight reduction, reduced dietary sodium intake, reduced alcohol intake, and increased physical activity. Weight loss averaged 2.6 kg after 4 years of intervention. This was approximately one-half of the weight loss attained after 1 year of intervenion, which is consistent with the recidivism that has been seen in all weight loss trials. Participants reduced urinary sodium excretion by almost 5 mmol/l from entry and reduced alcohol by an average of 1 drink. In this study, the group who received pharmacologic treatment as well had improved clinical outcomes. The authors felt that although lifestyle change as defined by their study was a reasonable start to those with stage I hypertension, failure to achieve this goal by 3 to 6 months of sustained effective counseling might warrant the addition of an antihypertensive drug to the lifestyle regimen (91).

Recent data suggest that weight loss with a fat-modified diet plus increased exercise produces favorable long-term effects not only on blood pressure but also on the plasma lipid fractions of adults with stage I hypertension (92). In the placebo group in this trial, there was a 5.1 mg/dl change in total cholesterol and a 3.6 mg/dl change in LDL-C. This amount of change in cholesterol levels has been shown to be associated with almost a 10% decline in coronary disease events (93). Since approximately 36 million American have stage I (mild) hypertension, the potential impact of nutritional therapy alone is considerable.

Important lifestyle and behavioral correlates of change in CHD risk factors were measured 8 years apart in the young adult offspring of the Framingham Heart Study cohort. The attribute most strongly and consistently related to lipoprotein and blood pressure changes in both sexes was change in BMI (94). In addition to weight gain, increases in alcohol consumption in men and beginning oral contraceptive use in women were associated with increases in blood pressure over the study period. In addition, weight loss, stopping or decreasing cigarettes, increasing alcohol intake, and, in women, discontinuing oral contraceptives, were independently related to improvements in lipoprotein profiles during follow-up .

Yet in addition to weight loss and sodium reduction in the diet, other interventions should be considered as well. One of these is dietary calcium intake. Three recent analyses of calcium supplementation provide a superb overview of the field. In the first, data from 28 active treatment arms or strata from 22 randomized clinical trials were pooled to yield a weighted average (95). Although there was a statistically significant decrease in systolic blood pressure with calcium supplementation, the effect was too small to recommend the use of calcium for preventing or treating hypertension. Additional pooled analyses of normotensives, hypertensives, and pregnant women confirmed that there is a small, definite effect of calcium on blood pressure (96,97). Furthermore, McCarron has pointed out that many adults have inadequate intakes of calcium; for example, American men over age 40 have median calcium intakes of < 750 mg/day (98). He suggested that calcium supplementation may then be of particular benefit to the elderly, the obese, people of African origin, and pregnant women. When advising individuals regarding calcium intakes, ethic differences in food sources must be considered. For example, although dairy foods were the main source of calcium for Hispanics, corn tortillas were important sources of calcium among Mexican-Americans (99).

V. ANTIOXIDANTS AND CHD

The prevention of CHD by antioxidants is plausible, as oxidized LDL appears to play a key role in atherosclerosis (100). Moreover, vitamin E is a potent lipid-soluble antioxidant which is carried on LDL. When added to plasma, vitamin E seens to make LDL more resistant to oxidation (101). This is not the case when vitamin C, a potent, water-soluble antioxidant, is given alone. Likewise, beta-carotene supplementation does not increase LDL's resistance to oxidation in vitro. Yet observational studies suggested that people who consumed higher dietary levels of fruits and vegetables containing beta-carotene might have a lower risk for certain cancers as well as cardiovascular disease (102,103). In the EURAMIC study (European Community Multicenter Study on Antioxidants, Myocardial Infarction [MI] and Breast Cancer), adipose tissue levels of beta-carotene and alpha tocophoerol in cases of MI were compared with controls (104). The authors felt that their data suggested that consumption of beta-carotene-rich foods such as carrots and green leafy vegetables might reduce the risk of MI. Dietary considerations regarding antioxidants might be particularly important to cigarette smokers. In particular, cigarette smoking may contribute to atherosclerosis by depleting natural antioxidants such as vitamin C, vitamin E, and beta-carotene, and enhancing LDL oxidation (105).

Two prospective cohort studies, one in female nurses and the other in male health professionals, intensified interest in antioxidants in general and vitamin E in particular. These were not double-blind, randomized clinical trials, but they did forcibly suggest that vitamin E supplements reduced risk of CHD (106,107). This risk reduction was substantial in both studies. When women in the top fifth of the distribution with respect to vitamin E intake were compared to those in the bottom, there was a reduction of 34% in risk of CHD. Women who used vitamin E supplements for < 2 years derived little benefit. The findings persisted after adjustment for carotene, vitamin C, and use of multivitamins. Among men followed prospectively, those in the top fifth for vitamin E intake had an age-adjusted risk of CHD of 0.59, suggesting a 41% reduction in risk. Beta-carotene consumption showed a highly significant association which was strongest among current and past cigarette smokers.

More recently, a prospective sample of postmenopausal women from Iowa showed that the intake of vitamin E from foods is inversely associated with the risk of death from CHD. Although simply an observational trial, these data suggested that women could lower their risks without using vitamin supplements (108). In this study, intake of vitamins A and C was not associated with risk of death from CHD.

Much confusion developed as clinical trial data have not corroborated inferences made from observational studies on the benefits of supplementation of antioxidant vitamins. Although many proceeded to take supplements of vitamins A, E, and C, Steinberg pleaded for clinical trial data to determine both efficacy and long-term toxicity of vitamin E in primary or secondary prevention (109). He noted that selection bias might figure heavily in observation studies where intake of vitamins is highly correlated with so many healthy behaviors. That advice was well taken. Three carefully done trials showed that there was a lack of effect on long-term supplementation with beta-carotene on both cancer and cardiovascular disease (110–112). Moreover, the fact that the combination of beta-carotene and vitamin A not only had no benefit, but may have had an adverse effect on lung cancer and the risk of death from lung cancer, cardiovascular disease, and on any cause in cigarette smokers and workers exposed to asbestos, is indeed sobering for those who recommended these vitamins before clinical trial data were at hand (111).

Studies of vitamin E continue to remain suggestive of a beneficial effect. Participants in the Alpha Tocopherol, Beta Carotene Cancer Prevention study were followed up for the incidence of angina pectoris by Rose questionnaire (113). During a median follow-up time of 4.7 years, there was a minor but statistically significant decrease in incidence with the relative risk of 0.91 (P = .04). Beta-carotene supplementation had no preventive effect. The use of supplementary and dietary vitamin E and C intake (nonrandomized) was determined in subjects in the Cholesterol Lowering Atherosclerosis Study (114). Among these middle-aged men who had undergone previous coronary bypass surgery and had been randomized to either cholestyramine resin and niacin or placebo, subjects with vitamin E intake from supplements of 100 IU or greater demonstrated less coronary artery progression than did subjects with vitamin E intake below 100 IU. This was true for all lesions and particularly so for mild to moderate lesions (P = .01). This benefit only accured to those within the active treatment group. No benefit was seen for supplementary vitamin C exclusively or in conjunction with vitamin E. While not completely conclusive, the Cambridge Heart Antioxidant Trial (CHAOS) did show a significant decrease in nonfatal MI for those taking 400 IU of alpha tocopherol daily for 1 year as compared to placebo (115). This was not a conclusive study because there was a nonsignificant excess of total deaths in the intervention group.

Although not a vitamin, flavonoid intake may affect risk of CHD. One of the best studies was in Zutphen, Netherlands, where 900 elderly men were followed and their flavonoid intake was related to CHD mortality and total CHD events (116). The major sources of flavonoid intake were black tea (61%), onions (13%), and apples (10%). This amounted to approximately 15 oz. of tea/day. Flavonoid intake was inversely related to CHD mortality. Of interest, the risk of mortality from CHD was decreased by approximately 50% in men in the highest tertile of flavonoid intake (compared with the lowest tertile). Importantly, all-cause mortality was also decreased with increased flavonoid intake. Flavonoids appear in vitro to act as "free radical" scavengers that inhibit LDL oxidation and subsequent toxcity. They also inhibit cyclooxygenases which, via decreased platelet aggregation, may reduce thrombosis.

Taken as a whole, these studies on antioxidants suggest that supplementation with antioxidant vitamins is still far from proven. A prudent diet to reduce risk from cancer as well as heart disease would still include at least five servings of fruits and vegetables daily. Physicians should remember that recommending interesting but unproved therapy may unknowingly limit use of other therapies of proven efficacy.

VI. EXERCISE

It is hard to think of lifestyle change without focusing on recreational exercise. As a barometer of how recreational time is used in a community setting, the self-reported leisure time physical activity was analyzed for 1598 men and 1762 women aged 20 to 69 years in Framingham (117). The most common physical activity for both sexes throughout the year was walking for pleasure. The results showed improved risk factor profiles for those who exercised regularly with higher HDL-C, lower heart rate, lower BMI, and fewer cigarettes smoked per day across four quartiles of increasing physical activity levels ($P < .01$). Men who participated in at least 1 hour of conditioning activities per week had significantly different mean levels for these four risk factors than men who reported less than 1 hour of such activities per week ($P < .001$). For those aged 65 and over, the benefits of leisure-time physical activity are also seen with lower all-cause as well as CHD mortality (118–120). Among older adults, however, the prevalence of regular physical activity is only 37% among older men and 24% among older women (121). The two major activities were walking and gardening.

How does exercise confer benefit? First are its salutary effects on longevity and CHD. Paffenbarger studied Harvard alumni aged 35 to 74 and showed that those who expended the least energy on such activities as walking, stair climbing, and sports play had the highest rates of death on follow-up (122). Moreover, the protection of high physical activity was enjoyed only by those who were active as adults; youthful athleticism alone was not enough (123). Blair and colleagues used graded treadmill exercise test duration as a quantitative measure of whether individuals were physically active or not. Fitness level strikingly predicted survival, even after correction for all of the typical risk factors such as age, smoking habit, cholesterol level, systolic blood pressure, and fasting blood sugar level (124). Moreover, when Blair and co-workers looked at previously unfil individuals who became fit over a

2-year period, they noted a reduced risk of mortality as contrasted with those who remained unfit (125). In the Lipid Clinic Trial, the heart rate during stage 2 of such a submaximal exercise test was also used (126). In both studies, fitness level strikingly predicted survival, even after correction for all of the typical risk factors such as age, smoking habit, cholesterol level, systolic blood pressure, and fasting blood sugar level. The highest risk for death or cardiovascular disease was seen in those who were among the bottom 20% for fitness. Interestingly, the Multiple Risk Factor Intervention Trial (MRFIT) also confirmed the reduction in total mortality and risk from CHD with leisure-time physical activity, but did not find that participating beyond an hour a day was associated with any further risk reduction (127).

Second, there is evidence that exercise can reduce obesity, which is associated with the risk of CHD risk factors such as diabetes, hypertension, and hyperlipidemia. Mann and colleagues demonstrated that young men consuming high-fat diets were able to maintain constant body weight and not raise serum blood fats by exercising vigorously (128). When they stopped exercising, they gained weight! A review of the exercise and obesity literature more than a decade old came to these conclusions (129):

1. Overweight persons are characterized by underexercising more than overeating.
2. Exercise produces reliable effects on weight loss, with those who exercised 4 to 5 times weekly, losing more weight than those who exercised three times a week.
3. Heavy persons lose more weight at the same exercise intensity than their lighter counterparts.
4. People do not lose as much weight as expected by their exercise intensity; this discrepancy was largest for light people.

Wood and co-workers compared the effects of diet and supervised exercise in a carefully planned trial (130). After 1 year, dieters had significant losses of total body weight, fat weight, and lean, nonfat weight as compared to controls. The exercisers did not lose as much total weight, but, in contrast to the diet-only group, did not have significant losses of lean weight. Both weight loss groups increased HDL-C with no significant changes in the total cholesterol and the LDL-C.

These observations were extended by a carefully controlled trial in obese subjects comparing 1 year of diet and exercise versus diet alone (131). The BMI for men was 28 to 34 and the BMI for premenopausal women was 24 to 30, which means they used subjects in the approximately 20% to 30% overweight group. The diet group was on a calorie-controlled step I diet. Those assigned to the diet and exercise group engaged in aerobic exercise 3 days per week at 60% to 80% of their maximal heart rate for at least 25 min initially and then gradually increased to 45 min by the fourth month. There was significantly more weight lost when diet and exercise were combined. Moreover, this loss was primarily fat weight and resulted in a greater improvement in the waist-to-hip ratio in men who also exercised. In women, the ratio was reduced in those assigned to the exercise group, but not to those who underwent diet alone. This is an important point due to the strong association of the waist/hip ratio with total mortality, mortality from coronary heart disease, and likelihood of diabetes (132,133). In both intervention groups, there was improvement in both the systolic and diastolic blood pressure. Moreover, the diet and exercise group had significantly lower triglycerides and elevated HDL-C values. LDL-C/HDL-C ratios changed favorably as compared to the control group with a better response seen in the men who were on diet and exercise rather than on diet alone. Among women, changes in this ratio were less striking, and the LDL-C/HDL-C ratio improved only in women who were on both diet and exercise. These studies corroborate the experience of weight control clinics that there is greater success long-term if the program includes exercise as a component (134,135).

Third, beneficial changes in lipids and lipoproteins are seen with regular exercise. Aerobic exercise will lower triglyceride levels due to increased utilization or disposal triglyceride (136). In addition, reduced fasting and postprandial levels of triglyceride-rich lipoproteins are seen with an average of 15.2 miles per week in one small but carefully done study (137). The changes in triglycerides are accompanied by increases in HDL-C. Kokkinos noted that when men were stratified based on miles run per week, a gradual increase in HDL-C was seen averaging about 0.308 mg/dl increase in HDL-C per mile (138). Most changes were noted in those who jogged 7 to 14 miles per week at mild to moderate intensities. Other studies have considered that a threshold level (10 miles per week jogged) was required (139) For women, using cross-sectional data, plasma HDL-C levels were higher for every additional mile run per week, by an amount nearly identical with that previously reported for men (140). Certainly changes in HDL-C with exercise do not occur quickly. It may take as long as 4 months to 1 year of regular exercise before significant changes in HDL-C are seen (131,141).

Importantly, men with CHD and low HDL-C can increase their HDL-C with exercise training even if they are on a beta-blocking drug (142). A study of men with a recent history of MI noted that those on a nonselective beta blocker did not demonstrate a significant change in HDL-C after exercise as compared to those who were not on such a drug. Nonetheless, for patients who had an initial HDL-C < 35, there was a significant increase in HDL-C despite the beta blocker therapy. On the other hand, a 9-week program of moderate exercise did not raise HDL-C in young, nonobese, nonsmoking, sedentary men with HDL-C < 40 (143). In more detailed and longer studies,

Thompson and colleagues concluded that 8 to 11 months of exercise training in eight previously sedentary men enhanced fat tolerance and increased HDL-C (144). They noted that the changes in HDL-C were not large and suggested that the potential for exercise-related changes in HDL-C may be modest in many subjects. Finally, regular exercise may exert beneficial effects on concentrations of small LDL, the most atherogenic of the LDL particles (145).

Fourth, studies suggest that exercise may be useful in both preventing and treating those with insulin resistance, glucose intolerance, or non-insulin-dependent diabetes mellitus (NIDDM). Physical training, even in the absence of weight loss, can increase insulin sensitivity and improve glucose tolerance in both nondiabetics and those with NIDDM (146). Moreover, it appears that being physically active may either prevent or delay the onset of NIDDM. In the nurses' cohort study, women who engaged in vigorous exercise had two-thirds the risk of NIDDM compared with those who did not (147). This was as true in the obese as in the nonobese. A survey of University of Pennsylvania graduates showed a similar trend in men (148). These investigators found that those who expended the most calories per week in activities like walking, stair climbing, and sports were least likely to develop NIDDM. Moreover, they found the protective effect of physical activity was strongest in those at highest risk for NIDDM—namely, the obese as defined by a high BMI, a history of hypertension, or a parental history of diabetes.. This was also seen in a recent report from Finland which noted a 64% reduction in the risk of NIDDM in similarly high risk men who engaged in moderately intensive physical activities above the 40 min per week (149).

Fifth, there are substantial psychological benefits to a regular exercise program. Stunkard has emphasized the negative psychological aspects of dieting (150). Exercise may prove useful in combating this with less perceived stress and anxiety reported from a 12-month study on psychological outcomes in adults 50 to 65 years of age (151). Reductions in stress were particularly notable in smokers. Regardless of program assignment, greater exercise participation was significantly related to less anxiety and fewer depressive symptoms, independent of changes in fitness or body weight. A not unexpected finding is that those who derive the greatest benefit from exercise are usually the least fit (152). Nonetheless, the scientific evidence linking exercise and reduced depression is not conlusive with studies both supporting and denying the beneficial relationship (153).

Sixth, physically inactive persons have a 35% to 52% greater risk of developing high blood pressure than those who exercise (154,155). This observation may be linked to those above, as hyperinsulinism is clearly an important risk factor for hypertension. In the nonobese patient with hypertension, exercise alone is less useful. A randomized, control trial of exercise in

Table 2 Exercise Goals for Americans Based on the NIH Concensus Development Panel on Physical Activity and Cardiovascular Health (160)

---

1. All Americans should engage in regular physical activity at a level appropriate to their capacity, needs, and interest.
2. Children and adults alike should set a goal of accumulating at least 30 min of moderate-intensity physical activity on most, and preferably all, days of the week.
3. For those with known cardiovascular disease, cardiac rehabilitation programs that combine physical activity with reduction in other risk factors should be more widely used.

---

patients with untreated mild hypertension—systolics (140 to 180) and diastolics (90 to 105)—did not show benefits after 4 months (156). What is not known is whether a longer duration of exercise would have proven useful. On the other hand, the value of exercise as part of a complete program is highlighted by the Stanford Coronary Risk Intervention Project (SCRIP), where patients were provided individualized programs involving a low-fat and low-cholesterol diet, exercise, weight loss, smoking cessation, and medications to favorably alter lipoprotein profiles (157). This study used serial angiography to show multifactorial risk reduction favorably reduced the rate of luminal narrowing in coronary arteries of men and women with coronary artery disease and decreased hospitalizations for clinical cardiac events.

Also in the fight against CHD, exercise is an important, but certainly not exclusive, component of the entire risk prevention program. Runners who feel that exercise alone is all that is needed should be cautioned that coronary fatalities have been recorded in those who exercise at a very high level—marathon runners (158). Marathon runners, especially those with a family history of heart disease and other coronary risk factors, should seek medical advice immediately if they develop any symptoms suggestive of CHD. Thompson has noted that the overall risk of exercise is very low with appromxately 0.75 and 0.13 deaths per 100,000 young male and female athletes and 6 per 100,000 middle-aged men per year (159). He cautioned that physicians should perform routine screening on young athletes and carefully evaluate those with exercise-induced symptoms. Also, physicians needed to inform middle-aged adults regarding the symptoms that suggest coronary ischemia.

Finally, the recommendations of the NIH Consensus Development Panel on Physical Activity and Cardiovascular Health are worthy of emphasis to conclude this section (160). The goal is to include exercise as a regular part of every day for all Americans. See Table 2.

VII. CIGARETTE SMOKING

Although more than 30 years have passed since the Surgeon General's report indicating the health hazards of cigarette smoking, it remains the single greatest preventable cause of illness and premature death in the United States. One in every five deaths in the United States can be attributed to tobacco use, and 48 million Americans considered "current users" of tobacco (161). More than 90% of adults who smoke cigarettes start their habit when they are still in their teenage years (162). After high school graduation, approximately one-third of young people are considered "current" users of tobacco, and nearly one in five are frequent smokers. Rates of teen smoking have remained essentially constant while rates of adult smoking have dropped. A survey among students at two vocational high schools in Virginia listed the need to relax and reduce tension or stress, satisfy a self-defined addiction to nicotine, and cope with boredom as the major reasons. Girls were more likely than boys to say that they smoked to control their weight (38% versus 7%).

Detailed reviews such as the one by Fielding have elaborated the economic costs of cigarette smoking and its effects on CHD, peripheral vascular disease, cerebrovascular disease, cancer of the lung, and cancer of the larynx (163). Active smoking is associated with an earlier age at onset of first infarctions, with a striking inverse dose-response effect (164). Stopping smoking appears to reduce the premature occurrence of coronary events and to decrease CHD mortality. The degree of risk reduction is determined by the length of time after cessation, the amount smoked, and the duration of smoking before cessation. After 1 year the CHD risk is halved in the patient who quits, although it takes a decade or more to approach the risk of a nonsmoker (165). Recent data suggest that the risk for stroke falls very quickly after a person quits smoking (166). Of note, the absolute benefit of quitting smoking on risk of stroke is most marked in hypertensive subjects. This likely is due to the fact that cigarette smoking decreases insulin sensitivity (167).

Unfortuately, quitting smoking, like getting over any addiction, is very difficult. Fiore and colleagues noted that most smokers who successfully quit, do so on their own (168). Moreover, quit rates (smoking abstinence for ≥ 1 year) are twice as high for those who do so on their own as for those who participate in a cessation program. These observational data could be self-fulfilling in that those who cannot quit have to enter cessation programs. Also, smokers who quit "cold turkey" are more likely to remain abstinent than those who try various ways to reduce gradually their consumption of tobacco products. Finally, heavy (≥ 25 cigarettes per day), more addicted smokers are much more likely to participate in an organized cessation program than persons who smoke less. Even after an MI, when motivation would be predicted to be high, smoking quit rates are still less than ideal. Exercise training may

Table 3 The Clinical Practice Guideline on Smoking Cessation Contains Six
Major Recommendations

1. Every person who smokes should be offered smoking cessation treatment at every office visit.
2. Clinicians should ask and record the tobacco use status of every patient.
3. Cessation treatment even as brief as 3 min is effective.
4. The more intense the treatment, the more effective it is in producing long-term abstinence from tobacco.
5. Nicotine replacement therapy (nicotine patches or gum), clinician-delivered social support, and skills training are effective components of smoking cessation treatment.
6. Health care systems should be modified to routinely identify and intervene with all tobacco users at every visit.

help, but plasma thiocyanate levels collected on a random sample suggest that 19% of patients who quit smoking after MI fail to continue to do so (169). A more detailed review of smoking and atherogenesis is presented in Chapter 4.

What should the physician do? In a systematic review of stop smoking interventions from 188 randomized controlled trials, it was estimated that 2% of all smokers stopped and did not relapse for 1 year following the personal advice and encouragement given by their physician during a single routine consultation (170). Behavioral modification techniques in group or individual sessions led by a psychologist have a statistically significant effect that is regrettably no greater than the simple advice of the physician. Hypnosis is unproven. Nicotine replacement is effctive in approximately 13% of smokers who seek help with quitting, with its greatest effects in those who are nicotine-dependent. An important caveat is that nicotine gum used long-term is associated with hyperinsulinemia and insulin resistance, so nicotine replacement therapy should be of limited duration (171).

Advice and encouragement are particularly effective for smokers at special risk such as pregnant women and patients with CHD. The cost of saving a life through the physician's routine advice to smokers is about $1500—clearly a bargain in terms of lifestyle interventions (167). As a result Lewis and Fiore suggest the four A's as a routine part of a physician's practice: Ask about smoking at every opportunity, advise patients to stop, assist patients in quitting, and arrange follow-up (172). They emphasized that nicotine replacement therapy can potentially double the long-term success rate of those who attempt to quit smoking. (For current Agency for Health Care Policy and Research Guidelines, see Table 2.)

Finally, in the United States it is estimated that 37,000 CHD deaths per year are attributed to environmental tobacco smoke exposure. A careful review suggests that nonsmokers are more sensitive to smoke including cardiovascular effects and sidestream smoke contains higher concentrations of gas constituents including carbon monoxide (173). This needs to be considered carefully by those nonsmokers who fail to see that the deleterious effects of tobacco smoke reach out to smokers and nonsmokers alike.

VIII. CONCLUSION

This chapter has detailed the evidence for lifestyle interventions as a means of reducing atherosclerotic vascular disease. The striking contrasts as described by Ravussin and co-workers of the Pima Indians in Arizona and their relatives in the highlands of Mexico are worth considering (174).

Despite a common heritage, the former are obese, hypertensive, and diabetic, while the latter are not. The difference seems to be due to the more demanding lifestyle with more strenuous work and less abundant food for the Pima residing in Mexico. Extensive studies beginning with Reaven's description of Syndrome X have confirmed that hyperinsulinemia related to abdominal obesity may explain the clustering of hypertension, dyslipidemia, and glucose intolerance as well as abnormalities of fibrinolysis (175,176). The answer then seems to be a dietary style low in fat and calories designed to prevent obesity, regular aerobic exercise, avoidance of cigarette smoking, and treatment of hypertension with pharmacologic means if nonpharmacologic means are not successful. These preventive efforts are more important now more than ever, since treatment of atherosclerotic vascular disease has become so expensive for both the average person and society.

REFERENCES

1. Walker A. Diabetes in Europe and Beyond. BMJ 1991; 302:1231.
2. Frank E, Winkleby M, Fortmann SP, Farquhar JW. Cardiovascular disease risk factors: improvements in knowledge and behavior in the 1980s. American Journal of Public Health 1993; 83(4):590–593.
3. Kuczmarski RJ, Flegal KM, Campbell SM, Johnson CL. Increasing prevalence of overweight among US adults. The National Health and Nutrition Examination Surveys, 1960 to 1991. JAMA 1994; 272(3):205–211.
4. Yusuf S, Anand S. Cost of prevention. The case of lipid lowering. Circulation 1996; 93:1774–1776.
5. Stamler J. Lectures on Preventive Cardiology. New York: Grune and Stratton, Inc., 1967; 434.

6. Summary of the Second Report of the National Cholesterol Education Program (NCEP) Expert Panel on Detection, Evaluation, and Treatment of High Blood Cholesterol in Adults (Adult Treatment Panel II). JAMA 1993; 269:3015–3023.

7. Daily Dietary Fat and Total Food-Energy Intakes—NHANES III, Phase I, 1988–91 MMWR 1994; 43:116–117,123–125.

8. Report of the Expert Panel on Population Strategies for Blood Cholesterol Reduction. US Dept of Health and Human Services, National Cholesterol Education Program. NIH Publication No. 90–3046, Washington: U.S. Government Printing Office, Nov. 1990.

9. Keys A, Anderson JT, Grande F. Serum cholesterol response to changes in the diet. II. The effect of cholesterol in the diet. Metabolism 1965; 14:759–765.

10. Hegsted DM. Serum-cholesterol response to dietary cholesterol: a re-evaluation. Am J Clin Nutr 1986:44:299–305.

11. McNamara DJ, Kolb R, Parker TS, et al. Heterogeneity of cholesterol homeostasis in man. Response to changes in dietary fat quality and cholesterol quantity. J Clin Invest 1987; 79:1729–1739.

12. Edington JD, Geekie M,Carter R, Benfield L, Ball M, Mann J. Serum lipid response to dietary cholesterol in subjects fed a low-fat, high-fiber diet. Am J Clin Nutr 1989; 50:58–62.

13. Kestin M, Clifton PM, Rouse IL, Nestel PJ. Effect of dietary cholesterol in normolipidemic subjects is not modified by nature and amount of dietary fat. Am J Clin Nutr 1989; 50:528–532.

14. Fielding CJ, Havel RJ, Todd KM, et al. Effects of dietary cholesterol and fat saturation on plasma lipoproteins in an ethnically diverse population of healthy young men. J Clin Invest 1995; 95(2):611–618.

15. Retzlaff BM, Walden CE, Dowdy AA, Tsunehara CH, Knopp RH. Effects of two eggs per day versus placebo in moderately hypercholeseterolemic and combined hyperlipidemic subjects consuming an NCEP Step One Diet. Circulation 1995; 92(I):I–350.

16. Kesaniemi YA, Einholm C, Miettinen TA. Intenstinal cholesterol absorption efficiency in man is related to apoprotein E phenotype. J Clin Invest 1987; 80:578–581.

17. McCombs RJ, Marcadis DE, Ellis J, Weinberg RB. Attenuated hyperchol- esterolemic response to a high cholesterol diet in subjects heterozygous for the apolipoprotein A-IV-2 allele. N Engl J Med 1994; 331:706–710.

18. Tikkanen MJ, Xu C-F, Hamalainen T, et al. XbaI polymorphism of the apolipoprotein B gene influences plasma lipid response to dietary intervention. Clin Genet 1990; 37:327–334.

19. Shekelle RB, Shyrcck AM, Paul O, et al. Diet, serum cholesterol, and death from coronary heart disease: The Western Electric Study. N Engl J Med 1981; 304:65–70.

20. Stamler J, Shekelle R. Dietary cholesterol and human coronary heart disease. Arch Pathol Lab Med 1988; 112:1032–1040.

21. Woolett LA, Spady, DK, Dietschy JM. Mechanisms by which saturated triacylglycerols elevate the plasma low density lipoprotein-cholesterol concentration in

hamsters. Differential effects of fatty acid chain length. J Clin Invest 1989; 84:119–128.

22. Kromhout D, Menotti A, Bloemberg B, et al. Dietary saturated and trans fatty acids and cholesterol and 25–year mortality from coronary heart disease: the Seven Countries Study. Prev Med 1995; 24(3):308–315.

23. Grundy SM. Influence of stearic acid on cholesterol metabolism relative to other long-chain fatty acids. Am J Clin Nutr 1994; 60(6 suppl):986S–990S.

24. Denke MA. Role of beef and beef tallow, an enriched source of stearic acid, in a cholesterol-lowering diet. Am J Clin Nutr 1994; 60(6 suppl): 1044S–1049S.

25. Ginsberg HN, Barr SL, Gilbert A, et al. Reduction of plasma cholesterol levels in normal men on an American Heart Assocation Step 1 diet or a Step 1 diet with added monounsaturated fat. N Engl J Med 1990; 322:574–579.

26. Reaven P, Parthasarathy S, Grasse BJ, Miller E, Steinberg D, Witztum JL. Effects of oleate-rich and linoleate-rich diets on the susceptibility of low density lipoprotein to oxidative modification in mildly hypercholesterolemic subjects. J Clin Invest 1993; 91(2):668–676.

27. Parthasarathy S, Khoo JC, Miller E, Barnett J, Witztum JL, Steinberg D. Low-density lipoprotein enriched in oleic acid is protected against oxidative modification: implications for dietary prevention of atherosclerosis. Proc Natl Acad Sci USA 1990; 87:3894–3898.

28. Reaven PD, Grasse BJ, Tribble DL. Effects of linoleate-enriched and oleate-enriched diets in combination with alpha-tocopherol on the susceptibility of LDL and LDL subfractions to oxidative modification in humans. Arterioscler Thrombos 1994; 14(4):557–566.

29. Garg A, Grundy SM, Koffler M. Effect of high carbohydrate intake on hyperglycemia, islet function, and plasma lipoproteins in NIDDM. Diabetes Care 1992; 15(11):1572–1580.

30. Willett WC, Ascherio A. Trans fatty acids: are the effects only marginal? Am J Public Health 1994; 84(5):722–724.

31. Mensink RP, Katan MB. Effect of dietary trans fatty acids on high-density and low-density lipoprotein cholesterol levels in healthy subjects. N Engl J Med 1990 Aug 16; 323(7):439–445.

32. van Tol A, Zock PL, van Gent T, Scheek LM, Katan MB. Dietary trans fatty acids increase serum cholesterylester transfer protein activity in man. Atherosclerosis 1995; 115(1):129–134.

33. Mensink RP, Zock PL, Katan MB, Hornstra G. Effect of dietary cis and trans fatty acids on serum lipoprotein(a) levels in humans. J Lipid Res 1992; 33(10): 1493–1501.

34. Willett WC, Ascherio A. Trans fatty acids: are the effects only marginal? Am J Public Health 1994; 84(5):722–724.

35. Trans fatty acids and coronary heart disease risk. Report of the expert panel on trans fatty acids and coronary heart disease. Am J Clin Nutr 62(3):655S–708S.

36. Sturdevant RAL, Pearce ML, Dayton S. Increased prevalence of cholelithiasis in men ingesting a serum cholesterol lowering diet. New Engl J Med 1973; 288:24–27.

37. Meydani SN, Lichtenstein AH, White PJ, et al. Food use and health effects of soybean and sunflower oils. J Am Coll Nutr 1991; 10(5):406–428.
38. Ullmann D, Connor WE, Hatcher LF, Connor SL, Flavell DP. Will a high-carbohydrate, low-fat diet lower plasma lipids and lipoproteins without producing hypertriglyceridemia?. Arterioscler Thrombos 1991; 11(4):1059–1067
39. Anderson
40. Davidson MH, Dugan LD, Burns JH, Bova J, Story K, Drennan KB. The hypocholesterolemic effects of b glucan in oatmeal and oat bran. A dose-controlled study. JAMA 1991; 265:1833–1839.
41. Anderson JW, Zettwoch N. Cholesterol-lowering effects of psyllium hydrophilic mucilloid for hypercholesterolemic men. Arch Intern Med 1988; 148:292–296.
42. Jenkins DJA, Wolever TMS, Venketeshwer R, et al. Effect of blood lipids of very high intakes of fiber in diets low in saturated fat and cholesterol. N Engl J Med 1993; 329:21–26.
43. Edington JD, Geekie M, Carter R, Benfield L, Ball, Mann J. Serum lipid response to dietary cholesterol in subjects fed a low-fat high fiber diet. Am J Clin Nutr 1989; 50:58–62.
44. Hunninghake et al. Am J Med 1994:97:501–503.
45. Warshafsky S, Kamer RS, Sivak SL. Effect of garlic on total serum cholesterol. A meta-analysis. Ann Intern Med 1993; 119(7 Pt 1):599–605
46. Phelps S, Harris WS. Garlic supplementation and lipoprotein oxidation susceptibility. Lipids 1993; 28(5):475–477.
47. Barnard. Arch Intern Med 1991; 151:1389.
48. Ornish D, Brown SE, Scherwitz LW, et al. Can lifestyle changes reverse coronary heart disease? The Lifestyle Heart Trial. Lancet 1990 Jul 21; 336(8708):129–133.
49. Grundy, S. Critique of short term lifestyle change Arch Intern Med 1991; 151: 1275–1276.
50. Lichtenstein AH, Ausman LM, Carrasco W, Jenner JL, Ordovas JM, Schaefer EJ. Short-term consumption of a low-fat diet beneficially affects plasma lipid concentrations only when accompanied by weight loss. Hypercholesterolemia, low-fat diet, and plasma lipids. Arterioscler Thrombos 1994; 14(11):1751–1760
51. Dyerberg J, Bang HO, Stoffersen E, Moncada S, Vane JR. Eicosapentaenoic acid and prevention of thrombosis and atherosclerosis? Lancet 1978; 2(8081):117–119
52. Connor WE, DeFrancesco CA, Connor SL. N-3 fatty acids from fish oil. Effects on plasma lipoproteins and hypertriglyceridemic patients. Ann NY Acad Sci 1993; 683:16–34.
53. Zambon S, Friday KE, Childs MT, Fujimoto WY, Bierman EL, Bierman EL, Ensinck JW. Effect of glyburide and omega 3 fatty acid dietary supplements on glucose and lipid metabolism in patients with non-insulin-dependent diabetes mellitus. Am J Clin Nutr 1992; 56(2):447–454.
54. Connor WE, Prince MJ, Ullman D, et al. The hypotriglyceridemic effect of fish oil in adult-onset diabees without adverse glucose control Ann NY Acad Sci 1993; 683:337–440.
55. Westerveld HT, de Graaf JC, van Breugel HH, et al. Effects of low-dose EPA-E on glycemic control, lipid profile, lipoprotein(a), platelet aggregation, viscosity,

and platelet and vessel wall interaction in NIDDM. Diabetes Care 1993; 16(5): 683–688.

56. Meydani SN, Lichtenstein AH, Cornwall S, et al. Immunologic effects of a National Cholesterol Education Panel step-2 diets with and without fish-derived N-3 fatty acid enrichment. J Clin Invest 1993; 92:105–113.

57. Walsh BW, Sacks FM. Effects of low dose oral conraceptives on very low density and low density lipoprotein metabolism. J Clin Invest 1993; 91:2126–2132.

58. Chait A, Mancini M, February AW, Lewis B. Clinical and metabolic study of alcoholic hyperlipidaemia. Lancet 1972; 2:62–64.

59. Hartung GH, Lawrence SJ, Reeves RS, Foreyt JP. Effect of alcohol and exercise on postprandial lipemia and triglyceride clearance in men. Atherosclerosis 1993; 100(1):33–40.

60. Hegstedt DM, Ausman LM. Diet, alcohol, and coronary heart disease in men. J Nutr 1988; 1184–1189.

61. Langer RD, Criqui MH, Reed DM. Lipoproteins and blood pressure as biological pathways for effect of moderate alcohol consumption on coronary heart disease. Circulation 1992; 85(3):910–915.

62. Renaud S, de Lorgeril M. Wine, alcohol, platelets, and the French paradox for coronary heart disease. Lancet 1992; 339(8808):1523–1526.

63. Elwood PC, Renaud S, Sharp DS, Beswick AD, O'Brien JR, Yarnell JW. Ischemic heart disease and platelet aggregation. Caerphilly Collaborative Heart Disease Study. Circulation 1991; 83(1):38–44.

64. Meade TW, Mellows S, Brozovic, et al. Haemostatic function and ischaemic heart disease: principle results of the northwick park heart study. Lancet 1986; 2:533–537.

65. Criqui MH, Ringel BL. Does diet or alcohol explain the french paradox? Lancet 1994; 344:1719–1723.

66. Cutler JA, Kuller LH. Alcohol use and mortality from coronary heart disease: the role of high-density lipoprotein cholesterol. The Multiple Risk Factor Intervention Trial Research Group. Ann Intern Med 1992; 116(11):881–887.

67. Manolio TA, Levy D, Garrison RJ, Castelli WP, Kannel WB. Relation of alcohol intake to left ventricular mass: the Framingham Study. JACC 1991; 17(3):717–721.

68. Holme I. An analysis of randomized trials evaluating the effect of cholesterol reduction on total mortality and coronary heart disease incidence. Circulation 1990; 82:1916–1924.

69. Hjermann I, Holme I, Velve Byre K, Leren. Effect of diet and smoking intervention on the incidence of coronary heart disease. Lancet 1981; 2:1303–1310.

70. Dayton S, Pearce ML, Hashimoto S, et al. A controlled clinical trial of a diet high in unsaturated fat in preventing complications of atherosclerosis Circulation 1969; 39–40(suppl 20):1–63.

71. Turpeinen O, Karvonen MJ, Pekkarinen M, Miettinen M, Elosuo R, Paavilainen E. Dietary prevention of heart disesae: the Finnish mental hospital study. Int J Epidemiol 1979; 8:99–118.

72. Frantz ID, Dawson EA, Ashman PL, et al. Test of effect of lipid lowering by diet on cardiovascular risk. The Minnesota Coronary Survey. Arteriosclerosis 1989; 9:129–135.
73. Hjermann I, Holme I, Leren P. Oslo study diet and antismoking trial results after 102 months. Am J Med 1986; 80(suppl 2A):7–12.
74. World Health Organization Collaborative Group. Multifactorial trial in the prevention of coronary heart disease, III: incidence and mortality results. Eur Heart J 1983; 4:141–147.
75. Wilhelmsen L, Berglund G, Elmfeldt D, et al. The Multifactor Primary Prevention Trial in Goteborg, Sweden. Eur Heart J 1986; 7(4):279–288.
76. Multiple Risk Factor Intervention Trial Research Group. Multiple risk factor intervention trial risk factor changes and mortality results. JAMA 1982; 248: 1465–1477.
77. Arntzenius AC, Kromhout D, Barth JD, et al. Diet, lipoproteins, and the progression of coronary atherosclerosis. The Leiden Intervention Trial. N Engl J Med 1985; 312:805–811.
78. Blankenhorn DH, Johnson RL, Mack WJ, El Zein HA, Vailas LI. The influence of diet on the appearance of new lesions in the human coronary arteries. JAMA 1990; 263:1646–1652.
79. Schuler G, Hambrecht R, Schlierf G, et al. Regular physical exercise and low-fat diet. Effects of progression on coronary artery disease. Circulation 1992; 86:1–11.
80. Ornish D, Brown SE, Scherwitz LW, et al. Can lifestyle changes reverse coronary heart disease? The Lifestyle Heart Trial. Lancet 1990; 335:129–133.
81. Watts GF, Lewis B, Brunt JNH, et al. Effects of coronary artery disease of lipid lowering diet, or diet plus cholestyramine in the St. Thomas Atherosclerosis Regression Study (STARS). Lancet 1992; 339:563–569.
82. Leung W-H, Lau C-P, Wong C-K. Beneficial effect of cholesterol-lowering therapy on cronary endothelium-dependent relaxation in hypercholesterolemic patients. Lancet 1993; 341:1496–1500.
83. Stamler R, Stamler J, Grimm R, et al. Nonpharmacological control of hypertension. Prev Med 1985 May; 14(3):336–45.
84. Stamler R, Stamler J, Gosch FC, et al. Primary prevention of hypertension by nutritional-hygienic means. Final report of a randomized, controlled trial. JAMA 1989; 262(13):1801–1807
85. Cutler JA. Prevention of hypertension. Curr Opin Nephrol Hypertens 1993; 2(3): 404–414.
86. Law MR, Frost CD, Wald NJ. By how much does dietary salt reduction lower blood pressure? III. Analysis of data from trials of salt reduction. BMJ 1991; 302:819–824.
87. Midgley JP, Matthew AG, Greenwood CM, Logan AG. Effect of a reduced dietary sodium on blood pressure: a meta-analyis of randomized controlled trials. JAMA 1996; 275:1590–1597.
88. Kotchen TA, Krauss RM. Letter to the editor. JAMA 1996.

89. Elliott P, Stamler J, Nichols R, et al. Intersalt revisted: further analyses of 24 hour sodium excretion and blood pressure within and across populations. BMJ 1996; 312:1249–1253.

90. Intersalt Cooperative Reserach Group. Intersalt: an international study of electrolyte excretion and blood pressure. Results for 24 hour urinary sodium and potassium. BMJ 1988; 297:319–328.

91. Neaton JD, Grimm RH, Prineas RJ, et al. Treatment of mild hypertension study. Final results. JAMA 1993; 270:713–724.

92. Grimm RH, Flack JM, Grandits GA, et al. Long-term effects on plasma lipids of diet and drugs to treat hypertension. JAMA 1996; 275:1549–1556.

93. Lipid Research Clinics Coronary Primary Prevention Trial Results II. The relationship of reduction in incidence of coronary heart disease to cholesterol lowering. JAMA 1984; 251:365–374.

94. Hubert HB, Eaker ED, Garrison RJ, Castelli WP. Life-style correlates of risk factor change in young adults: an eight-year study of coronary heart disease risk factors in the Framingham offspring. Am J Epidemiol 1987; 125(5):812–831.

95. Allender PS, Cutler JA, Follmann D, Cappuccio FP, Pryer J, Elliott P. Dietary calcium and blood pressure: a meta-analysis of randomized clinical trials. Ann Int Med 1996; 124:825–831.

96. Bucher HC, Cook RJ, Guyatt GH, et al. Effects of dietary calcium supplementation in blood pressure: a meta-analysis of randomized controlled trials. JAMA 1996; 275:1016–1022.

97. Bucher H, Guyatt GH, Cook RJ, et al. Effect of calcium supplementation on pregnancy-induced hypertension and preeclampsia. a meta-analysis of randomized controlled clinical trials. JAMA 1996; 275:1113–1117.

98. McCarron DA. Dietary calcium and lower blood pressure. We can all benefit. JAMA 1996:275:1128–1129.

99. Looker AC, Loria CM, Carroll MD, McDowell MA, Johnson CL. Calcium intakes of Mexican Americans, Cubans, Puerto Ricans, non-Hispanic whites, and non-Hispanic blacks in the United States. JADA 1993; 93:1274–1279.

100. Steinberg D, Parthasarathy S, Carew TE, Khoo JC, Witzum JL. Beyond cholesterol: modifications of low-density lipoprotein that increase its atherogenicity. New Engl J Med 1989; 320:915–924.

101. Princen HMG, van Poppel G, Vogelzang C, Buytenhek R, Kok FJ. Supplementation with vitamin E but not β carotene in vivo protects low density lipoprotein from lipid peroxidation in vitro. Arterioscler Thrombos 1992; 12:554–562.

102. Peto R, Doll R, Buckley JD, Sporn MB. Can dietary beta-carotene materially reduce human cancer rates? Nature 1981; 290:201–208.

103. Gaziano JM, Manson JE, Buring JE, Hennekens CH. Dietary antioxidants and cardiovascular disease. Ann NY Acad Sci 1992; 669:249–259.

104. Kardinaal AF, Kok FJ, Ringstad J, ct al. Antioxidants in adipose tissue and risk of myocardial infarction: the EURAMIC study. Lancet 1993; 342:1379–84.

105. Princen HMG, van Poppel G, et al. Supplementation with vitamin E but not beta-carotene in vivo protects low density lipoprotein from lipid peroxidation in vitro: effect of cigarette smoking. Arterioscler Thrombos 1992; 12:554–562.

106. Stampfer MJ, Hennekens CH, Manson JE, Colditz GA, Rosner B, Willett WC. Vitamin E consumption and the risk of coronary disease in women. N Engl J Med 1993; 328:1444–1449.

107. Rimm EB, Stampfer MJ, Ascherio A, Giovannucci E, Colditz GA, Willett WC. Vitamin E consumption and the risk of coronary heart disease in men. N Engl J Med 1993; 328:1450–1456.

108. Kushi LH, Folsom AR, Prineas RJ, Mink PJ, Wu Y, Bostick RM. Dietary antioxidant vitamins and death from coronary heart disease in postmenopausal women. N Engl J Med 1996; 334:1156–1162.

109. Steinberg, D. N Engl J Med 1993; 328.

110. Hennekens CH, Buring JE, Manson JE, et al. Lack of effect of long-term supplementation with beta carotene on the incidence of malignant neoplasms and cardiovascular disease. N Engl J Med 1996; 334:1145–1149.

111. Omenn GS, Goodman GE, Thornquist MD, et al. Effects of a combination of beta carotene and vitamin A on lung cancer and cardiovascular disease. N Engl J Med 1996; 334:1150–1155.

112. α Tocopherol, β Carotene Prevention Study Group. The effect of vitamin E and beta carotene on the incidence of lung cancer and other cancers in male smokers. N Engl J Med 1994; 330:1029–1035.

113. Rapola JM, Virtamo J, Haukka JK, et al. Effect of vitamin E and beta carotene on the incidence of angina pectoris. A randomized, double-blind, controlled trial. JAMA 1996; 275:693–698.

114. Hodis HN, Mack WJ, LaBree L, et al. Serial coronary angiographic evidence that antioxidant vitamin intake reduces progression of coronary artery atherosclerosis. JAMA 1995; 273:1849–1854.

115. Stephans NG, Parsons A, Schofield PM, et al. Randomized controlled trial of vitamin E in patients with coronary disease: Cambridge Heart Antioxidant Study (CHAOS). Lancet 1996; 347:781–786.

116. Hertog MGL, Feskens EJM, Hollman PCH, Katan MB, Kromhout D. Dietary antioxidant flavonoids and risk of coronary heart disease: the Zutphern elderly study. Lancet 1993; 342:1007–1011.

117. Dannenberg AL, Keller JB, Wilson PW, Castelli WP. Leisure time physical activity in the Framingham Offspring Study. Am J Epidemiol 1989; 129(1):76–88.

118. Chaplain GA, Seaman TEN, Cohen RD, Knudsen LP, Guralnik J. Mortality among the elderly in the Alameda County Study: behavioral and demographic risk factors. Am J Public Health 1987; 77:307–312.

119. Simonsick EM, Lafferty ME, Phillips CL, et al. Risk due to inactivity in physically capable older adults. Am J Public Health 1993; 83:1443–1450.

120. Donahue RP, Abbott RD, Reed DM, Yano K. Physical activity and coronary heart disease in middle aged and elderly men: the Honolulu Heart Program. Am J Public Health 1988; 78:683–685.

121. Yusuf HR, Croft JB, Giles WH, et al. Leisure-Time Physical Activity Among Older Adults. United States 1990. Arch Intern Med 1996; 156: 1321–26.

122. Paffenbarger RS, Hyde RT, Wing AL, Hsieh C. Physical activity, all-cause mortality, and longevity of college alumni. N Engl J Med 1986; 314:605–613.

123. Paffenberger RS Jr, Hyde RT, Wing AL, et al. Physical activity, all-cause mortality, and longevity of college alumni. N Engl J Med 1986; 314(10):605–613.
124. Blair SN, Kohl HW, Paffenbarger RS, Clark DG, Cooper KH, Gibbons LW. Physical fitness and all-cause mortality. JAMA 1989; 262:2395–2401.
125. Blair SN, Kohl HW, Barlow CE, Paffenbarger RS, Gibbons LW, Macera CA. Changes in physical fitness and all-cause mortality: a prospective study of healthy and unhealthy men. JAMA 1995; 273:1093–1098.
126. Ekelund L, Haskell WL, Johnson JL, Whaley FS, Criqui MH, Sheps DS. Physical fitness as a predictor of cardiovascular mortlaity in asymptomatic north american men. The Lipid Research Clinics Mortality followup study. N Engl J Med 1988; 319:1379–1384.
127. Leon AS, Connett J, Jacobs DR Jr, Rauramaa R. Leisure-time physical activity levels and risk of coronary heart disease and death: the Multiple Risk Factor Reduction Trial. JAMA 1987; 258:2388–2395.
128. Mann GV, Teel K, Hayes O, McNally A, Bruno D. Exercise in the disposition of dietary calories. Regulation of serum lipoproteins and cholesterol levels in human subjects. N Engl J Med 1955; 253:349–355.
129. Epstein LH, Wing RR. Aerobic exercise and weight. Addict Behav 1980; 5:371–378.
130. Wood PD, Stefanick ML, Dreon DM, et al. Changes in plasma lipids and lipoproteins in overweight men during weight loss through dieting as compared with exercise. N Engl J Med 1988; 319:1173–1179.
131. Wood PD, Stefanick ML, Williams PT, Haskell WL. The effects on plasma lipoproteins of a prudent weight-reducing diet with or without exercise, in overweight men and women. N Engl J Med 1991; 325:461–466.
132. Larsson B, Svardsudd K, Welin L, Wilhelmsen L, Bjorntorp P, Tibblin G. Abdominal adipose tissue distribution, obesity, and risk of cardiovascular disease and death: 13 year followup of participants in the study of men born in 1913. Br Med J 1984; 288:1401–1404.
133. Lapidus L, Bengtsson C, Larsson B, et al. Distribution of adipose tissue and risk of cardiovascular disease and death: a 12 year followup of participants in the population study of women in Gothenberg, Sweden. Br Med J 1984; 289:1257–1261.
134. Gormally J, Rardin D, Black S. Correlates of successful response to a behavioral weight control clinic. J Couns Psychol 1980; 27:179–191.
135. Miller PM, Sims KL. Evaluation and component analysis of a comprehensive weight control program. Int J Obes 1981; 5:57–65.
136. Thompson PD, Cullinane EM, Sady SPK, Flynn MM, Chenevert CB, Herbert PN. High density lipoprotein metabolism in endurance athletes and sedentary men. Circulation 1991; 84:140–152.
137. Weintrabu MS, Rosen Y, Otto R, Eisenberg S, Breslow JL. Physical exercise conditioning in the absence of weight loss reduces fasting and postprandial triglyceride-rich lipoprotein levels. Circulation 1989; 79:1007–1014.
138. Kokkinos PF, Holland JC, Narayan P, Colleran JA, Dotson CO, Papademetriou V. Miles run per week and high-density lipoprotein cholesterol levels in healthy,

middle-aged men. A dose-response relationship. Arch Intern Med 1995; 155(4): 415–420.

139. Williams PT, Wood PD, Haskell WL, Vranizan K. The effects of running mileage and duration on plasma lipoprotein levels. JAMA 1982; 2476:6274–6279.

140. Wiliams PT. High-density lipoprotein cholesterol and other risk factors for coronary heart disease in female runners. N Engl J Med 1996; 334:1298–1303.

141. Huttunen JK, Lansimies E, Voutilainen E, et al. Effect of moderate physical exercise in serum lipoproteins: a controlled clinical trial with special reference to serum high density lipoproteins. Circulation 1979; 6:1220–1229.

142. Arvan S, Rueda BG. Nonselective beta-receptor blocker effect on high density lipoprotein cholesterol after chronic exercise. J Am Coll Cardiol 1988; 12:662–668.

143. Raz I, Rosenbilt H, Kark JD. Effect of moderate exercise on serum lipids in young men with low high density lipoprotein cholesterol arteriosclerosis. 1988; 8:245–251.

144. Thompson PD, Cullinane EM, Sady SP, et al. Modest changes in high-density lipoprotein concentration and metabolism with prolonged exercise training. Circulation 1988; 78:25–34.

145. Williams PT, Krauss RM, Vranizan KM, Albers JJ, Terry RB, Wood PDS. Effects of exercise-induced weight loss on low density lipoprotein subfractions in healthy men. Arteriosclerosis 1989; 9:623–632.

146. Schneider SH, Amorosa LF, Khachadurian AK, Ruderman NB. Studies on the mechanism of improved glucose control during regular exercise in Type 2 (non-insulin dependent) diabetes. Diabetologia 1984; 26:355–360.

147. Manson JE, Rimm EB, Stampfer MJ, et al. Physical activity and incidence of non-insulin-dependent diabetes mellitus in women. Lancet 1991; 338:774–778.

148. Helmrich SP, Ragland DR, Leung RW, Paffenbarger RS. Physical activity and reduced occurrence of non-insulin-dependent diabetes mellitus. N Engl J Med 1991; 325:147–152.

149. Lynch J, Helmrich SP, Lakka TA, et al. Moderately intensive physical activities and high levels of cardiorespiratory fitness reduce the risk of non-insulin-dependent diabetes mellitus in high risk men. Arch Intern Mcd 1996; 156:1307–1314.

150. Stunkard AJ, Rush J. Dieting and depression reexamined. A critical review of reports of untoward responses during weight reduction for obesity. Ann Int Med 1974; 81:526–533.

151. King AC, Taylor CB, Haskell WL. Effects of differing intensities and formats of 12 months of exercise training on psychological outcomes in older adults. Health Psychol 1993; 12(4):292–300

152. Folkins CH, Amsterdam, EA. Control and modification of stress emotions through chronic exercise in exercise. In: Cardiovascular Health and Disease, Amsterdam EA, Wilmore JH, DeMaria AN, eds. New York: Yorke Medical Books, 1977; 280–295.

153. Dunn, AL, Dishman RK. Exercise and the neurobiology of depression. In: Exercise and Sport Sciences Reviews, Holloszy JO, ed. Baltimore: Williams and Wilkins, 1991.

154. Blair SN, Goodyear NN, Gibbons LW, Cooper KH. Physical fitness and incidence of hypertension in healthy normotensive men and women. JAMA 1984; 252:487–490.
155. Paffenbarger RS Jr, Wing AL, Hyde RT, Jung DL. Physical activity and incidence of hypertension in college alumni. Am J Epidemiol 1983; 117:245–257.
156. Blumenthal JA, Siegel WC, Appelbaum M. Failure of exercise to reduce blood pressure in patients with mild hypertension. Results of a randomized controlled trial. JAMA 1991; 266:2098–2104.
157. Haskell WL, Alderman EL, Fair JM, et al. Effects of intensive multiple risk factor reduction on coronary atherosclerosis and clinical cardiac events in men and women with coronary artery disease. The Stanford Coronary Risk Intervention Project (SCRIP). Circulation 1994; 89(3):975–990.
158. Noakes TD. Heart disease in marathon runners: a review. Med Sci Sports Exercise 1987; 19(3):187–94.
159. Thompson PD. The cardiovascular complications of vigorous physical activity. Arch Intern Med 1996; 156:2297–2302.
160. NIH Consensus Development Panel on Physical Activity and Cardiovascular Health. Physical activity and cardiovascular health. JAMA 1996; 276(3):241–246.
161. Centers for Disease Control. Cigarette smoking among adults—United States 1992 and changes in the definition of current cigarette smoking. MMWR Morb Mortal Wkly Rep 1994; 43:342–346.
162. Schwartz R. Let's help young smokers quit. Patient Care 1996; 30:45–51.
163. Fielding JE. Smoking: health effects and control. New Engl J Med 1995:313:491–498, 313:555–561.
164. Gottlieb S, Fallavollita J, McDermott M, Brown M, Eberly S, Moss AJ. Cigarette smoking and the age at onset of a first non-fatal myocardial infarction. Coron Artery Dis 1994; 5(8):687–694.
165. Department of Health and Human Services. The Health Consequences of Smoking: Cardioavascular Disease. A Report of the Surgeon General. Rockville, MD: U.S. Government Printing Office, 1983.
166. Wannamethee SG, Shaper AG, Whincup PH, Walker M. Smoking cessation and the risk of stroke in middle-aged men. JAMA 1995; 274(2):155–160.
167. Attvall S, Fowelin J, Lager I, Von Schenck H, Smith U. Smoking induces insulin resistance: a potential link with the insulin resistance syndrome. J Intern Med 1993; 233:327–332.
168. Fiore MC, Novotny TE, Pierce JP, et al. Methods used to quit smoking in the United States: do cessation programs help? JAMA 1990; 263:2760–2765.
169. Taylor CB, Houston-Miller N, Haskell WL, Debusk RF. Smoking cessation after acute myocardial infarction: the effects of exercise training. Addict Behav 1988; 13(4):331–335.
170. Law M, Tang JL. An analysis of the effectiveness of interventions intended to help people stop smoking. Arch Intern Med 1995; 155:1933–1941.
171. Eliasson B, Taskinen M-R, Smith, U. Long-term use of nicotine gum is associated with hyperinsulinemia and insulin resistance. Circulation 1996; 94:878–881.
172. Lewis SF, Fiore MC. Smoking cessation: What works? What doesn't? J Respir Dis 1995; 16(5):497–510.

173. Kritz H, Schmid P, Sinzinger H. Passive smoking and cardiovascular risk. Arch Intern Med 1995; 155:1942–1948.

174. Ravussin E, Valencia ME, Esparza J, Bennett PH, Schulz LO. Effects of a traditional lifestyle on obesity in Pima Indians. Diabetes Care 1994; 17:1067–1074.

175. Reaven GM. Role of insulin resistance in human disease. Diabetes 1988; 37: 1595–1601.

176. Laws A, Reaven G. Insulin resistance, hyperinsulinemia, dyslipidemia and cardiovascular disease. In: E. Braunwald, W.B. ed. Heart Disease, Update 1, 4th ed., Philadelphia: Saunders Co., 1992; 1–7.

6

Effects of Gonadal Hormones on Atherogenesis

Robert H. Knopp
Northwest Lipid Research Clinic; University of Washington School of Medicine; and Harborview Medical Center, Seattle, Washington

Bartolome Bonet* and Xiaodong Zhu
Northwest Lipid Research Clinic, and University of Washington School of Medicine, Seattle, Washington

I. INTRODUCTION

Gonadal hormones are assuming an increasingly important role in the understanding of atherosclerosis pathophysiology as well as the treatment and prevention of atherosclerosis. The purpose of this chapter is to review the basic science mechanisms whereby sex hormones alter the pathogenesis of arteriosclerosis, give examples of medical conditions where the effect of gonadal hormones is known to alter the natural history of the disease, and, finally, to give examples where gonadal hormones can be used for therapeutic benefit, or, in some cases, are found to have unwanted effects.

The gonadal hormones with the best-known effects on atherogenesis are the estrogens. These provide a basis for comparison with other categories of sex steroid hormones in which metabolic effects are recognized and the atherogenic process is influenced. In general, the progestins and androgens have effects that oppose estrogenic effects, and this physiological pattern offers a basis for predicting the effects of these hormones on atherogenesis where studies are not available.

---

* *Current affiliation*: University of San Pablo, Madrid, Spain

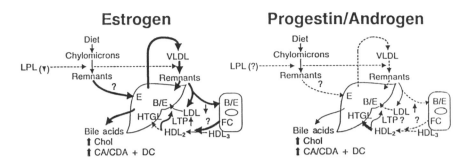

Figure 1 Effects of sex steroids on lipoprotein metabolism. Width of the lines indicates the rate of cholesterol traffic under influence of estrogen (left) or progestin/androgen (right). Question marks indicate effects for which documentation is uncertain or limited. From Knopp (4), with permission.

II. EFFECTS ON LIPOPROTEIN METABOLISM

The longest history of known effects of gonadal hormones on atherogenesis is related to their influence on lipoprotein metabolism. These studies provide the basis for much of our current understanding about atherosclerosis as related to gonadal hormones and also current therapeutic interventions.

A. Estrogenic Effects on Lipoprotein Metabolism

The effects of estrogens on lipoprotein metabolism have been recently reviewed (1–4) and the lipoprotein pathways affected are shown in Figure 1 (1–4). The main point from the illustration is that estrogen enhances the metabolic traffic of cholesterol transport in virtually every pathway except one. The pathways are discussed in detail below.

1. *Plasma Triglyceride Elevations*

Probably the best-recognized effect of estrogen treatment is an increase in plasma triglycerides, one example of which is shown in Table 1. This effect is greatest when estrogen is given orally and less when given systemically by injection, patch, or natural ovarian secretion (1–4). The increase in plasma triglyceride concentrations is due to an increased hepatic triglyceride secretion in the form of increased entry of very low density lipoprotein (VLDL) into the circulation. Such an effect has been demonstrated by Schaefer and associates (5) and Walsh and associates (6) as well as in vitro models (1–4). The natural estrogen dominant condition is pregnancy, and here again, increased

Table 1 Effects of 1 μg/kg Ethinylestradiol Given Daily for 1 Month in Six Women Fed a High-Cholesterol Diet

	Diet	Diet + ethinylestradiol
Triglyceride	98	154[*]
Cholesterol	255	225[*]
VLDL cholesterol	14	13
LDL cholesterol	173	130[*]
HDL cholesterol	68	82[*]
HDL$_2$	33	46[*]
HDL$_3$	35	36
Apo-E	6.84	4.60[*]
Apo-B	125	111[*]
Apo-A-I	155	212[*]
Apo-A-II	34.5	37.5[*]
LPL	125[a]	94[a]
HTGL	162[a]	51[a*]
LCAT	5.4[b]	5.1[b]

Source: Applebaum-Bowden et al. (9).
VLDL = very low density lipoprotein; HDL = high-density lipoprotein; LPL = lipoprotein lipase; HTGL = hepatic triglyceride lipase; LCAT = lecithin:cholesterol acetyltransferase.
Values are given in mg/dl, except [a]mmol/min/ml; [b]ng/ml.
* $P < .05$.

entry of triglyceride-rich lipoproteins in the blood stream has been shown in an animal model of pregnancy (7). Thus, it is very clear that plasma triglyceride concentrations increase largely because of increased entry into the circulation.

Very early, the question was asked whether the hypertriglyceridemic effect of estrogen was due to a reduction in the activity of lipoprotein lipase (LPL) activity, the enzyme system predominantly responsible for the removal of circulating triglycerides from the bloodstream. The first measurement of this effect was performed by Appelbaum and associates in 1977 and repeated in 1989 with similar results, showing that estrogen is associated with a wide variation in lipoprotein lipase activity but with no net increase or decrease that is statistically significant (8,9). On the other hand, Iverius and Brunzell found that endogenous estrone levels in postmenopausal women were inversely related to lipoprotein lipase activity (10). However, in this instance, intra-abdominal obesity could be, in common, a cause of low LPL activity and increased estrone formation, rather than estrone being the cause of the lower LPL activity. While this hypothesis deserves further research, the main point is that prospective studies show no effect on estrogen on LPL activity (1–4,8,9).

The question has often been raised about whether the triglyceride rise in estrogen-treated women is associated with an increased risk for arteriosclerosis. While this matter is discussed in a later section, the short answer is that overall, estrogen is believed to inhibit atherogenesis. In this setting it would seem unlikely that the triglyceride rise would alter this picture substantially. In fact, a physiological explanation is available for the lack of an atherogenic effect associated with estrogen-induced hypertriglyceridemia. Walsh and Sacks (11) have shown that estrogen alters the nature of the triglyceride-rich VLDL particles to become large, buoyant, and cholesterol-poor. Such large particles are thought to have less access to the arterial intima, unlike smaller, more cholesterol-rich low-density lipoprotein (LDL). An example of this effect is seen in Table 1, in the experiments of Appelbaum and associates, where ethinylestradiol (EE), 1 μg/kg, was given daily for 1 month to six postmenopausal women (9). In the experiment, plasma triglyceride concentrations nearly doubled but the VLDL cholesterol concentration was actually unchanged, a feature of a large VLDL particle. The large size of such particles, as well as their relatively diminished cholesterol content, renders them less atherogenic. Admittedly, this scenario could benefit from a direct experimental proof.

LPL provides for the removal of chylomicron triglyceride as well as VLDL triglyceride, as shown in Figure 1. When VLDL concentrations are high, LPL activity is occupied or saturated by VLDL particles, leaving less available LPL activity for chylomicron triglyceride removal. Thus, it is common in hypertriglyceridemic states associated with endogenous VLDL overproduction from the liver, as in oral estrogen therapy, that exogenous absorbed triglyceride-rich particles, chylomicrons, can be delayed in their removal. The accumulation of chylomicrons in plasma begins at plasma triglyceride levels between 500 and 1000 mg/dl (5.6 to 12.2 mM). Thus, hyperchylomicronemia can be a consequence of estrogen treatment, not directly, but because VLDL is competing for LPL removal along with the chylomicron particle, and to the disadvantage of chylomicron removal. Intestinal fat absorption per se, as far as is known in humans, is not altered by estrogen therapy.

2. Remnant Metabolism

The next step in lipoprotein metabolism is the removal of chylomicron and VLDL remnants, as pictured in Figure 1. Information on the effect of estrogen on the removal of endogenous VLDL remnants is the most extensive. Remnants are recognized by the presence of apoprotein E-3 or E-4 on the surface of the remnant particle by the LDL receptor, largely in the liver. In the illustration, the LDL receptor is shown as the B/E receptor, indicating that apoproteins B and E are recognized by this receptor. Individuals who lack the apoprotein E-3 or E-4 phenotype and have either the common defective type apoprotein E-2, or other, rarer types, have remnant accumulation. This disorder is known as remnant removal disease, which in the original Fredrickson typing system was known as type III hyperlipidemia (12). Estrogen enhances the removal of remnant lipoprotein by upregulating the LDL receptor, which may explain in part the low content of cholesterol in the VLDL fraction as well as the LDL fraction (see below), since remnants overlap the VLDL and LDL ranges. The estrogen effect on the LDL receptor is related to an increase in transcription of LDL-mRNA from the LDL receptor gene, as initially shown by Ma and associates (13). Decreases in remnant lipoprotein levels and enhanced remnant catabolism have been observed in type III hyperlipidemic females treated with estrogen (12,14).

Clinical experience indicates that more women present with estrogen-induced hypertriglyceridemia and concomitant type III hyperlipidemia than are successfully treated with estrogen. This apparent discrepancy with estrogen research described above probably reflects a dual etiology of type III hyperlipidemia which involves an excessive entry of VLDL into the circulation usually as a consequence of familial combined hyperlipidemia together with the remnant removal impairment associated with the abnormality of apoprotein E. It is our experience that the majority of hypertriglyceridemic type III women aggravated by oral estrogen administration are successfully treated by discontinuing oral estrogen and its first-pass hepatic effect on triglyceride production and substituting for it the more physiological, systemically administered estrogen patch. The main point is that clinicians need to be alert to either possibility—that estrogens may improve or aggravate type III hyperlipidemia.

Still another step in the remnant removal process is the removal of triglyceride from the remnant by hepatic lipase prior to its uptake by the LDL receptor (8,9). This uptake process appears to be impaired by the downregulation of hepatic lipase under the influence of estrogen (8,9). So it is conceivable that in a given case, the balance between the upregulation of the LDL receptor and the downregulation of the hepatic lipase enzyme might modify the effect of estrogen in unexpected ways. In addition, what is known about hepatic lipase action is largely obtained from studies of orally administered estrogen; the effect of the more physiological route of systemic administration has not been adequately investigated. The functional importance of hepatic lipase as a route for terminal triglyceride removal from remnants, LDL and high-density lipoprotein (HDL), is borne out by the fact that these lipoproteins are triglyceride-enriched in the plasma of estrogen-treated, oral-contraceptive-treated, and pregnant women (15,16).

With respect to the effect of estrogen on the clearance of the chylomicron remnant, the matter has not been directly studied. However, women treated with an oral contraceptive (OC) containing a moderately androgenic progestin have an enhanced clearance of retinylpalmitate-labeled fatty acids. Thus, enhanced clearance of the chylomicron remnant under the influence of estrogen is plausible as shown in Figure 1, although not perfectly documented (17).

3. LDL Metabolism

The reduction in LDL cholesterol concentrations with estrogen treatment is seen primarily with orally administered estrogen formulations and is related to increased LDL receptor activity (13). A lesser LDL reduction is seen with patch formulations, as shown by Walsh and Sacks (11), due to the lack of a high-dose estrogen exposure in the liver obtained with oral administration. Very recently, it has been reported that estrogen enhances LDL receptor independent catabolism of LDL in an animal model (18). Thus, oral administration of estrogen replacement therapy appears to be preferable to patch or systemic administration for effects on LDL (and HDL; see below) if there are no contraindications such as the hypertriglyceridemias associated with VLDL overproduction, lipoprotein lipase deficiency, impaired remnant removal, or a history of venous thrombosis. A possible adverse effect of estrogen treatment is the formation of small, dense LDL. However, this effect, along with the rise in triglyceride, does not seem to negate the overall sense of benefit to the circulation since the reduction in LDL is one of the major mechanisms of estrogen efficacy in atherosclerosis prevention.

4. Lipoprotein(a) Metabolism

Associated with LDL and exaggerating its inherent atherogenicity is apoprotein(a), a plasminogen homolog that is synthesized in the liver and associates with LDL in the plasma, forming lipoprotein(a), i.e., Lp(a) (19). According to most authorities, Lp(a) is a strong cardiovascular risk factor, commonly seen in individuals with elevated LDL cholesterol levels and premature coronary artery disease (20). Lp(a) appears to be associated with greater penetration and/or retention of LDL in the arterial wall as well as inhibition of plasminogen-mediated thrombolysis. The basis for the inhibition of plasminogen-mediated thrombolysis is the striking homology between Lp(a) and plasminogen. The main point for this review is that estrogen in moderate to high doses reduces Lp(a) levels (21–23). Even the estrogen antagonist with an estrogenic effect of its own, tamoxifen, will lower Lp(a) (24). The molecular mechanism for the estrogenic reduction in Lp(a) plasma concentration is unknown.

5. HDL Metabolism

Another well-known effect of estrogen is to increase plasma HDL cholesterol concentrations, an example of which is also shown in Table 1. In this case, the HDL increase is confined to the more buoyant, or lipid-rich HDL_2 (9). HDL_3 cholesterol concentrations are unchanged (9). Because HDL_2 cholesterol concentrations are also selectively increased with hygienic measures such as exercise, it was originally thought that HDL_2 was the only beneficial fraction of HDL. This conclusion no longer appears to be valid, but an increase in HDL_2 is nonetheless associated with a reduction in cardiovascular disease risk.

The mechanism of the increase in HDL_2 cholesterol concentration is multifactorial but is due in part to an increase in apoprotein A-I secretion from the liver, an effect supported by a majority of recent metabolic studies (25–27). (The effect of hepatic lipase reduction is discussed below.) Apoprotein A-I is the principal apoprotein of HDL, and its plasma concentrations are associated with diminished risk from cardiovascular disease. In contrast, apoprotein A-II, a related HDL apoprotein, is present in lower concentrations than apoprotein A-I and appears not to be estrogen-sensitive. Recent studies indicate that apoprotein A-II is proatherogenic in animal models (28). Likewise, HDL_3 is associated more predominantly with HDL particles containing both apoproteins A-I and A-II (29,30) and is thought to be less efficient in reverse cholesterol transport and less protective against arteriosclerotic vascular disease (31). Particles containing apo-A-I only are more associated with HDL_2 and are higher in women compared to men (30).

Recent studies by Oram and associates have indicated that a cell surface recognition mechanism is necessary for apoprotein A-I to pick up free cholesterol and phospholipid from cells (32). In this investigation, apoprotein A-I-mediated cholesterol and phospholipid uptake from cells was impaired in individuals with Tangier's disease, which is characterized by a lack of the cellular apoprotein A-I recognition system and very low HDL levels. Apoprotein A-II had no effect in this system. The effect of estrogen on apo-A-I recognition has not been studied to our knowledge.

After free cholesterol is taken up from cells onto the surface of HDL, it is esterified and then incorporated into the neutral lipid core of the HDL particle. This esterification process is accomplished by the enzyme lecithin-cholesterolacyltransferase, or L-CAT, where a fatty acid is transferred from lecithin to form cholesterol ester with the formation of lysolecithin as a result. This enzyme activity appears not to be appreciably altered by estrogen therapy, as shown in Table 1 (9). However, hepatic lipase activity, as noted above, is significantly reduced (9,33). While earlier studies indicated that HDL cholesterol concentrations are inversely associated with hepatic lipase concentrations when estrogens are given (8), this reduction does not appear to reduce the rate of clearance of whole HDL particles containing either A-I or A-I plus A-II (33). This observation is consistent with what is known about the terminal steps in HDL metabolism—namely, that the clearance of the apoproteins A-I and A-II contained in HDL particles is not dependent on hepatic lipase activity whereas the removal of HDL cholesterol and, probably, phospholipid is. The main point is that an estrogen-induced reduction in hepatic lipase contributes to the increase in HDL cholesterol and phospholipid levels.

Two other steps in HDL catabolism deserve mention. One is the transfer of cholesterol from HDL to LDL or VLDL via the lipid transfer protein (LTP), also known as cholesterol ester transfer protein (CETP). It appears that LTP is under hormonal control as its activity is increased in the plasma of pregnant women (34). This LTP effect in combination with the reduction in hepatic lipase activity (8,9,33) appears to favor a recycling of cholesterol to LDL and VLDL by the transfer protein in exchange for triglyceride. This effect may further contribute to the triglyceride elevation in HDL and LDL initiated by a reduction in hepatic lipase activity under the influence of estrogen, as mentioned above. The net effect of estrogen on reverse cholesterol transport is to conserve the supply of cholesterol in the bloodstream by recycling it through the lipoprotein cascade.

The final effect of estrogen on cholesterol metabolism and distal to its transport in lipoproteins is the enhanced excretion of cholesterol in the bile. Cholic acid excretion in relation to the excretion of chenodeoxycholic acid plus deoxycholic acid is also increased (Fig. 1). The increased cholesterol content of the bile may enhance the susceptibility of women to gallstone disease. Whether gallstones form depends on the solubility of cholesterol in the bile which in turn depends on the bile acid and phospholipid content of the bile.

In summary, the effect of estrogen is to increase the transport of cholesterol in the body. This effect applies to both the exogenous and endogenous pathways, from the enhanced secretion of lipoprotein from the liver and increased uptake by both liver and peripheral cells to the recycling of cholesterol from peripheral cells back to LDL and VLDL via HDL and the reverse cholesterol transport pathway. Protection from arteriosclerotic vascular disease would not be expected to be a direct effect of this enhancement in cholesterol traffic, but a reduction in LDL-C levels and an increase in reverse cholesterol transport via HDL appear to have this effect. Perhaps more closely linked to survival of the species is the enhanced availability of cholesterol to the placenta provided by the increase in cholesterol transport induced by estrogen. As much as 30% or 40% of daily cholesterol balance is consumed in the formation of the sex steroids of pregnancy—primarily progesterone, and to a lesser extent estrogen (35). The effects of sex steroids on the regulatory steps of lipoprotein metabolism are summarized in Table 2.

Table 2 Effects on Female Sex Steroids and Androgens on Lipoprotein Metabolism

	Estrogen	Estrogen + androgenic progestin	Androgen
Cholesterol absorption	=[a]	?	?
LPL activity	=, ↓	?	=, ? ↑
Chylomicron remnant clearance	↑ ?	↑	? ↓
VLDL secretion	↑	↓	↓
VLDL remnant clearance			
Hepatic lipase-mediated	↓	↑	↑
B/E receptor-mediated	↑	↓	↓
LDL formation	↑	? ↑	?
LDL removal	↑	↓	↓
HDL transport	↑	↓	↓
LCAT activity	↓	?	?
Hepatic lipase activity	↓	↑	↑
Lipid transfer protein activity	↑	?	?
Lp(a) concentration	↓	=	↓

Source: modified with permission from Ref. 1.

[a] The equals sign indicated no change. LPL = lipoprotein lipase; VLDL = very low density lipoprotein; B/E = LDL receptor; HDL = high-density lipoprotein; LCAT = lecithin:cholesterol acetyltransferase.

B. Effects of Progestins and Androgens vs. Estrogens on Lipoprotein Metabolism

As mentioned earlier, progestins, including natural progesterone, tend to oppose the effect of estrogen in a number of systems. Probably the most fundamental biological example is the upregulation of the progestin receptor in the endometrium by estrogen and the downregulation of this receptor by progesterone in the same system (35). In fact, the entire morphology of the endometrium changes from a proliferative to a secretory form in the second half of the menstrual cycle as a result of this interaction (35). Similarly, androgens oppose estrogen effects in many systems, including the lipoprotein transport system. As shown in Figure 1, each of the key steps of lipoprotein metabolism enhanced by estrogen administration appears to be reduced by progestins—in particular, androgenic progestins or androgens themselves. The net effect is to diminish cholesterol transport throughout the body, sometimes to increase the steady-state concentration of LDL depending on dose and type of agent, and to lower the concentration of HDL. Oxandrolone, an anabolic androgenic steroid, for example, given to male subjects, halves plasma VLDL concentrations, the major triglyceride-bearing lipoprotein; increases LDL concentrations from 179 to 211 mg/dl (4.63 to 5.46 mM); and drops HDL cholesterol concentrations from 43 to 28 mg/dl (1.11 to 0.72 mM) (36).

Mechanistically, androgens diminish VLDL secretion (37), downregulate the LDL receptor (38), and lower HDL cholesterol levels at least in part by increasing hepatic lipase activity (39). Surprisingly, androgens such as stanozolol and testosterone lower Lp(a) (40,41). The mechanism and teleologic significance of this effect, which is paradoxically similar to estrogen are unknown.

In terms of clinical significance, individuals with a predisposition to hyperlipidemia or those with hypercholesterolemia might be expected to be adversely affected in LDL and HDL by administration of high doses of anabolic steroids. On the other hand, advantage can be taken of the triglyceride-lowering effect of androgens such as oxandrolone or stanozolol when severe hypertriglyceridemia cannot be treated any other way.

III. ESTROGEN-PROGESTIN EFFECTS ON LIPOPROTEINS; ORAL CONTRACEPTIVE STEROIDS

Examples of the interplay of estrogen and progestin on lipoprotein levels are seen with oral contraception. High-dose oral contraceptive formulations (42) are associated with a moderate to marked increase in LDL concentration (see Knoopp et al. [1] for more details). Formulations with the most androgenic progestin, levonorgestrel, reduce HDL-C reduction the most. All of these formulations elevate triglyceride 40% to 90% from baseline, suggesting a high estrogenic effect. The high dose, estrogen-dominant oral contraceptives create an effect similar to late-gestation pregnancy where triglyceride increases two- to fourfold, LDL 25% to 50% and HDL 25% (1,16).

The lower-dose, second-generation oral contraceptives (43,44) are not associated with as great an LDL cholesterol increase, but tend to have slight reductions in HDL cholesterol concentrations. Plasma triglyceride concentrations are increased to a lesser extent (4% to 15%) than with the high-dose oral contraceptives. Effects in the triphasic oral contraceptive series using the progestins levonorgestrel or norethindrone show similar, less marked LDL effects than in the low-dose monophasic formulations, reflecting further reductions in hormone dose. Overall, the second generation of OCs has a lesser estrogen effect relative to the progestin effect.

The new, or third-generation of oral contraceptives (45–48) make use of the synthetic progestins norgestimate, desogestrel, or gestodene, three relatively nonandrogenic progestins, which are associated with essentially no increase in LDL cholesterol concentrations and modest increases in HDL concentration. The triglyceride elevations with these formulations are not as great (20% to 50%) as with the earlier, high-dose formulations and are similar to the low-dose formulations, again reflecting the 30 to 40 μg doses of EE within the oral contraceptive estrogen administered, but now the HDL-raising effect of the estrogen can be seen in the absence of an androgenic progestin effect. Probably the absence of an LDL cholesterol rise in users of the third-generation OCs can be explained in the same way.

Clinical applications from these generalizations are several. One is that if a woman with high plasma triglycerides takes an OC, the potential always exists for serious hypertriglyceridemia to develop and result in acute pancreatitis. Therefore, a triglyceride measurement before or soon after starting OC is a good idea. A second caveat is that individual HDL-C and LDL-C changes in response to oral contraceptive steroid use can vary markedly. Therefore, women using oral contraceptive steroids need to be checked once, probably 3 months after commencing, to see if marked changes in any important fraction are occurring, particularly if there is a prior history of triglyceride elevations, LDL-C elevations, HDL-C reductions, and a family history of coronary disease. On the other hand, the average beneficial effect of third-generation oral contraceptives on lipoproteins may lead to their selected use to remedy lipoprotein abnormalities and conceivably ameliorate coronary disease risk (see below).

IV. SEX STEROID EFFECTS ON LIPOPROTEINS IN POSTMENOPAUSAL WOMEN

Observationally, the higher LDL-C level in postmenopausal women compared to younger women is likely due in part to the relative deficiency of endogenous estrogen in post-postmenopausal women (1–4). When women have been studied through the menopause and estrogen deficiency develops, the LDL-C level increases by 12.0 mg/dl (0.31 mM) and HDL-C decreases by 3.5 mg/dl (0.09 mM) (49). These differences reflect the absence of endogenous ovarian estrogen secretion into the systemic circulation. It is also noteworthy that plasma insulin, glucose, and body weight all increase more in women becoming menopausal than in those not becoming menopausal (49).

When hormone users are compared to non-hormone users, estrogen treatment raises the HDL cholesterol level as much as 8 mg/dl (0.2 mM) (42). Compared to the smaller difference associated with menopause, the greater difference with hormone replacement may be due to subject selection, higher doses of estrogen that were used in the 1970s or the oral route of administration. On the other hand, the recently published double-blind, randomized Postmenopausal Estrogen-Progestin Intervention trial (PEPI) showed a lesser HDL

Table 3 Results of the PEPI Trial

| | | | | Change from baseline | | | | | | |
	TG (mg/dl)	LDL-C (mg/dl)	HDL-C (mg/dl)	Glucose (mg/dl) 0 hr	2 hr	IRI pmol/L) 0 hr	2 hr	Fibrinogen (mg/dl)	Weight (kg)	Waist-hip ratio
Premarin 0.625 mg	13.7	−14.5	5.6	−2.8	2.0	−1.7	−8.0	−20	0.4	0.003
Premarin, micronized Pg (cyclic)	13.4	−14.8	4.3	−2.5	3.0	−3.5	−25.1	1	0.6	0.007
Premarin, Provera 10 (cyclic)	12.7	−17.7	1.6	−2.7	7.5	1.3	13.4	6	0.8	0.010
Premarin, Provera 2.5 (continuous)	11.4	−16.5	1.2	−2.1	6.9	−3.8	1.2	1	0.6	0.007
Placebo	−3.2	−4.1	−1.2	−0.5	−0.1	3.8	−13.7	10	1.3	0.010

Source: Adapted from ref. 50; from the Writing Group for the PEPI Trial.
Breast cancer incidence equal among groups (8 total cases) (total n = 875, ~175/group). TG = triglyceride; LDL-C = low-density lipoprotein cholesterol; HDL-C = high-density lipoprotein cholesterol; IRI = immunoreactive insulin.

cholesterol increase in women given Premarin 0.625 mg daily, as shown in Table 3 (50). In this case, the HDL-C increase is about 5.6 mg/dl (0.14 mM) above control. Premarin given with medroxyprogesterone acetate, either 10 mg given cyclically or 2.5 mg given continuously, diminishes the HDL increase to 1.6 and 1.2 mg (0.04 and 0.03 mM) above baseline during the course of therapy, respectively. Most interestingly, when micronized natural progesterone is given cyclically with Premarin, the Premarin effect on HDL cholesterol is almost entirely preserved (4.3 mg/dl or 0.11 mM increase above baseline).

On the other hand, all of the postmenopausal hormonal formulations examined were associated with reductions in LDL cholesterol concentrations of about 14.5 to 17.7 mg/dl (0.37 to 0.45 mM) without any distinctions among the groups. It is unclear why an antiestrogenic effect of any of the progestogins used would not antagonize the LDL-lowering effect of Premarin alone. It may be that the effects of progestins on LDL and HDL are mechanistically different. Another possibility is that the progestin dose was not sufficient to alter LDL metabolism, though it was sufficient for HDL. In any case, the triglyceride elevations were minor, ranging from 11.4 to 13.7 mg/dl (0.13 to 0.15 mM), and less than the 20% to 50% triglyceride elevations associated with third-generation oral contraceptives.

V. EFFECTS OF GONADAL HORMONES ON NONLIPID CARDIOVASCULAR DISEASE RISK FACTORS

Postmenopausal hormone replacement therapy, either estrogen alone or estrogen plus progestin, affects cardiovascular disease risk factors other than lipoproteins. These include clotting factors and indices of carbohydrate metabolism and vascular wall physiology and pathophysiology.

A. Plasma Glucose Levels

Nabulsi and associates compared nonusers and current users of postmenopausal hormones in the Arteriosclerosis Risk factors In Community (ARIC) (Table 4) (22), and a more recent and very similar study of the question has been reported from Finland in the FINRISK study (51). In both the ARIC and FINRISK studies, plasma glucose concentrations are generally lower among hormone users, as originally reported by Barrett-Connor (52). Lower fasting glucose levels are also seen among oral contraceptive users (53). Finally, a reduction in fasting glucose concentrations 2.1 to 2.8 mg/dl (0.12 to 0.16 mM) is seen in the prospective PEPI study on all estrogen-progestin combinations used (Table 3) (50).

Table 4 Adjusted Physiological Cardiovascular Disease Risk Factors in Women Using Different Postmenopausal Replacement Hormones

	Nonusers		Current		P
	Past	Never	Estrogen	E_2 + Pg	Users vs. nonusers
TG	123	120	141	131	< .001
LDL-C	141	141	125	127	< .001
HDL-C	58	58	67	66	< .001
HDL_2-C	17	16	21	21	< .001
ap-A-1	141	140	159	156	< .001
ap-B	95	95	91	92	< .015
Lp(a)	114	116	101	101	< .006
Fibrinogen	3.1	3.2	3.0	3.0	< .001
Factor VII	126	125	136	127*	< .001
Factor VIII	133	136	134	132	NS
Von Willebrand	119	121	119	118	NS
Antithrombin III	114	115	110	113	< .001
Protein C	3.3	3.3	3.5	3.3	NS
Glucose	99	99	97	95	< .001
Insulin	11.7	11.3	10.0	10.5	< .001
BP					
Systolic	121	122	121	120	NS
Diastolic	72	72	72	71	NS

Source: Nabulsi et al. (22).
E_2 = estradiol; Pg = progestin; TG = triglyceride; LDL-C = low-density cholesterol; HDL-C = high-density lipoprotein cholesterol; NS = not significant; BP = blood pressure.
$P < .001$ estrogen vs. estrogen + progestin.

    Postprandially, glucose concentrations in the PEPI study tend to be slightly higher than control with ethinylestradiol and EE plus micronized progesterone (2.0 and 3.0 mg/dl, 0.11 and 0.17 mM, respectively). The highest postprandial concentrations are associated with EE plus MPA at 10 or 2.5 mg daily, 7.5 and 6.9 mg/dl, respectively (0.42 and 0.38 mM) ($P < .01$ in both instances). On the other hand, in the FINRISK study, postprandial glucose concentrations are not different among hormone users vs. nonusers, but of course this is a weaker, case-control design than the prospective PEPI study (50,51). Glucose intolerance induced by progestins appears to be generalizable because the greatest glucose elevation is seen with high-dose oral contraceptives with androgenic progestins (54), but is also seen with natural progesterone given alone (55).

B. Plasma Insulin Levels

As to whether postmenopausal hormone replacement enhances insulin sensitivity, the PEPI study (Table 4) shows that fasting immunoreactive insulin levels (IRI) are lowest among women using Premarin, Premarin plus micronized progesterone, and Premarin plus Provera 2.5 mg continuously (50). A slight insulin increase is observed in women using Premarin plus Provera 10 mg, and the highest increase was among placebo users. These data suggest that, at least in the overnight fasting condition, a slightly lower glucose concentration is maintained at a lower insulin concentration, but a higher progestin dose opposes the heightened insulin sensitivity attained with estrogen alone. Impaired glucose tolerance, insulin resistance, and elevated insulin levels have been seen most clearly among the old, high-dose, progestin-dominant oral contraceptives (54) but have also been seen with natural progesterone (55) and with testosterone given to women (56). Similar trends are seen in the 2-hour postprandial insulin levels of the PEPI study. In summary, a relatively nonandrogenic combined hormone regimen such as Premarin plus micronized progesterone appears to be the ideal replacement program from the standpoint of both lipoprotein and carbohydrate metabolism. The estrogen-induced improvement in insulin sensitivity should be an additional mechanism of reduced cardiovascular disease risk associated with estrogen.

The above improvements in carbohydrate metabolism with postmenopausal estrogen replacement therapy or nonandrogenic oral contraceptive therapy may benefit the obese older woman or the insulin-resistant hyperandrogenic premenopausal female with polycystic ovary syndrome (PCO) (see Talbott et al. [57] for review). Indeed, PCO is another example of how estrogen deficiency and androgen excess are associated with obesity, insulin resistance, and a coronary disease-prone lipid profile. Recently it has been found that PCO can be ameliorated with metformin therapy, which diminishes insulin resistance and plasma insulin levels (58).

C. Clotting Factors

With respect to clotting factors, both the ARIC (22) and FINRISK (51) studies have shown diminished concentrations of fibrinogen among postmenopausal hormone users, regardless of progestin use (Table 4). This result contrasts with oral contraceptive users where the estrogen doses are two or three times that of postmenopausal replacement and where the fibrinogen concentrations are elevated (48,59). On the other hand, other clotting factors, even in postmenopausal women appear to be increased, including Factor VII, as seen in the ARIC study (22) and confirmed in the FINRISK study, and plasminogen, seen in the FINRISK study (51). Antithrombin III was measured in the ARIC study and was found to be depressed, an unfavorable effect. Other factors measured, including Factor VIII, Von Willibrand factor, and protein C, were not significantly altered in the ARIC survey. In the prospective PEPI study (50), fibrinogen levels decreased 20 mg/dl (0.2 g/L) with Premarin alone, were intermediate with combined hormone therapy and increased 10 mg/dl (0.1 g/L) in the placebo group. These results indicate that progestins can oppose the effect of estrogen on the clotting system.

We have also seen this effect in oral contraceptive users using formulations containing androgenic vs. nonandrogenic progestins (unpublished data). Whether the changes in clotting factors described here are material to the cardiovascular risk factor status of pre- or postmenopausal women is unclear. In previous publications regarding oral contraceptive use, these changes have also been regarded as minor (48,59). However, as discussed below, coronary artery disease, although infrequent, can be increased among oral contraceptive users, especially those with risk factors. Whether inborn errors predisposing to venous thrombosis such as Factor V resistance to protein S have an effect on arterial thrombosis, remains to be determined (60).

D. Arterial Wall

Regarding the effect of estrogen on the physiology of the arterial wall, studies of Wagner and associates (61) have demonstrated that there is diminished penetration of LDL and/or less arterial wall retention, as suggested by Haarbo et al. (62). In addition, estrogen is a powerful antioxidant in the physiological range of estrogen concentrations in plasma (63–65). This antioxidant effect opposes oxidative stress on lipoproteins including LDL oxidation and in turn favors vasodilatation of coronary arteries in the presence of acetylcholine (66,67). Acetylcholine causes release of the endothelium-derived relaxation factor (EDRF), or nitric oxide, which is destroyed by pro-oxidant forces but preserved by estrogen (67), but endothelium-independent relaxation may also be mediated by estrogen (68).

A clinical application of the ability of estrogen to reverse inappropriate vasoconstriction in arteriosclerosis is the reversal of cardiologic Syndrome X—i.e., a coronary artery vasospasm and angina disorder without angiographically evident coronary artery disease (69,70). This benefit could be mediated through augmentation of nitric oxide release at the endothelial surface, since circulating nitric oxide levels in blood are increased with postmenopausal estrogen therapy (71). Interestingly, progestin appears to oppose EDRF-mediated vasodilatation (72). Whether other factors are involved, such as reduction in plasma endothelin levels, which are powerful vasoconstrictors, remains to be seen, but lower endothelin levels are seen in women than in men (73). In summary, if women present with angina pectoris, without obvious

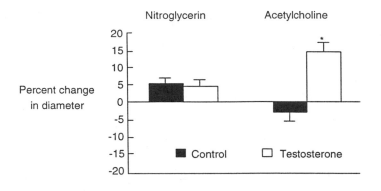

Figure 2 Arterial vasomotion in response to testosterone administration in female cholesterol-fed cynomolgus monkeys. Acetylcholine favors vasodilation in the presence of testosterone but not in its absence. $^*P$ = .05 from baseline. From Adams et al. (78), with permission.

or major arterial narrowing, estrogen could be tried as a therapeutic option. A recent report indicates this benefit can be attained with transdermal as well as oral estrogen replacement (74).

Contrary to the antioxidant and vasodilatory effect of estrogen, progesterone and testosterone have a modest pro-oxidant effect (64,75), and progesterone can cause vasoconstriction (72) in the systemic circulation albeit with vasodilatation in the uterine arterial bed (76). This progestin effect suggests a survival benefit for the developing fetus. While the mechanism of the vasoconstriction is yet unclear, we have found the pro-oxidant effect of testosterone and progesterone on LDL repeatedly in the absence as well as the presence of cultured cells including cultured macrophages (derived from placenta) and placental trophoblasts themselves (75). A pro-oxidant effect of certain synthetic progestins in the presence of copper ion, and LDL has also been seen (Zhu, unpublished data) although the in vivo significance of this observation is also unclear. In contrast to the vasoconstrictive effect of progesterone, testosterone is a vasodilator, another logical survival adaptation (Fig. 2) (77,78). This result indicates that the estrogen vs. progestin/androgen antagonism seen in so many systems may be modified, possibly by a receptor-specific mechanism.

Another way in which sex hormones affect arterial wall physiology is through the thromboxane/prostacyclin system, which can favor vasoconstriction and platelet aggregation if thromboxane formation is dominant, and vasodilatation and diminished platelet aggregation if prostacyclin is dominant (79). Consistent with its effects on nitric oxide metabolism and probably arterial wall redox state, estrogen favors prostacyclin dominance (80) while testosterone favors thromboxane formation (79,81), diminishes prostacyclin formation (82), and enhances platelet thromboxane receptor binding on platelets (83). Again, the estrogen-androgen antagonism is borne out in another physiological system.

Sex hormones also affect the arterial response to injury. Estrogen inhibits the inflammatory response to arterial wall balloon injury (84), though testosterone was without adverse effect in this system. Androgen and estrogen receptors are present on human macrophages (85), and estrogen inhibits the formation of the monocyte chemoattractant protein MCP-1 in cultured rodent fibroblasts (86). This inhibition is blocked by tamoxifen, pointing toward an estrogen receptor-mediated mechanism (86). Also noteworthy is the presence of estrogen receptors in most healthy arteries and their virtual absence in arteriosclerotic arteries (87). It appears that arterial damage destroys the ability of the artery to protect itself via an estrogen receptor-mediated mechanism, potentially aggravating the atherosclerotic cycle.

Finally, sex hormones affect cardiac function. The QT interval is longer in women than men. This effect may be related to downregulation of potassium channel protein expression, as recently demonstrated in the hearts of rabbits treated with estrogen (88).

VI. ORAL CONTRACEPTIVES AND CORONARY DISEASE

Regarding the question whether oral contraceptive hormone use is associated with myocardial infarction, the high-dose oral contraceptive formulations were associated with an approximately threefold increase in cardiovascular disease risk (89). This effect is synergistic with a number of cardiovascular disease risk factors, including hypertension, hypercholesterolemia, smoking, and diabetes leading to much higher degrees of risk (90,91). With the advent of the use of lower-estrogen-dose oral contraceptive formulations, the incidence of myocardial infarction in healthy young women without risk factors appears to be quite low and little or no different from nonusers (92–94). However, individuals who continue to smoke can have extraordinarily high multiples of cardiovascular risk, as much as 20-fold, as shown in studies by Rosenberg et al. and Croft and Hannaford (91,94). The mechanism whereby the CVD risk of cigarette smoking multiplies in the presence of oral contraceptive hormone therapy is unknown. The consensus is that the myocardial infarction-promoting effect of the oral contraceptive is associated with the thrombotic effect of the estrogen, since no carryover effect of coronary disease among oral contraceptive-using women is seen after women stop using the

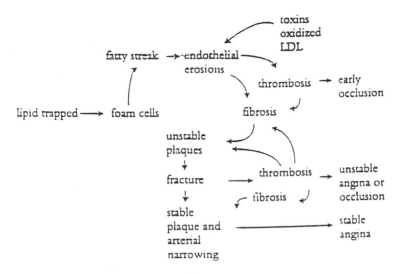

Figure 3 Vicious cycle of arterial injury and occlusion. In smoking oral contraceptive users, two mechanisms are possible. Early endothelial erosions can lead to thrombosis. Later, acute vasoconstriction could lead to plaque rupture and thrombosis. In each instance estrogen in supraphysiologic amounts can further promote thrombosis. From Ref. 123, with permission.

oral contraceptive pill (95). An earlier report of Slone et al. found a coronary disease association with oral contraceptive use and duration postdiscontinuation (96). However, this study was a case-control rather than a prospective cohort design study, and none of the prospective studies have confirmed this observation (95).

The nature of the interaction between smoking and oral contraceptive hormone use may have to do with the arterial injury associated with the oxidative stress of smoking and consequent susceptibility to thrombosis, which is enhanced by supraphysiological doses of estrogen. An additional mechanism is the vasoconstrictive effect of smoking, due in part to the oxidative destruction of nitric oxide, which progestin-dominant oral contraceptives might actually aggravate. Thrombosis might again ensue, particularly if plaque rupture occurs. This sequence of events is illustrated in Figure 3. What is clinically important is that the coronary disease risk associated with the use of hormones and cigarettes alike disappears upon discontinued use.

Regardless of mechanism, the important point for patient care is to discourage cigarette smoking among oral contraceptive-using females as strongly as possible. The easiest clinical algorithm to remember is that women over 35 who smoke should not use oral contraceptive steroids and vice versa. The

Table 5 Risk Factors for Myocardial Infarction in Women

---

* The "metabolic syndrome" (X)
  - insulin resistance
  - obesity
  - hypertension[*]
  - diabetes[*]
  - combined hyperlipidemia
  - low HDL-C (< 35 mg/dl)[*]
  - polycystic ovary syndrome (amenorrhea, hirsutism, infertility)
* Smoking[*]
* Inactivity
* Age
* Increased triglyceride, low HDL, high LDL
* Homocystine
* Family history of premature disease: age < 55 in men and < 65 in women (first degree relatives)

Source: Adapted from Ref. 97.
[*] Official National Cholesterol Education Program risk factor.

same may be said for women with other cardiovascular disease risk factors, including marked hypercholesterolemia, such as LDL cholesterol > 190 mg/dl (4.9 mM), a history of premature coronary artery disease, uncontrolled hypertension and age > 35. Pertinent risk factors are listed in Table 5. A decision-making approach to oral contraceptive prescription is given in Table 6 (97). Again, marked hypertriglyceridemia greater than approximately 300 mg/dl (3.38 mM) is also a contraindication to oral contraceptive use, but for a different reason, the prevention of acute pancreatitis.

In light of the above, oral contraceptive choices in the insulin-dependent diabetic are difficult. Most IDDM women are encouraged to complete their families early and then undergo permanent sterilization. In the meantime, plausible choices for oral contraception run the gamut from low-dose, third-generation oral contraceptive formulations, 20 µg ethinylestradiol oral contraceptive formulations, to very low dose progestin-only formulations that do not inhibit normal menstrual cyclicity or ovulation. The major objective would be to avoid hormonal augmentation of thrombotic or vasoconstrictor potential in such vascular disease-prone individuals. Again, prescription of oral contraceptives with an appreciation of cardiovascular disease risk factors among high-risk individuals such as older smokers appears to be extremely important.

Regarding the question whether lipoprotein abnormalities induced by oral contraceptives will in fact alter human risk for cardiovascular disease is

Table 6 Suggested Guidelines for OC Use on the Basis of LDL-C Level, Number of Heart Disease Risk Factors, and Age

	Risk factors			
	< 35 yr		≥ 35 yr	
LDL-C (mg/dl)	0–1	2 or more	0–1	2 or more
< 130	Yes	Yes	Yes[a]	Yes[a]
130–160	Yes	Yes with diet	Yes with diet[a]	No
160–190	Yes with diet	No	No	No
> 190	No	No	No	No

Source: With permission from Ref. 97.
[a] By established practice, smoking precludes OC use in women > 35 years in age.

difficult to say since most of the evidence is from animal models of atherosclerosis. The argument appeared to end when no carryover effect of oral contraceptive use on cardiovascular disease was seen after discontinuation (95) and when Adams and associates found that an ethinylestradiol/levonorgestrel combination given to female macaques inhibited arteriosclerosis induced by an atherogenic diet (98). On the other hand, levonorgestrel given alone in these experiments was associated with an acceleration of arteriosclerotic disease—that is, a loss of the female protective effect (98). More recently, the same workers have found that testosterone can accelerate the progression of anatomically demonstrable atherosclerosis associated with cholesterol feeding (78). Finally, the same group (99) has found that medroxyprogesterone acetate is associated with a loss of the protective effect of replacement doses of estrogen in female macaques. Thus, the possibility remains open that oral contraceptive steroids have unfavorable effects on lipoprotein levels and may in fact promote susceptibility to coronary artery disease, particularly in high-risk individuals. The inhibitory effect of an oral contraceptive on arteriosclerosis in the presence of an androgenic progestin in the early macaque studies appears to be due to the content in the contraceptive of a high dose of estrogen (98).

The animal studies suggest that sex hormone influences on coronary artery disease susceptibility could be unfavorable or favorable, depending on the nature of the lipoprotein change induced and effects on other physiological parameters as well. For instance, if LDL cholesterol levels remain normal but HDL cholesterol concentrations increase, as observed with the third-generation oral contraceptives, one might predict a diminished arteriosclerotic disease susceptibility. In fact, European studies investigating the effects of the third-generation oral contraceptives on venous thrombosis (reportedly slightly increased) (100–102), also find trends toward reductions in the occurrence of arteriosclerotic vascular disease. While not definitive, these data provide preliminary support for the use of nonandrogenic progestins with oral contraceptives for the purpose of minimizing CVD risk. If the dose of estrogen is low enough, the time may come when such formulations will be used in arteriosclerosis-prone individuals. In fact, an investigation of the effect of a third-generation oral contraceptive on the LDL-C/HDL-C ratio in women with elevated LDL-C levels is currently under way. As to the reported effect of third-generation oral contraceptives to increase venous thrombosis, the effect appears to be due to the prothrombotic effect of estrogen, now less opposed in the presence of less androgenic progestin. This observation invites development of oral contraceptive formulations with lower doses of estrogen in conjunction with a nonandrogenic progestin.

VII. POSTMENOPAUSAL HORMONE USE AND CORONARY DISEASE

Postmenopausal hormone replacement therapy induces favorable lipoprotein changes (described above) which can be used to predict the extent to which coronary disease can be prevented. When the changes in LDL and HDL observed in postmenopausal, hormone-treated subjects are projected onto Framingham risk projections, a 50% reduction in CAD is predicted, with approximately 13% from the LDL-C decrease and 36% from the HDL-C increase. Using correlative change measurements, Bush et al. estimated about a 50% benefit from the lipoprotein change, later revised even lower. As discussed above, clearly there are other mechanisms of cardiovascular benefit besides lipoproteins, and the relative contributions of each remain speculative (Table 7).

Table 7 Benefits of Estrogen to the Arterial Wall

- Beneficial lipoprotein effects
- Diminished insulin and glucose levels
- Diminished fibrinogen (postmenopausal)
- Diminished arterial wall penetration/retention
- Diminished LDL oxidation
- Favorable effect on arterial wall nitric oxide
- Improved vasomotion
- Diminished response to injury

Table 8 Relative Risk of Postmenopausal Hormone
Use for Coronary Artery Disease

	Major CAD	Fatal CVD	Stroke
No use	1.0	1.0	1.0
Current use	0.56	0.61[a]	0.97
Former use	0.83	0.79	0.99

Source: From Ref. 104.
[a] Confidence interval at 1.0 (0.37–1.00).

Regarding clinical observations, as many as 30 case-controlled and prospective cohort studies have been performed over the past 20 years (1–4,103–105). An example of one of the most recent is presented in Table 8 (104). These indicate that the incidence of coronary artery disease among women on ERT is approximately half that among nonusers. It is uncertain if this effect can be entirely ascribed to the beneficial effects of estrogen or whether there is a healthy user effect in all of these analyses. Barrett-Connor and associates (106) have estimated that half of the reduction in coronary artery disease among estrogen users might be ascribed to this selection bias. For this reason, two large prospective randomized trials are under way to directly determine whether estrogen therapy in postmenopausal women will benefit women from the standpoint of preventing coronary artery disease and whether there are other unwanted side effects in the course of this treatment.

The first of the randomized trials is the Heart Estrogen-Progestin Replacement Study (HERS), in which women taking 0.625 mg Premarin and 2.5 mg medroxyprogesterone acetate continuously are compared to placebo, with all of the women having had a previous occurrence of coronary artery disease characterized by myocardial infarction, angina pectoris, revascularization surgery, angioplasty, or coronary artery narrowing > 50% by angiography. The results of this study are expected in 1999. Approximately 2500 women with coronary disease have been randomized to the two arms of this study. Unfortunately, this trial will not answer the question of whether estrogen alone is beneficial, but it will give the earliest information about heart disease prevention by a postmenopausal hormone regimen.

A much longer-term prospective randomized trial of estrogen and estrogen plus progestin hormone replacement therapy is being conducted by the Women's Health Initiative (WHI) in at least 40 centers nationwide. A much larger study involving many more subjects is required because of the much lower incidence of coronary disease in a primary prevention setting such as the WHI. Thus a study duration of at least 10 years is required for this investigation. This study will be more informative on possible unwanted effects of complications such as breast cancer (107,108). On the question of cancer in postmenopausal hormone replacement therapy, it is interesting that in a recent prospective cohort study, Ettinger and associates (105) found a trend toward reduction in lung cancer among postmenopausal estrogen users in a study from Kaiser-Permanente in California, suggesting possible offsetting causes of cancer mortality. Nonetheless, unrecognized selection biases could be operating, as in all such epidemiological surveys.

In the meantime, what do we tell patients? It does not seem possible to dogmatically recommend estrogen replacement therapy, given the lack of prospective randomized trials. On the other hand, many reasons can be given for offering or suggesting estrogen replacement hormone therapy, including sense of well-being, prevention of osteoporosis, preservation of skin turgor, prevention of senility and even Alzheimer's disease (108), preservation of vaginal mucosa, metabolic benefits (see below), and even higher intellectual functions. Most women come to this decision aware of at least some of these benefits as well as some of the side effects and often have their own viewpoints well established. If a woman wants hormone replacement therapy, there are certainly enough indications (108). The place of the practitioner seems primarily to instruct patients in the available evidence and on the potential for cardiovascular disease reduction, including beneficial effects on metabolism in human studies and consistent arteriosclerosis prevention in animal models (see example in Table 9) (98,109,110). Unfortunately, a conclusive case cannot be made in humans in the absence of double-blind, randomized trials.

Regarding the question of whether combined estrogen/progestin replacement therapy reduces cardiovascular disease risk, a recent publication from the Nurses' Health Study indicates preservation of benefit in a prospective cohort with a risk ratio of 0.39 compared to nonusers (111). Estrogen-only users had a risk ratio of 0.60. Psaty et al. have found equivalent reductions in CVD among estrogen and estrogen plus progestin users—0.69% and 0.68%, respectively (112). The fact that a contrary result has been seen in cholesterol-fed equine estrogen, medroxyprogesterone acetate-treated macaques (99) underscores the necessity for prospective, randomized clinical trials in humans.

As to the epidemiological surveys of the capacity of estrogen to prevent recurrent heart attack, a recent study by Newton supports this possibility (113). In her study, subjects using estrogen had less recurrent coronary disease (risk ratio 0.64, confidence interval 0.25 to 1.0) than in non-hormone users. It seems likely that the greater risk of antecedent coronary disease, the greater the benefit based on up to 10 years of follow-up from Sullivan and associates (114). In this study, the greater antecedent coronary disease by angiography (none, < 70% narrowing, > 70% narrowing), the less the survival rate at 10

Table 9 Efect of Estrogen and Progesterone Replacement in Cholesterol-Fed Oviarectomized Monkeys

	Control	E_2/Pg^a	E_2
mg/dl			
Total cholesterol	463	433	448
HDL-C	34.9	35.2	35.9
Arteriosclerosis (mm^2)			
Coronary artery plaque area	0.227	0.101[b]	0.099[b]
Thoracic aortic area	1.32	0.89	1.04
Abdominal aortic area	0.82	0.53	0.62
Carotid	1.45	1.11	1.07
Femoral	0.24	0.15[b]	0.11[b]

Source: Adams et al. (109).
[a] E_2 and Pg given as silastic implants.
[b] Significantly different from control

years (91%, 85%, and 60%, respectively). In contrast, benefit was seen in all estrogen user groups with 98%, 96%, and 97% survival, respectively, after 10 years! Again, this study is not a randomized trial; nonetheless, it suggests a greater proportional benefit in higher-risk situations.

VIII. EFFECTS OF ANDROGENS ON ARTERIOSCLEROSIS

With respect to the effect of androgens on arteriosclerotic vascular disease, testosterone has an atherogenic effect in the cholesterol-fed monkey (78) (Fig. 4). Likewise, the androgenic progestin, levonorgestrel, is atherogenic in the monkey model (98). Both hormone effects are largely independent of lipoprotein changes in cholesterol-fed macaques (78,98). The cellular and molecular mechanism of this atherogenic effect is unknown, but both testosterone and progesterone are weak pro-oxidants, possibly favoring oxidation of LDL, as mentioned above (64,75).

Human studies of androgen and cardiovascular disease are somewhat conflicting. In one study, testosterone levels were inversely associated with plasma insulin and glucose and PAI-I levels (115); that is, low testosterone levels were associated with increased cardiovascular disease risk factors. Even more paradoxical is the observation that estradiol levels tend to be higher in men with coronary artery disease (116). A possible mechanism for this effect

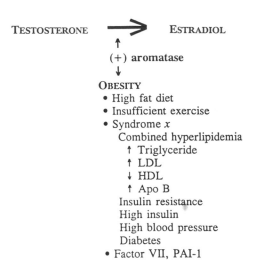

TESTOSTERONE ⟶ ESTRADIOL
                    ↑
              (+) aromatase
                    ↓
              OBESITY
              • High fat diet
              • Insufficient exercise
              • Syndrome *x*
                  Combined hyperlipidemia
                      ↑ Triglyceride
                      ↑ LDL
                      ↓ HDL
                      ↑ Apo B
                  Insulin resistance
                  High insulin
                  High blood pressure
                  Diabetes
              • Factor VII, PAI-1

Figure 4   Diet-induced atherosclerotic plaque in coronary arteries of female cynomolgus monkeys treated with androstenedione or testosterone. From Adams et al. (78), with permission.

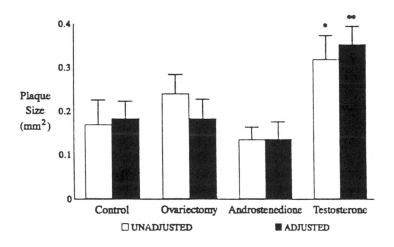

Figure 5   Hypothetical explanation of the relationship of low testosterone and high estradiol levels with coronary artery disease and its risk factors in men, mediated by an increased conversion of testosterone to estradiol by steroid hormone aromatase activity in adipose tissue. From Ref. (117) with permission.

is the effect of abdominal obesity, which favors the formation of estradiol from testosterone and could diminish the concentration of testosterone (Fig. 5) (117). Thus, abdominal obesity could be the underlying risk factor for coronary disease, and low testosterone and high estrogen a consequence thereof (Fig. 5). Whether this scenario actually exists remains to be established, since no one to our knowledge has examined these relationships simultaneously quantifying abdominal obesity. Another point to keep in mind is that even in normal men, testosterone administration has little effect on HDL unless conversion to estrogen is blocked and the endogenous testosterone secretion is suppressed (see Knopp et al. [117] for review).

Other interesting effects of testosterone have been described, including a tendency to promote platelet aggregation (81,82) but favor vasodilation in vitro (83) as well as in vivo (78). This effect may confer a male survival benefit during physical stress. Thus, some but not all mechanisms of testosterone action on the arterial wall physiology may favor arteriosclerosis.

As to applications to human atherosclerosis, more than 20 case reports of coronary artery disease have been reported among androgen-taking athletes (118). This clinical experience, as well as atherogenic effects of androgens in animal models, continues to argue against the use of excessive or pharmacologic amounts of androgen in young athletes.

The adrenal and ovarian androgen precursor dehydroepiandrosterone (DHEA) has a divergent association with arteriosclerotic disease, depending on gender. In males, it has been shown that DHEA levels decline with age and are lower in male subjects prone to have coronary artery disease (119). On the other hand, in female subjects, higher DHEA levels are associated with overproduction of testosterone by the ovary in association with obesity, insulin resistance, and the polycystic ovary syndrome (57,58,120) and are not associated with diminished CVD risk in women (121). At the very best, in female subjects DHEA seems to be a marker of the obesity/insulin resistance syndrome, which is associated with ovarian dysfunction (57,58,120). In contrast, in male subjects DHEA may actually be beneficial. When given to animal models fed cholesterol to cause atherosclerosis, DHEA prevents arteriosclerotic progression (122). DHEA synthesis, at least in women, is favored by insulin availability or action (117). Most recently in females, it has been reported that diminished plasma insulin concentrations and diminished insulin resistance in metformin-treated women with the polycystic ovarian syndrome results in a reductions in 17α OH progesterone and testosterone but no decrease in DHEA plasma levels (58). The reduction in androgens might further diminish insulin resistance.

The clinical implication of these developing observations suggests that DHEA may protect against arteriosclerosis, at least in men. However, this hypothesis requires much more research and does not justify the almost black-market commerce in DHEA use. On the other hand, any hygienic step such as weight loss and exercise that can lower insulin levels, at least in females, and reduce arteriosclerotic disease risk in association with reductions in circulating androgen, appears to be beneficial. As to whether a reduction in circulating androgen can reduce atherosclerosis in women, no one knows, but certainly reducing plasma insulin concentration and insulin resistance in any setting, male or female, seems reasonable.

IX.   SUMMARY AND CONCLUSIONS

In general, estrogen is associated with favorable effect on lipoprotein metabolism, arterial wall penetration of LDL, insulin sensitivity, plasma glucose concentrations, and some clotting factors at replacement hormone levels. The best available information from cross-sectional and cohort epidemiologic surveys indicates that estrogen can reduce coronary artery disease about 50%, but a healthy-user selection bias has not been ruled out. Progestins and androgens, varying in degree of androgenicity, oppose the estrogenic effects on lipoprotein levels, glucose and insulin metabolism, and clotting factors, and some cases, in their own right, accelerate atherogenesis in animal models. Whether these effects are the result of changes in lipoprotein metabolism, glucose and insulin levels, diminished clotting tendency, diminished lipoprotein penetration of the arterial wall or vascular wall motion, or a less damaging response to injury remains to be seen (Table 7).

What is well known is that high-dose oral contraceptive hormone given to women with CVD risk factors, in particular smoking, can aggravate arteriosclerotic vascular disease as much as 20-fold. Postmenopausally, combined estrogen-progestin use generally has little deleterious effect compared to estrogen alone, based on epidemiologic surveys. Caution is still justified based on the report of an adverse effect of medroxyprogesterone acetate on the estrogen prevention of atherosclerosis in the experimental monkey. Estrogen seems appropriate to use in women with cardiovascular Syndrome X—i.e., coronary spasm without visible atherosclerosis by angiography. Caution is advised to clinicians in giving estrogen in any condition where individuals have an underlying hypertriglyceridemia. Should hypertriglyceridemia result from estrogen administration, or if the subjects at baseline have plasma triglyceride levels > 300 mg/dl (3.38 mM), patch estrogen regimens should be used as a substitute. The future appears bright for the use of sex hormones for disease prevention and therapy using the knowledge reviewed here as a base.

REFERENCES

1. Knopp RH, Zhu X-D, Lau J, Walden C. Sex hormones and lipid interactions: implications for cardiovascular disease in women. Endocrinologist 1994; 4:286–301.
2. Knopp RH, Zhu X, Bonet B. Effects of estrogens on lipoprotein metabolism and cardiovascular disease in women. Atherosclerosis 1994; 110:S83–S91.
3. Sacks FM, Gerhard M, Walsh BW. Sex hormones, lipoproteins, and vascular reactivity. Curr Opin Lipidol 1995; 6:161–166.
4. Knopp RH. The effects of oral contraceptives and postmenopausal estrogens on lipoprotein physiology and atherosclerosis. In: Halbe HW, Rekers H, eds. Oral Contraception Into the 1990's. Carnforth, UK: Parthenon Publishing, 1989:31–45.
5. Schaefer EJ, Foster DM, Zech LA, Lindgren FT, Brewer HB Jr, Levy RI. The effects of estrogen administration on plasma lipoprotein metabolism in premenopausal females. J Clin Endocrinol Metab 1983; 57:262–267.
6. Walsh BW, Schiff I, Rosner B, Greenberg L, Ravnikar V, Sack FM. Effects of postmenopausal estrogen replacement on the concentrations and metabolism of plasma lipoproteins. N Engl J Med 1991; 325:1196–1204.
7. Humphrey JL, Childs MT, Montes A, Knopp RH. Lipid metabolism in pregnancy. VII. Kinetics of chylomicron triglyceride removal in fed pregnant rat. Am J Physiol 1980; 239 (Endocrinol Metab 2):E81–E87.
8. Applebaum DM, Goldberg AP, Pykalisto OJ, Brunzell JD, Hazzard WR. Effect of estrogen on post-heparin lipolytic activity: selective decline in hepatic triglyceride lipase. J Clin Invest 1977; 590:601–608.
9. Applebaum-Bowden D, McLean P, Steinmetz A, et al. Lipoprotein, apolipoprotein, and lipolytic enzyme changes following estrogen administration in postmenopausal women. J Lipid Res 1989; 30:1895–1906.
10. Iverius PH, Brunzell JD. Relationship between lipoprotein lipase activity and plasma sex steroid level in obese women. J Clin Invest 1988; 82:1106–1112.
11. Walsh BW, Sacks FM. Effects of low oral dose contraceptives on very low density and low density lipoprotein metabolism. J Clin Invest 1993; 91:2126–2132.
12. Hazzard WR. Primary Type III in hyperlipoproteinemia. In: Rifkind BM, Levy RI, eds. Hyperlipidemia: Diagnosis and Therapy. New York: Grune & Stratton, Inc, 1977:137–175.
13. Ma PTS, Yamamoto T, Goldstein JL. Increased binding of low density lipoprotein receptor in livers of rabbits treated with 17 alpha-ethinyl estradiol. Proc Natl Acad Sci USA 1986; 83:792–796.
14. Chait A, Brunzell JD, Albers JJ, Hazzard WR. Type III hyperlipoproteinemia ("remnant removal disease"): insight into the pathogenic mechanism. Lancet 1977; 1:1176–1178.
15. Gustafson A, Svanborg A. Gonadal steroid effects on plasma lipoproteins and individual phospholipids. J Clin Endocrinol Metab 1972; 35:203.
16. Knopp RH, Bergelin RO, Wahl PW, Walden CE. Effects of pregnancy, postpartum lactation and oral contraceptive use on the lipoprotein cholesterol/triglyceride ratio. Metabolism 1985; 34:893–899.

17. Berr F, Eckel RH, Kern F Jr. Contraceptive steroids increase hepatic uptake of chylomicron remnants in young women. J Lipid Res 1986; 27:645–51.

18. Colvin PL Jr. Estrogen increases low-density lipoprotein receptor-independent catabolism of apolipoprotein B in hyperlipidemic rabbits. Metabolism 1996; 45: 889–896.

19. Callow MJ, Stoltzfus LJ, Lawn RM, Rubin EM. Expression of human apolipoprotein B and assembly of lipoprotein(a) in transgenic mice. Proc Natl Acad Sci USA 1994; 91:2130–2134.

20. Bostom AG, Cupples A, Jenner JL, et al. Elevated plasma lipoprotein(a) and coronary heart disease in men aged 55 years and younger. JAMA 1996; 276:544–548.

21. Henriksson P, Angelin B, Berglund L. Hormonal regulation of serum Lp(a) levels: opposite effects after estrogen treatment and orchidectomy in male prostatic carcinoma. J Clin Invest 1992; 89:1166–1171.

22. Nabulsi AA, Folsom AR, White A, et al. Association of hormone-replacement therapy with cardiovascular risk factors in postmenopausal women. N Engl J Med 1993; 328:1069–1075.

23. Sacks FM, McPherson R, Walsh BW. Effect of postmenopausal estrogen replacement on plasma Lp(a) lipoprotein concentrations. Arch Intern Med 1994; 154: 1106–1110.

24. Shewmon DA, Stock JL, Abusamra LC, Kristan MA, Baker S, Heiniluoma KM. Tamoxifen decreases lipoprotein (a) in patients with breast cancer. Metabolism 1994; 43:531–532.

25. Kushwaha RS, Foster DM, Murthy VN, Carey KD, Bernard MG. Metabolic regulation of apoproteins in high-density lipoproteins by estrogen and progesterone in the baboon. Metabolism 1990; 39:544–552.

26. Tam SP, Archer T, Deeley RG. Effects of estrogen on apolipoprotein secretion by the human hepatocarcinoma cell line HepG2. J Biol Chem 1985; 260:1670–1675.

27. Walsh BW, Li H, Sacks FM. Effects of postmenopausal hormone replacement with oral and transdermal estrogen on HDL metabolism. J Lipid Res 1994; 35:2083–2093.

28. Warden CH, Hedrick CC, Qiao J-H, Castellani LW, Lusis AJ. Atherosclerosis in transgenic mice overexpressing apolipoprotein A-II. Science 1993; 261:469–472.

29. Cheung MC, Albers JJ. Characterization of lipoprotein particles isolated by immunoaffinity chromatography: particles containing A-I and A-II and particles containing A-I but no A-II. J Biol Chem 1984; 259(19):12201–12209.

30. Duverger N, Rader D, Brewer HB Jr. Distribution of subclasses of HDL containing apo A-I without apo A-II (LpA-I) in normolipidemic men and women. Arterioscler Thromb 1994; 14:1594–1599.

31. Pieters MN, Schouten D, Van Berkel TJC. In vitro and in vivo evidence for role of HDL in reverse cholesterol transport. Biochim Biophys Acta 1994; 1225:125–134.

32. Francis GA, Knopp RH, Oram JF. Defective removal of cellular cholesterol and phospholipids by apolipoprotein A-I in Tangier disease. J Clin Invest 1995; 96(1):78–87.

33. Brinton A. Oral estrogen replacement therapy in postmenopausal women selectively raises levels and production rates of lipoprotein A-I and lowers hepatic lipase activity without lowering fractional catabolic rate. Arterioscler Thromb Vasc Biol 1996; 16:431–440.

34. Silliman K, Tall AR, Kretchmer N, Forte TM. Unusual high-density lipoprotein subclass distribution during late pregnancy. Metabolism 1993; 42(12):1592–1599.

35. Knopp RH, Magee MS. Pregnancy and Partuition. In: Patten HD, Fuchs A, Hille B, Scher A, Steiner R, eds. Textbook of Physiology. 21st ed. Vol. 2. Philadelphia: W.B. Saunders; 1989:1380–1407.

36. Olsson AG, Orö L, Rossner S. Effects of oxondrolone on plasma lipoproteins and the intravenous fat tolerance in man. Atherosclerosis 1974; 19:337–346.

37. Wolfe BM, Huff MW. Effects of low dose progestin-only administration upon plasma triglyceride and lipoprotein metabolism in postmenopausal women. J Clin Invest 1993; 92:456–461.

38. Khokha R, Huff MW, Wolfe BM. Divergent effects of d-norgestrel on the metabolism of rat very low density and low density apolipoprotein B. J Lipid Res 1986; 27:699–705.

39. Tikkanen MJ, Nikkilä EA, Kuusi T, Sipenen S. High-density lipoprotein-2 and hepatic lipase: reciprocal changes produced by estrogen and norgestrel. J Clin Endocrinol Metab 1982; 54:1113–1117.

40. Albers JJ, Taggart HM, Applebaum-Boeden D, Haffner S, Chestnutt CH III, Hazzard WR. Reduction of lecithin-cholesterol acyltransferase, apolipoprotein D and the Lp(a) lipoprotein with the anabolic steroid stanozolol. Biochim Biophys Acta 1984; 795:293–296.

41. Zmuda JM, Thompson PD, Dickenson R, Bausserman LL. Testosterone decreases lipoprotein(a) in men. Am J Cardiol 1996; 77:1244–1247.

42. Wahl PW, Walden CE, Knopp RH, Wallace R, Rifkind B. The effect of estrogen/progestin potency on lipid/lipoprotein cholesterol. N Engl J Med 1983; 308:862–867.

43. Burkman RT, Robinson JC, Kruszon-Moran D, Kimball AW, Kwiterovich P, Burford RG. Lipid and lipoprotein changes associated with oral contraceptive use: a randomized clinical trial. Obstet Gynecol 1988; 71:33–38.

44. Krauss RM, Roy S, Mishell DR Jr, Casagrande J, Pike MC. Effects of two low-dose oral contraceptives on serum lipids and lipoproteins: differential changes in high-density lipoprotein subclasses. Am J Obstet Gynecol 1983; 145:446–452.

45. Magee MS, Knopp RH, Pierce C, Kranz J, Fish B, Walden CE. Effects of low-dose multiphasic oral contraceptives over one year on total and LDL-C in comparison to preceding and succeeding normal menstrual cycles. Program of the 71st Annual Meeting of the Endocrine Society, Seattle, WA, June 21–24 1989, Abstract #1637.

46. Notelovitz M, Feldman EB, Gillespy M, Gudat J. Lipid and lipoprotein changes in women taking low-dose triphasic oral contraceptives: a controlled, comparative, 12–month clinical trial. Am J Obstet Gynecol 1989; 160:1269–1280.

47. Patsch W, Brown SA, Gotto AM, Young RL. The effect of triphasal oral contraceptives on plasma lipids and lipoproteins. Am J Obstet Gynecol 1989; 161:1396–1401.

48. Speroff L, DeCherney A, Advisory Board for the New Progestins. Evaluation of a new generation of oral contraceptives. Obstet Gynecol 1993; 81:1034–1047.

49. Matthews KA, Mailahn E, Kuller LH, Kelsey SF, Caggiula AW, Wing RR. Menopause and risk factors for coronary heart disease. N Engl J Med 1989; 321:641–646.

50. The Writing Group for the PEPI Trial. Effects of estrogen or estrogen/progestin regimens on heart disease risk factors in postmenopausal women: the Postmenopausal Estrogen/Progestin Intervention Trial. JAMA 1995; 273:199–208.

51. Salomaa C, Rasi V, Pekkanen J, et al. Association of hormone replacement therapy with hemostatic and other cardiovascular risk factors: the FINRISK hemostasis study. Arterioscler Thromb Vasc Biol 1995; 15:1549–1555.

52. Barrett-Connor E, Laakso M. Ischemic heart disease risk in postmenopausal women: effects of estrogen use on glucose and insulin levels. Arteriosclerosis 1990; 10:531–534.

53. Knopp RH, Bergelin RO, Wahl PW, Walden CE, Chapman MB. Clinical chemistry alterations in pregnancy and oral contraceptive use. Obstet Gynecol 1985; 66:682–690.

54. Spellacy WN. Carbohydrate metabolism during treatment with estrogen, progestogen, and low-dose oral contraceptives. Am J Obstet Gynecol 1982; 142:732–734.

55. Kalkhoff RK. Metabolic effects of progesterone. Am J Obstet Gynecol 1982; 142:735–738.

56. Polderman KH, Gooren LJG, Asscheman H, Bakker A, Heine RJ. Induction of insulin resistance by androgens and estrogens. J Clin Endocrinol Metab 1994; 79:265–271.

57. Talbott E, Guzick D, Clerici A, et al. Coronary heart disease risk factors in women with polycystic ovary syndrome. Arterioscler Thromb Vasc Biol 1995; 15:821–826.

58. Nestler JE, Jakubowicz DJ. Decreases in ovarian cytochrome P450c17a activity and serum free testosterone after reduction of insulin secretion in polycystic ovary syndrome. N Engl J Med 1996; 335:617–623.

59. Comp PC, Zacur HA. Contraceptive choices in women with coagulation disorder. Am J Obstet Gynecol 1993; 168:1990–1993.

60. Bloemenkamp KWM, Rosendaal FR, Helmerhorst FM, Büller HR, Vanderbroucke JP. Enhancement by factor V Leiden mutation of risk of deep-vein thrombosis associated with oral contraceptives containing a third-generation progestogen. Lancet 1995; 346:1593–1596.

61. Wagner JD, Clarkson TB, St Clair RW, Schwenke DC, Shively CA, Adams MR. Estrogen and progesterone therapy reduces low density lipoprotein accumulation

in the coronary arteries of surgically postmenopausal monkeys. J Clin Invest 1991; 88:1995–2002.

62. Haarbo J, Nielson LB, Stander S, Christiansen C. Aortic permeability to LDL during estrogen therapy: a study in normocholesterolemic subjects. Arterioscler Thromb 1994; 14:243–247.

63. Mazière C, Auclair M, Ronveaux MF, Salmon S, Santus R, Maziere JC. Estrogens inhibit copper and cell-mediated modification of low density lipoprotein. Atherosclerosis 1991; 89:175–182.

64. Zhu X, Meekins D, Bonet N, et al. Effects of sex hormones on susceptibility of low density lipoprotein to copper mediated oxidative modification. Clin Res 1993; 41:26A. Submitted.

65. Sack MN, Rader DJ, Cannon RO, III. Oestrogen and inhibition of oxidation of low density lipoproteins in postmenopausal women. Lancet 1994; 343:269–270.

66. Williams JK, Adams MR, Klopfenstein HS. Estrogen modulates responses of atherosclerotic coronary arteries. Circulation 1990; 81:1680–1687.

67. Herrington DM, Braden GA, Williams JK, Morgan TM. Endothelial-dependent coronary vasomotor responsiveness in postmenopausal women with and without estrogen replacement therapy. Am J Cardiol 1994; 73:951–952.

68. Mügge A, Riedel M, Barton M, Kuhn M, Lichtlen PR. Endothelium independent relaxation of human coronary arteries by 17β-oestradiol ion vitro. Cardiovasc Res 1993; 27:1939–1942.

69. Gerhard M, Ganz P. How do we explain clinical benefits of estrogen? From bedside to bench. Circulation 1995; 92:5–8.

70. Guetta V, Cannon RO III. Cardiovascular effects of estrogen and lipid-lowering therapies in postmenopausal women. Circulation 1996; 93:1928–1937.

71. Rosselli M, Imthern B, Keller PJ, Jackson EK, Dubey RK. Circulating nitric oxide (nitrite/nitrate) levels in postmenopausal women substituted with 17β-estradiol and norethisterone acetate: a two-year follow-up study. Hypertension 1995; 25(part 2):848–853.

72. Miller VM, VanHoutte PM. Progesterone and modulation of endothelin dependent responses in canine coronary arteries. Am J Physiol 1991; 261:R1022–R1027.

73. Polderman KH, Stehouwer CDA, van Kamp GJ, Dekker GA, Verheugt FWA, Gooren LJG. Influence of sex hormones on plasma endothelin cells. Ann Intern Med 1993; 118:429–432.

74. Albertsson PA, Emanuelsson H, Milsom I. Beneficial effect of treatment with transdermal estradiol-17-β on exercise-induced angina and ST depression in Syndrome X. Int J Cardiol 1996; 54:13–20.

75. Zhu X-D, Bonet B, Knopp RH. 17β-estradiol, progesterone and testosterone inversely modulate low-density lipoprotein oxidation and cytotoxicity in cultured placental trophoblast and macrophages. Am J Obstet Gynecol 1997; 177:196–209.

76. Omar HA, Ramirez R, Gibson M. Properties of a progesterone-induced relaxation in human placental arteries and veins. J Clin Endocrinol Metab 1995; 80:370–373.

77. Yue P, Chatterjee K, Beale C, Poole-Williams PA, Collins P. Testosterone relaxes rabbit coronary arteries and aorta. Circulation 1995; 91:1154–1160.
78. Adams MR, Williams JK, Kaplan JR. Effect of androgens on coronary artery atherosclerosis and atherosclerosis-related impairment of vascular responsiveness. Arterioscler Thromb Vasc Biol 1995; 15:562–570.
79. Practico D, FitzGerald GA. Testosterone and thromboxane: of muscles mice and men. Circulation 1995; 91:2694–2698.
80. Bar J, Tepper R, Fuchs J, Pardo Y, Goldberger S, Odavia J. The effect of estrogen replacement therapy on platelet aggregation and adenosine triphosphate release in postmenopausal women. Obstet Gynecol 1993; 81:261–264.
81. Weyrich AS, Rejeski WJ, Brubaker PH, Parks JS. The effects of testosterone on lipids and eicosanoids in cynomolgus monkeys. Med Sci Sports Exerc 1992; 24:333–338.
82. Nakao J, Change WC, Murota SI, Orimo H. Testosterone inhibits prostacyclin production by rat aortic smooth muscle cells in culture. Atherosclerosis 1981; 39:203–209.
83. Ajayi AAL, Mathur R, Halushka PV. Testosterone increases human platelet thromboxane A_2 receptor density and aggregation responses. Circulation 1995; 91: 2742–2747.
84. Chen S-J, Li H, Durand J, Oparil S, Chen Y-F. Estrogen reduces myointimal proliferation after balloon injury of rat carotid artery. Circulation 1996; 93:577–584.
85. Cutolo M, Accardo S, Villaggio B, et al. Androgen and estrogen receptors are present in primary cultures of human synovial macrophages. J Clin Endocrinol Metab 1996; 81:820–827.
86. Kovacs EJ, Faunce DE, Ramer-Quinn DS, Mott FJ, Dy P-WW, Frazer-Jessen MR. Estrogen regulation of JE/MCP-1 mRNA expression in fibroblasts. J Leuk Biol 1996; 59:562–568.
87. Losordo DW, Kearney M, Kim EA, Jekanowski J, Isner JM. Variable expression of the estrogen receptor in normal and atherosclerotic coronary arteries of premenopausal women. Circulation 1994; 89:1501–1510.
88. Drici MD, Burklow TR, Haridasse V, Glazer RI, Woosley RL. Sex hormones prolong the QT interval and downregulate potassium channel expression in the rabbit heart. Circulation 1996; 94:1471–1474.
89. Mann JI, Vessey MP, Thorogood M, Doll R. Myocardial infarction in young women with special reference to oral contraceptive practice. BMJ 1975; 2:241–245.
90. Mann JI, Inman WHW. Oral contraceptives and death from myocardial infarction. BMJ 1975; 2:245–248.
91. Croft P, Hannaford PC. Risk factors for acute myocardial infarction in women: evidence from the Royal College of General Practitioner's oral contraception study. BMJ 1989; 298:165–168.
92. Porter JB, Hunter JR, Jick H, Stergachis A. Oral contraceptives and non-fatal vascular disease: recent experience. Obstet Gynecol 1985; 66:1–4

93. Porter JB, Hershel J, Walker AM. Mortality among oral contraceptive users. Obstet Gynecol 1987; 70:29–32.0

94. Rosenberg L, Kaufman DW, Helmrich SP, Miller DR, Stolley POD, Shapiro S. Myocardial infarction and cigarette smoking in women younger than 50 years of age. JAMA 1985; 253:2965.

95. Stampfer MJ, Willett WC, Colditz GA, Speizer FE, Hennekens CH. A prospective study of past use of oral contraceptive agents and risk of cardiovascular diseases. N Engl J Med 1988; 319:1313–1317.

96. Slone D, Shapiro S, Kaufman DW, Rosenberg L, Miettinen OS, Stolley PD. Risk of myocardial infarction in relation to current and discontinued use of oral contraceptives. N Engl J Med 1981; 305:420–424.

97. Knopp RH, LaRosa J, Burkman R. Contraception and Dyslipidemia. Am J Obstet Gynecol 1993; 168:1994–2004.

98. Adams MR, Clarkson TB, Koritnik DR, Nash HA. Contraceptive steroids and coronary artery atherosclerosis in cynomolgus macaques. Fertil Steril 1987; 47: 101–108

99. Adams MR, Register TC, Golden DL, Wagner JD, Williams JK. Medroxyprogesterone acetate antagonizes inhibitory effects of conjugated equine estrogens on coronary artery atherosclerosis. Arterioscler Thromb Vasc Biol 1997; 17:217–221.

100. World Health Organization Collaborative Study of Cardiovascular Disease and Hormone Contraception. Effect of different progestogens in low oestrogen oral contraceptives on venous thromboembolic disease. Lancet 1995; 346:1582–1588.

101. Jick H, Jick SS, Gurewich V, Myers MW, Vasilakis C. Risk of idiopathic cardiovascular death and nonfatal venous thromboembolism in women using oral contraceptives with differing progestogen components. Lancet 1995; 346:1589–1593.

102. Lewis MA, Spitzer WO, Heinemann LAJ, et al. Third generation oral contraceptives and the risk of myocardial infarction: an international case-control study. BMJ 1996; 312:88–90.

103. Stampfer MJ, Colditz GA. Estrogen replacement therapy and coronary heart disease: a quantitative assessment of the epidemiologic evidence. Prev Med 1991; 20:47–63.

104. Stampfer MJ, Colditz GA, Willett WC, et al. Postmenopausal estrogen therapy and cardiovascular disease: ten year follow-up from the Nurses' Health Study. N Engl J Med 1991; 325:756–762.

105. Ettinger B, Friedman GD, Bush T, Quesenberry CP Jr. Reduced mortality associated with long-term postmenopausal estrogen therapy. Obstet Gynecol 1996; 87:6–12.

106. Barrett-Connor E. Brief report: postmenopausal estrogen and prevention bias. Ann Intern Med 1991; 115:455–456.

107. Colditz GA, Hankinson SE, Hunter DJ, et al. The use of estrogens and progestins and the risk of breast cancer in postmenopausal women. N Engl J Med 1995; 332:1589–1593.

108. Lobo RA. Benefits and risks of estrogen replacement therapy. Am J Obstet Gynecol 1995; 173:982–990.
109. Adams MR, Kaplan JR, Manuck SB, et al. Inhibition of coronary artery atherosclerosis by 17–beta estradiol in ovariectomized monkeys: lack of an effect of added progesterone. Arteriosclerosis 1990; 10:1051–1057.
110. Sulistiyani SJ, Adelman A, Chandrasekaran A, Jayo J, St Clair RW. Effect of 17 alphadihydroequilin sulfate, a conjugated equine estrogen, and ethinyl estradiol on atherosclerosis in cholesterol-fed rabbits. Arterioscler Thromb Vasc Biol 1995; 15:837–846.
111. Grodstein F, Stampfer MJ, Manson JE, et al. Postmenopausal estrogen and progestin use and the risk of cardiovascular disease. N Engl J Med 1996; 335:453–461.
112. Psaty BM, Heckbert SR, Atkins D, et al. The risk of myocardial infarction associated with the combined use of estrogens and progestins in postmenopausal women. Arch Intern Med 1994; 154:1333–1339.
113. Newton KM, LaCroix AZ, McKnight B, et al. Estrogen replacement therapy and prognosis after first myocardial infarction. Am J Epidemiol 1997; 145:269–277.
114. Sullivan JM, Vande Zwaag R, Hughes JP, Maddock C, Kroetz FW, Ramanathan KB, Mirvis DM. Estrogen replacement and coronary artery disease: effect on survival in postmenopausal women. Arch Intern Med 1990; 150:2557–2562.
115. Yang X-C, Jing T-Y, Resnick LM, Phillips GB. Relation of hemostatic risk factors to other risk factors for coronary heart disease and to sex hormones in men. Arterioscler Thromb 1993; 13:467–471.
116. Phillips GB, Castelli WP, Abbott RD, McNamara PM. Associations of hyperestrogenemia and coronary heart disease in men in the Framingham cohort. Am J Med 1993; 74:863–869.
117. Knopp RH, Zhu X, Bonet B, Bagatell C. Effects of sex steroid hormones on lipoproteins, clotting and the arterial wall. Semin Reprod Endocrinol 1996; 14: 15–27.
118. Glazer G. Atherogenic effects of anabolic steroids on serum lipid levels: a literature review. Arch Intern Med 1991; 151:1925–1933.
119. Barrett-Connor E, Khaw K-T, Yen SSC. A prospective study of dehydroepiandrosterone sulfate, mortality and cardiovascular disease. N Engl J Med 1986; 315:1519–1524.
120. Derman RJ. Effects of sex steroids on women's health: implications for practitioners. Am J Intern Med 1995; 98(suppl 1):IA-137S-1A-143S.
121. Barrett-Connor E, Goodman-Gruen G. Dehydroepiandrosterone sulfate does not predict cardiovascular death in postmenopausal women: the Rancho Bernardo study. Circulation 1995; 91:1757–1760.
122. Gordon GB, Bush DE, Weisman HF. Reduction of atherosclerosis by administration of dehydroepiandrosterone: study in the hypercholesterolemic New Zealand white rabbit with aortic intimal injury. J Clin Invest 1988; 82:712–720.

123. Knopp RH. Oral contraception in acute myocardial infarction. In: Cohen J, ed. Oral Contraceptives and Cardiovascular Disease. Carnforth, UK: Parthenon Publishing, 1996.

7

Adjunctive Nonlipid-Lowering Strategies for the Therapy of Atherosclerosis

Bertram Pitt

University of Michigan School of Medicine, Ann Arbor, Michigan

I. INTRODUCTION

Lipid lowering agents, especially the HMG CoA reductase inhibitors, have been shown to prevent the development of human atherosclerosis, reverse endothelial dysfunction and therefore reduce coronary vasomotor tone, and most importantly reduce the incidence of nonfatal myocardial infarction and death as well as the need for revascularization (1–13). The results of lipid lowering on clinical endpoints such as nonfatal myocardial infarction and death have been relatively consistent in the major secondary prevention trials of HMG CoA reductase inhibitors, ranging between 30–60% (6,11,14–16). Despite these beneficial clinically and statistically significant results, there remains an important need to explore the effectiveness of adjunctive non-lipid-lowering strategies in patients with atherosclerosis since a relatively large percentage of patients with angiographically significant coronary artery disease have serum LDL cholesterol values which are lower than those currently recommended for lipid-lowering therapy—i.e., an LDL cholesterol < 130 mg/dl in the National Cholesterol Education Program (NCEP) guidelines (17,18) and lower than the levels shown to be of benefit for lipid lowering in the 4S (6), pravastatin regression (11), WOSCOP (14), and CARE (16) studies.

In the CARE (16) study it was suggested that patients with a baseline LDL cholesterol < 125 mg/dl did not show clinical benefit from lipid lowering with an HMG CoA reductase inhibitor. Thus there remains a significant percentage of patients with angiographic evidence of coronary artery disease and other atherosclerotic vascular disease in whom there is no currently recommended or proven benefit of lipid lowering. There may also be a need for adjunctive therapy even in those with an LDL cholesterol > 125 to 130 mg/dl who are considered for lipid-lowering therapy. First, many of these patients do not tolerate or are noncompliant to lipid-lowering therapy with diet and/or an HMG CoA reductase inhibitor (19). Second, even with effective lipid-lowering therapy, with for example an HMG CoA reductase inhibitor, there remains a relatively high incidence of ischemic events (6,11,16). Perhaps even more important is the fact that in those who do receive an HMG CoA reductase inhibitor there is a lag phase of 1 to 3 years after beginning lipid-lowering therapy before one begins to see a reduction in clinical events (20). It is possible that adjunctive therapy by further altering atherosclerotic plaque development, the tendency for plaque rupture, or thrombosis after plaque rupture might decrease this lag phase and further reduce ischemic events. This chapter will review some of the adjunctive strategies under investigation to prevent atherosclerosis and its clinical consequences. Although many of these strategies are supported by encouraging experimental data and in some instances angiographic evidence for preventing the development of human coronary atherosclerosis, it should be emphasized that none of these strategies has as yet been shown to prevent the clinical consequences of atherosclerosis—i.e., nonfatal myocardial infarction, stroke, coronary heart disease, death, and most importantly total mortality. It should also be emphasized that the strategies discussed in this chapter are not the only or necessarily the most promising. The rapid advances in vascular biology and in the understanding of the atherosclerotic process suggest that in the future more targeted approaches are likely using conventional drug or gene therapy.

II. BETA ADRENERGIC RECEPTOR BLOCKING AGENTS

Catecholamine release may influence atherosclerosis through a number of potential mechanisms (21,22). They increase blood pressure, heart rate, contractility, and thus sheer stress on the vascular wall. Increased sheer stress and/or direct catecholamine-induced cytotoxicity could contribute to endothelial dysfunction or injury.

Catecholamines may also have a direct effect on lipid accumulation into the vascular wall by changing the affinity of LDL cholesterol for binding to proteoglycans and hence their uptake by macrophages in the vascular wall. They increase esterification and accumulation of cholesterol within plaques by acylcholesterol acyltransferase and increase vascular permeability to lipoproteins (23). Catecholamines increase vasomotor tone and therefore may also play an important role in plaque rupture as well as the risk of thrombosis after plaque rupture. Norepinephrine and epinephrine increase platelet aggregation, the release of thromboxane A_2, and decrease the formation of prostacyclin (24,25). The decrease in prostacyclin may in itself have important effects on the accumulation of lipids into the vascular wall (26).

Beta-adrenergic receptor blocking agents have been shown to attenuate lipid-induced atherosclerosis in hypertensive rabbits (27). This effect has been suggested to be due to a reduction in sheer stress and velocity of flow since hydralazine, which in these experiments reduced blood pressure to an even greater degree, was not as effective (27). However in other studies in rabbits with endothelial injury, propranolol has been shown to increase neointimal thickening, lipid accumulation, and cellular proliferation (28). Kaplan et al. (29) have shown an effect of propranolol in preventing atherosclerosis in male cynomolgus monkeys exposed to behavioral stress. The exaggerated atherosclerosis seen among dominant monkeys in disturbed social groups could be almost completely prevented by propranolol (29). This effect has also been attributed to a reduction in heart rate and sheer stress. Catecholamine-induced endothelial injury as a result of psychologic stress, smoking, or other factors may activate other neurohormonal systems such as the renin angiotensin aldosterone (RAA) system and could therefore be an important facilitating event for the development of atherosclerosis in patients with hyperlipidemia.

Metoprolol, a B_1-selective adrenergic blocking agent protects against endothelial injury (30). Carvedilol, a beta-adrenergic blocking agent with oxygen free radical scavenging and alpha-adrenergic blocking properties (31) also protects against endothelial injury (32) and may be of particular interest in patients with atherosclerosis. In isolated vascular strips exposed to an oxygen free radical generating system, evaluated by determining the effect of acetylcholine on vasodilatation, carvedilol was shown to protect against endothelial dysfunction whereas propranolol, a beta-adrenergic blocking agent without oxygen free radical scavenging properties, did not (32).

Beta-adrenergic receptor blocking agents have been shown to reduce the incidence of nonfatal myocardial infarction and death in patients post-infarction (33), likely through a reduction in the tendency toward plaque rupture and/or thrombosis after plaque rupture. They also reduce the likelihood of ventricular arrhythmias and sudden cardiac death (34). Their effects on the development of atherosclerosis and its progression are somewhat less certain. There have been no long-term prospective serial angiographic studies in man evaluating the effectiveness of a beta-adrenergic blocking agent in preventing the development or progression of atherosclerosis. There has in fact been some concern about the role of beta-adrenergic blocking agents without intrinsic sympathetic activity, since they tend to increase serum triglycerides and decrease HDL cholesterol (35). The failure of beta-adrenergic blocking agents to reduce coronary heart disease death in patients with hypertension to the degree predicted by their reduction in blood pressure (36) could be postulated to be due to their decrease in HDL cholesterol, and thus an increased tendency toward oxidation of LDL cholesterol with resultant atherosclerotic plaque development. When compared to diuretics in a randomized study of patients with hypertension, no significant difference could be demonstrated on the incidence of coronary events and stroke (37), whereas one might have postulated, based on the fact that diuretics release or at least do not suppress catecholamines, that beta blockers would have been more effective. In other trials, however, such as the Metoprolol Atherosclerosis Prevention in Hypertensives trial (MAPHY) (38), there were fewer deaths due to coronary heart disease and stroke in patients treated with metoprolol than with those on diuretics. There has also been a suggestion from subgroup analysis in several antihypertensive studies and from the MAPHY trial (38), as well as a long-term follow-up of patients in the Heart Attack Primary Prevention in the Hypertensive (39) (HAPPHY) trial that beta-adrenergic blocking agents may be particularly effective in smokers (40). Thus, although the net effect of beta-adrenergic receptor blocking agent use in patients appears beneficial and experimental studies support an antiatherosclerotic effect, their effect on the development and progression of atherosclerosis in man remains uncertain and requires further study.

III. CALCIUM CHANNEL BLOCKING AGENTS

Calcium channel blocking agents have been shown to have a beneficial effect on several important pathophysiological processes in the development of atherosclerosis (41 50). They have been shown to prevent experimental lipid-induced endothelial dysfunction and atherosclerosis in experimental models (51,52), inhibit cholesterol ester deposition, and prevent calcium uptake by macrophages (49). Calcium channel blocking agents also increase cholesterol esterhydolase activity (45), inhibit smooth muscle cell migration (47), reduce systemic blood pressure (41) and hence wall stress, as well as having an antithrombotic and antiplatelet effect (42,50).

Several studies have explored the effectiveness of calcium channel blocking agents on the development and progression of human atherosclerosis. Loaldi et al. (53) were the first to show that a calcium channel blocking agent could prevent the progression of coronary atherosclerosis in humans. They compared the calcium channel blocking agent nifedipine to the beta-adrenergic receptor blocking agent propranolol and to the nitrate isosorbide dinitrate. They found on serial angiographic study that patients on nifedipine had significantly less progression of their coronary atherosclerosis than those treated with either propranolol or isosorbide dinitrate. Their study was, however, relatively small and of short duration, and did not provide information on the consequences of coronary atherosclerosis.

Gottlieb et al. (54) investigated the role of nifedipine compared to placebo in patients undergoing CABG surgery. Serial angiographic studies showed that patients randomized to nifedipine had significantly more coronary artery bypass grafts that were free of atherosclerosis on follow-up than those randomized to placebo. These encouraging results were followed by the Intervention Nifedipine Trial on Antiatherosclerotic Therapy (INTACT) (55). In this study 425 patients with angiographic evidence of coronary artery disease were randomized to nifedipine or placebo and followed for 3 years with repeat coronary angiography. The patients randomized to nifedipine (55) had a significant reduction in the development of new coronary artery lesions, but, in contrast to the studies by Loaldi et al. (53) and Gottlieb et al. (54), no significant effect on the progression of existing coronary artery lesions. The Montreal Heart Institute study (56), which randomized 383 patients with angiographic evidence of coronary artery disease to the calcium channel blocking agent nicardipine or placebo with repeat coronary arteriography at 2 years, also showed a significant effect of the calcium channel blocking agent on new coronary artery lesion development but no effect on the progression of existing lesions. Calcium channel blocking agents have also been shown to prevent the progression of carotid atherosclerosis. The Multicenter Isradipine Diuril Atherosclerosis (MIDAS) (57) study randomized 383 patients with hypertension to isradipine or the diuretic hydrochlorothiazide and showed a significant benefit of isradipine on the intimal-media thickness of the carotid artery as measured by serial B mode ultrasound after a 3-year follow-up.

Diltiazem has shown an effect on the progression of coronary artery atherosclerosis, at least in the posttransplant patient (58). Schroder et al. (58) randomized patients postcardiac transplant to diltiazem or placebo and showed that those randomized to diltiazem had significantly less vascular disease than those randomized to placebo. The pathology of posttransplant atherosclerosis is, however, different from that of the usual coronary artery disease. Thus, the bulk of evidence from experimental models and human studies suggests that the calcium channel blocking agents, in particular the dihydropyridines, may have a beneficial effect on the development of new coronary artery lesions and possibly, although not consistently, the progression of existing lesions.

It is therefore disappointing that despite these beneficial effects on coronary and carotid artery atherosclerosis the calcium channel blocking agents have not been shown to have a beneficial effect on the consequences of atherosclerosis such as nonfatal myocardial infarction or death. In the INTACT (55), Montreal Heart Institute study (56), and MIDAS (57,59), there was in fact a trend toward a higher incidence of nonfatal myocardial infarction and death despite beneficial effects on atherosclerosis. Although not statistically significant, this trend is different from that seen with the lipid-lowering agents studied in angiographic progression trials with relatively similar criteria for patient inclusion and sample sizes. The trend toward an adverse effect of the calcium channel blocking agents (especially the dlhydropyridines) on myocardial infarction and death has received increased attention due to the retrospective hypertension cohort study by Psaty et al. (60) and the meta-analysis of all calcium channel blocking agents in the therapy of hypertension and ischemic heart disease by Furberg et al. (61). Of interest is the finding that the heart rate-limiting calcium channel blocking agents such as verapamil appear to have a lower risk of myocardial infarction and death than the dihydropyridines, despite their apparent lack of benefit on the development and/or progression of atherosclerosis. The explanation for the apparent failure of calcium channel blocking agents, at least the first- and second-generation dihydropyridines such as nifedipine, nicardipine, and isradipine to reduce nonfatal myocardial infarction and death, is unclear but possibly related to their tendency to cause catecholamine release. It could be postulated that calcium channel blocking agent-induced catecholamine release and possibly induction of other vasoactive mediators might predispose to plaque rupture and/or sudden cardiac death.

Further studies of calcium channel blocking agents are under way or being planned with the hypothesis that the use of a calcium channel blocking agent such as amlodipine, which has been shown to prevent experimental atherosclerosis in primates (62) and has less of a tendency to or does not release catecholamines (63), might prevent new atherosclerotic lesions without an adverse effect on clinical events. In contrast to most other calcium channel blocking agents studied to date, amlodipine has been well tolerated in patients with dilated cardiomyopathy and has been suggested to have a beneficial effect in those with idiopathic dilated cardiomyopathy (64). Due to its favorable properties amlodipine is currently under study in the Prospective Randomized Evaluation of the Vascular Effects of Norvasc Trial (PREVENT) (65). In this study over 700 patients with angiographic evidence of coronary artery disease have been randomized to amlodipine or placebo and are being followed for 3 years to determine the effect of amlodipine on the development and progression of coronary atherosclerosis. Although not powered to provide an answer as to its effect on nonfatal myocardial infarction or death, this study should nevertheless provide important insight into the clinical potential of calcium channel blocking agents in preventing coronary atherosclerosis and its consequences.

Further insight should be provided by the Antihypertensive and Lipid-Lowering Treatment to Prevent Heart Attack Trial (ALLHAT) (66) in which patients with hypertension have been randomized to amlodipine, lisinopril, chlorthalidone, and doxazosin and followed for 6 years to determine the effects of these strategies on the incidence of fatal coronary heart disease and nonfatal myocardial infarction. Other studies of calcium channel blocking ·agents in patients with hypertension, although not directly addressing the effect of calcium channel blocking agents on coronary atherosclerosis, should nevertheless provide important insight as to their effect on myocardial infarction, stroke, and death, at least in patients with hypertension. Thus, although the calcium channel blocking agents have been demonstrated to have benefits on several pathophysiologically important mechanisms in the development of experimental atherosclerosis, prevent experimental endothelial dysfunction, and prevent the development of human atherosclerosis, they have not been shown to prevent the consequences of atherosclerosis and therefore cannot at this time be recommended for the secondary prevention of ischemic heart disease. Further concern in regard to the long-term use of calcium channel blocking agents in patients with atherosclerosis comes from the study of Pahoor et al. (67). In a case-control study of elderly patients with hypertension they noted an increased risk of cancer in patients taking a calcium channel blocking agent. They attribute this increased cancer risk to the effect of calcium channel blocking agents on inhibiting apoptosis. Thus, until further data are available on their net effect on total mortality in long-term follow-up studies, one should be cautious in using calcium channel blocking agents as adjunctive therapy in patients with atherosclerosis.

IV. NITRATES

Organic nitrovasodilators relax vascular smooth muscle by stimulating soluble guanylatcyclase resulting in an increase in cyclic GMP and the release of NO (67–69). Release of NO, vasodilatation, and the response to endothelial-mediated vasodilators such as acetylcholine have been shown to be impaired in patients with atherosclerosis as well as in patients with risk factors for atherosclerosis but without angiographic evidence of atherosclerosis (70,71). The release of NO has antimitogenic and antioxidant effects which prevent LDL cholesterol oxidation and further cellular damage (72,73). The release of NO also effects monocyte and platelet adhesion. Thus, NO release directly or through organic nitrovasodilators may exert an antiatherosclerotic effect through several mechanisms.

In animal studies penterythritol-tetranitrate (PETN) has been shown to prevent lipid-induced endothelial dysfunction and atherosclerosis (74). Of interest was the finding in these experiments that isosorbide mononitrate (ISDN) was not effective. This has been attributed to the longer action of the metabolites of PETN, a pharmacokinetic effect rather than a different mechanism. There may, however, be other explanations for the difference in effect such as differences in oxygen free radical release. Oxygen free radical release does not occur with PETN, accounting for its relative lack of tolerance in comparison to other organic nitrates (75).

Although nitroglycerin and organic nitrates are frequently used in patients with atherosclerosis for the relief and prevention of angina pectoris, their effect on the atherosclerotic process and the consequences of atherosclerosis, nonfatal myocardial infarction, stroke, and death remain uncertain. Loaldi et al. failed to show a beneficial effect of isorbide dinitrate on the progression of coronary artery disease (53). A meta-analysis of several small trials of the use of nitrates postinfarction suggested a beneficial effect on nonfatal myocardial infarction and death (76). However, in the GISSI III (77) and ISIS 4 (78) studies, no significant benefit of nitrates could be shown. These large-scale multicenter trials are, however, difficult to interpret because of a relatively high incidence of open-label nitrate use in the placebo groups and the relatively short duration of these studies, at least in regard to the development of atherosclerosis. Nitrates, especially PETN, deserve further long-term study to determine their effectiveness on the development of atherosclerosis and its consequences. Until further data are available, nitroglycerin and organic nitrates should be considered for the symptomatic therapy of angina pectoris and myocardial ischemia but not for long-term prophylactic use in the prevention of atherosclerosis and its consequences.

V. ANGIOTENSIN-CONVERTING ENZYME INHIBITORS

Activation of the RAA system has been suggested to be a new and independent risk factor for myocardial infarction. Alderman et al. (79) found in patients with hypertension that the incidence of myocardial infarction was high in patients with an elevated renin level independent of standard risk factors such as smoking, hypercholesterolemia, and diabetes mellitus. Activation of the RAA system has also been suggested to play an important role in several pathophysiologically important mechanisms in the development of atherosclerosis and its consequences (80,81).

Angiotensin II stimulates various cytokines which causes migration of monocytes into the endothelium (82), increases the transport of LDL cholesterol into the vascular wall by forming a complex (83), and causes the oxidation of LDL cholesterol (84,85), foam cell formation, and the release of endothelin (86). Angiotensin II also causes the release of plasminogen activator inhibitor (PAI-i) (87), which could impede intrinsic fibrinolysis and therefore promote complete thrombus formation and infarction after plaque rupture. ACE inhibitors block these effects of angiotensin II and increase levels of bradykinin, which in itself may help to prevent against atherosclerosis and infarction (88). ACE inhibitors prevent experimental lipid-induced endothelial dysfunction and atherosclerosis in animal models, independent of an effect on serum lipids (89,90), possibly by reducing blood pressure and/or shear stress. In addition to the potential beneficial effects of ACE inhibitors in preventing angiotensin II-induced oxidation of LDL cholesterol (85), they increase antioxidant defense mechanisms, such as superoxide dismutase (SOD) (91). These effects and the increase in bradykinin and prostacyclin levels associated with ACE inhibitor administration likely account for their effectiveness in increasing microvascular NO release (92). NO may be critical in the atherosclerotic process by inhibiting neutrophil and platelet adhesion to the vascular wall and thereby preventing the release of various growth factors. Vascular release of NO could also be important in preventing plaque rupture. ACE inhibitors through their effect on NO release and/or by preventing PAI-i release or stimulating the production of plasminogen activator (TPA) (93) may also be important in preventing thrombosis after plaque rupture.

There is also clinical evidence suggesting that ACE inhibitors are effective in preventing the consequences of atherosclerosis in man. Patients randomized to an ACE inhibitor in the SOLVD (94) and SAVE (95) trials had a significant reduction in the incidence of myocardial infarction and ischemic events. The interpretation of these studies for the secondary prevention of ischemic heart disease is difficult, however, since these beneficial effects could be due to a reduction in ventricular volume, remodeling, and/or a decrease in the release of neurohormones associated with reduction in ventricular dilatation, such as norepinephrine.

The potential role of ACE inhibitors in preventing human atherosclerosis and its consequences has recently been strengthened by the finding that the ACE inhibitor quinapril at a dose of 40 mg daily significantly reversed endothelial dysfunction in patients with angiographically proven coronary artery disease over a period of 6 months. In the Trial on Reversing Endothelial Function (TREND) (96), patients were randomized to quinapril or placebo and followed for 6 months at which time the study medication was withdrawn for 72 hours and repeat determination of the coronary arterial response to acetyl choline and nitroglycerin was obtained. Quinapril was effective in reversing endothelial dysfunction in patients who had a left ventricular ejection fraction > 40%, were normotensive with or without antihypertensive medication, and who had a mean serum LDL cholesterol of ~ 130 mg/dl. It should be pointed out, however, that in other studies of endothelial dysfunction ACE inhibitors have not been shown to be effective. For example, in patients with hypertension Creager and his colleagues (97) were unable to show that either captopril or enalapril was effective in improving forearm-mediated vasodilatation, Similarly, Kiowski et al. (98) in patients with hypertension were unable to show a beneficial effect of the ACE inhibitor cilazipril. Serruys et al. (99) were also unable to demonstrate a beneficial effect of cilazipril in reversing coronary endothelial dysfunction. Whether these differences are related to the presence of hypertension, which may affect endothelial function differently than atherosclerosis, or to differences in ACE inhibitor properties remains to be determined. Quinapril, for example, is a highly lipophilic ACE inhibitor and is tightly bound to the vascular ACE enzyme in contrast to more hydrophilic agents such as enalapril (100).

Several trials are currently exploring the hypothesis that ACE inhibitors will prevent the development of atherosclerosis and thereby prevent myocardial infarction and death. These trials are exploring the role of ACE inhibitors in patients without systolic left ventricular dysfunction. The Quinapril Ischemic Event Trial (QUIET) (101) has randomized approximately 1750 patients with coronary artery disease to quinapril or placebo and followed them for 3 years. The HOPE trial (66) is randomizing approximately 9000 patients with coronary artery disease and a left ventricular ejection fraction > 40% to the ACE inhibitor ramipril and, in a factorial design, vitamin E and following them for 5 years. The PEACE trial (66) will randomize 14,000 patients to the ACE inhibitor trandelopril or placebo and follow them for 5 years to determine its effect on total mortality.

While the theoretical basis for the use of ACE inhibitors to prevent atherosclerosis and its consequences is no more compelling than that for calcium channel blocking agents, the trends from available clinical studies are favorable in contrast to the calcium channel blocking agents. One explanation for this potential difference is the finding that ACE inhibitors tend to decrease whereas calcium channel blocking agents cause norepinephrine release. A release of norepinephrine or induction of other vasoactive mediators by calcium channel blocking agents could predispose to sudden cardiac death and plaque rupture. We must, however, await the results of ongoing studies before reaching any firm conclusions concerning the relative or absolute effects of the ACE inhibitors in preventing atherosclerosis. We will also need to await further studies before we understand the potential role of other means of blocking the RAA system, such as angiotensin II type I receptor antagonists (102). An angiotensin II type I receptor blocking agent has been shown to prevent experimental endothelial dysfunction (103). In contrast to ACE inhibitors the angiotensin II type I receptor antagonists do not decrease PAI-i levels (87). It has been suggested that release of PAI-i is due to angiotensin IV, rather than to angiotensin II, and therefore would be blocked by an ACE inhibitor but not by an angiotensin II type I receptor antagonist. The relative importance of inhibiting PAI-i activation and bradykinin release by ACE inhibitors in comparison to an angiotensin II type I receptor antagonist must await further human study and likely direct comparative trials before we can feel confident about their relative benefits.

VI. ENDOTHELIN ANTAGONISTS

Endothelin, a potent coronary vasoconstrictor (104) produced by endothelial cells, has been shown to have chemoattractive (105) and mitogenic effects (106) which may be important in the development of atherosclerosis. Increased plasma endothelin levels (107) and messenger RNA for preproendothelin in atherosclerotic plaques have been detected in patients with atherosclerosis (108). Oxidized LDL cholesterol (109) and angiotensin II (86) are known to cause the release of endothelin, and therefore the interaction of these substances could lead to a vicious cycle accelerating the development and/or progression of the atherosclerotic process.

Studies with a selective endothelin A receptor antagonist have shown it to be effective in preventing the development of atherosclerosis in hamsters fed a lipid-rich diet (110). It was postulated that the endothelin A antagonist may have impeded monocyte chemotaxis and thereby decreased arterial foam cell formation and/or the uptake of oxidized LDL cholesterol into the endothelium by decreasing cholesterol ester synthetase or increasing cholesterol ester hydrolysis.

However, there have been no prospective long-term studies of an endothelin receptor antagonist on the development of atherosclerosis in man. This approach appears promising, and it is likely that further information will become available over the next several years as a number of selective and nonselective endothelin antagonists are introduced into clinical investigation.

VII. OXYGEN FREE RADICAL INHIBITORS

Oxidized LDL cholesterol has been demonstrated to play a critical role in the development of experimental atherosclerosis (111,112). Native LDL cholesterol even in high concentrations does not produce foam cells, an important component of the fatty streak, the earliest lesion in the experimental atherosclerotic process (113). The classic LDL cholesterol receptor is downregulated by an increase in serum cholesterol (114). The scavenger receptor, however, is not downregulated by high serum cholesterol levels and can facilitate cholesterol ester accumulation (114,115). Oxidized LDL cholesterol is taken up into the vascular wall by scavenger receptors resulting in foam cell formation. Once oxidized LDL cholesterol is taken up into the vascular wall, it exerts a number of potentially deleterious effects such as increased leukocyte and monocyte adhesion to the endothelium, a decrease in vascular NO release, increased levels of endothelin, thromboxane A_2, serotonin, plasminogen activator inhibitor (PAI-i), and cytotoxicity (116–121). Oxidized LDL cholesterol can also release interleukin-1 (122), which could promote smooth muscle cell proliferation. In addition to stimulating the release of PAI-i (119) oxidized LDL cholesterol also effects tissue factor, which is important in thrombosis (123).

The role of oxidized LDL cholesterol in impeding NO production and/or release from the endothelium may be a critical step in the development of endothelial dysfunction and atherosclerosis. Reducing LDL cholesterol by cholestyramine or HMG CoA reductase inhibitors and thereby preventing oxidation of LDL restores endothelial function in patients with atherosclerosis (124–126). The combination of the antioxidant probucol and the HMG CoA reductase inhibitor lovastatin has been more effective in restoring endothelial function in patients with hyperlipidemia and coronary artery disease than lovastatin alone (127). In patients with non-insulin-dependent diabetes mellitus antioxidant vitamins such as vitamin C have been shown to restore endothelial function (128). Oxygen free radical formation in this circumstance may, however, be from monocytes and granulocytes in addition to oxidized LDL cholesterol. Free radical formation, whether from monocytes or oxidized LDL cholesterol directly, may decrease NO formation and/or release and thereby contribute to the atherosclerotic process both in patients with and without diabetes mellitus.

Experimental studies, mainly in the hypercholesterolemic rabbit, support the role of oxidized LDL cholesterol in the development of atherosclerosis and of antioxidants in protecting against atherosclerosis. Several studies have shown the antioxidant probucol to be effective in preventing experimental atherosclerosis (129,130). The antioxidant BHT, which increases serum cholesterol, decreases the development of atherosclerosis in the lipid-fed rabbit associated with a decrease in the auto-oxidation products of cholesterol, 7–keto cholesterol, and cholesterol alpha epoxide (131). N,N'-diphenylphenylenediamine DPPD, an antioxidant, also decreases the extent of atherosclerosis in the hypercholesterolemic rabbit (132).

Experimental studies have also shown that all trans beta carotene inhibits the development of atherosclerosis in cholesterol-fed rabbits (133). However, this effect was seen despite the fact that the susceptibility of LDL cholesterol to oxidize was not impaired. Thus, it has been suggested that the effectiveness of all trans beta carotene may be due to factors other than the oxidation of LDL cholesterol (133). This points out the difficulty in ascribing a particular mechanism to the beneficial effects of an antioxidant vitamin such as carotene in experimental studies and the importance of the experimental model. The relevance of the cholesterol-fed rabbit for human atherosclerosis has been questioned since beta-VLDL, the major circulating lipoprotein in the rabbit, in contrast to native LDL, can convert macrophages into foam cells (133,134).

Oxidized LDL cholesterol has been found in rabbit and human atherosclerotic plaques, and the presence of autoantibodies against LDL cholesterol correlates with the progression of atherosclerosis (135,136). Patients with atherosclerosis and overt vascular disease have been found to have decreased antioxidant defense mechanisms such as glutathione peroxidase and high levels of Von Willibrand factor, suggesting endothelial damage (137).

Experimental studies suggest the importance of the role of oxidized LDL cholesterol in human atherosclerosis. In addition to the finding that auto antibodies against oxidized LDL cholesterol correlate with atherosclerosis (136), Reganstrom et al. (138) have shown an inverse correlation between the lag phase of oxidized LDL cholesterol and the extent of atherosclerosis at coronary angiography. Several epidemiological studies also show a correlation between antioxidant vitamin intake such as vitamins E, C, and beta carotene and the risk of coronary artery disease (139–144). Cigarette smoking, a major risk factor for coronary artery disease, causes the oxidation of LDL cholesterol (145). Cigarette smokers also have a relatively low intake of antioxidant vitamins such as vitamins E and C, which may also contribute to the risk of atherosclerosis in these individuals (141). The incidence of coronary artery disease in Europe has also been shown to be inversely related to plasma concentrations of antioxidant vitamins (139). The effectiveness of the Mediterranean diet in reducing the risk of ischemic heart disease has been attributed to a relatively high concentration of antioxidant vitamins E and carotene (146).

In a Dutch study the consumption of antioxidant flavonoids, contained in vegetables, fruit, tea, and wine, by elderly individuals has also been associated with a reduced incidence of coronary heart disease (143). The risk of developing angina pectoris has been correlated with a low intake of vitamins E and C (147). Prospective cohort studies, such as the nurses' health study of 87,245 nurses with no proven history of coronary heart disease, have also demonstrated a reduced risk of coronary artery disease in those with a high intake of vitamins E and beta carotene, although not vitamin C (148). Further support for a role of antioxidant vitamins in the development of atherosclerosis comes from the Atherosclerosis Risk in Communities (ARIC) study (149). The relationship between the intake of vitamin C, alpha tocopherol, and provitamin A carotenoids to carotid wall thickness was studied in 6318 female and 4987 male participants 45 to 64 years old in ARIC. There was a significant inverse relationship in both men and women between vitamin C intake and carotid wall thickness. There was also an inverse relationship for alpha tocopherol, but only for women, and carotene intake, but only in older men. The relationship of carotene to carotid wall thickness was, however, weakened after adjustment for potential confounders. A subgroup analysis from the Cholesterol Lowering Atherosclerosis Study (CLAS) has shown that patients taking supplemental vitamin E > 100 IU/day had less progression of coronary artery disease than those with lower levels (150). No benefit was found, however, for vitamin C, multivitamin use, or the increased dietary intake of vitamin E or C. The alpha tocopherol, beta carotene cancer prevention study, a prospective randomized trial in 29,000 male Finnish smokers has suggested, however, that vitamin E does not reduce the risk of coronary heart disease and that beta carotene actually has a deleterious effect (151). Further doubt concerning the importance of oxidized LDL cholesterol for the development of human atherosclerosis comes from the PQRST study of the antioxidant probucol (152). Probucol as mentioned above is a potent antioxidant that prevents the oxidation of LDL cholesterol (153). In the PQRST study (152) in 274 hypercholesterolemic patients, probucol had no significant effect on the progression of femoral artery atherosclerosis. This negative effect of probucol may, however, be explained by the fact that probucol also reduces HDL cholesterol and the absorption of antioxidant vitamins (154,155). The beneficial effects of probucol on preventing oxidation of LDL cholesterol may therefore have been counterbalanced by a reduction in antioxidant defense mechanisms.

Thus, the failure of probucol to demonstrate a beneficial effect should not be construed as evidence against the hypothesis that oxidized LDL cholesterol is pathophysiologically important in human atherosclerosis, but rather as an indication that it is the net effect of several processes that are important. The importance of oxidized LDL cholesterol in human atherosclerosis and the potential for antioxidant vitamins to protect against the consequences of atherosclerosis was examined in the CHAOS study (156). This study examined the role of vitamin E supplementation on the incidence of ischemic events in patients with known coronary artery disease and found that vitamin E supplementation reduced the incidence of nonfatal myocardial infarction. Although encouraging for the hypothesis that oxidized LDL cholesterol is important in human atherosclerosis, one should be cautious in the interpretation of this study since mortality, which would be expected to decrease in conjunction with a decrease in the incidence of nonfatal myocardial infarction, actually increased, although not, significantly.

In view of the conflicting results from the available prospective randomized studies examining the role of antioxidant vitamins and other strategies to prevent the oxidation of LDL cholesterol in humans, it would be prudent to be cautious in recommending the use of antioxidant vitamins for the prevention of atherosclerosis until further data are available. Steinberg and others have reviewed the experimental, epidemiologic, and clinical data supporting the role of oxidized LDL cholesterol in atherosclerosis, which is conflicting (157–160). Steinberg (157) points out that oxidized LDL cholesterol is likely responsible for the development of the fatty streak in man but that there may be a long lag phase, > 5 years, before these lesions become important and hence antioxidant strategies effective. In the interim, other factors relating to plaque rupture and/or thrombosis, which may or may not depend on oxidized LDL cholesterol, may determine the incidence of ischemic events. He suggests further long-term trials to evaluate the importance of oxidized LDL cholesterol in atherosclerosis. Regardless, until further data are available from prospective randomized studies showing a significant net benefit on total mortality of antioxidant vitamins and other antioxidant strategies, one should be cautious in recommending them for clinical use in the prevention of atherosclerosis.

VIII. ESTROGEN

Estrogen has been shown to have important effects on several mechanisms important in the atherosclerotic process. Estrogen increases serum HDL and decreases LDL cholesterol (161–165). It has, however, been suggested that these effects on serum lipids account for only 25% to 50% of its beneficial effects on the atherosclerotic process (166).

Estrogen restores and prevents lipid-induced endothelial dysfunction in both animals and humans (167–174). The prevention and reversal of endothelial dysfunction by estrogen has been explained by both receptor-mediated and receptor-independent mechanisms (175,176). Basal release of NO from the endothelium is greater in females than males (177). Estrogen is an antioxidant (178) and therefore tends to preserve vascular NO production and/or release. Estrogen may also act by an estrogen-dependent mechanism to stimulate NO synthesis (175). Hayashi et al. have shown that estrogen increases nitric oxide synthetase-3 activity via an estrogen receptor-dependent mechanism, which is altered by cell senescence (176). These changes in NO production and endothelial function could result in a decrease in monocyte and platelet adhesion to the vascular wall and thus account for a large percentage of the benefits of estrogen in preventing atherosclerosis. Estrogen may also affect vasomotor tone by increasing vasodilator prostaglandins such as prostacyclin PGI-2 and/or by decreasing vasoconstrictor prostaglandins such as thromboxane B_2, by inhibiting alpha adrenergic tone, or by inhibiting calcium flux within the vascular wall (179–185). Hormone replacement therapy with estradiol valerate and norethisterone administered to postmenopausal women for 6 months has been shown to reduce serum angiotensin-converting enzyme (ACE) levels by 20%, whereas untreated women had no change (186). Estrogen has also been shown to have angiogenic properties and thereby may be important in collateral vessel development (187). In existing high-grade obstructive coronary artery lesions complete occlusion is relatively common, but myocardial infarction less common, due in part to the development of collateral vessels (188). Estrogen has also been shown to cause a change in vascular extra cellular matrix and decrease collagen formation (189–191). It may also have an effect on thrombus formation and fibrinolysis. Estrogen can lower fibrinogen, antithrombin III, thromboxane A_2 and increase levels of factor VII prostacyclin and protein C. In the ARIC study women who used replacement hormone therapy had a lower mean level of tissue plasminogen activator (TPA) and plasminogen activator inhibitor-1 (PAI-i), suggesting an enhanced fibrinolytic potential (192). Estrogen has also been suggested to improve insulin sensitivity (193–195) which may also improve the potential for fibrinolysis and the prevention of thrombosis.

Epidemiological studies also suggest an important role of estrogen in the prevention of atherosclerosis (196,197). Before the age of 60, men develop cardiovascular disease more than twice as frequently as woman. However, after menopause, by the age of 75 years, the incidence of cardiovascular disease in men and woman is similar (197). The nurses' health study (199) demonstrated a 0.56 overall risk for coronary heart disease after adjustment for other risk factors in postmenopausal estrogen users. A recent meta-analysis by Grady et al. (200) estimated a relative risk of 0.65 for woman who had ever used estrogen compared to nonestrogen users for nonfatal and fatal coronary artery disease.

Experimental studies suggest that the beneficial cardiovascular effects of estrogen may be reduced by the addition of progesterone (201,202). There is also evidence that progestin decreases the rise in HDL cholesterol seen with estrogen alone. Thus, in the PEPI trial women randomized to congregated equine estrogen and continuous or cyclical medroxyprogesterone acetate had a smaller increase in HDL cholesterol than women receiving estrogen alone (203). In the Framingham offspring study postmenopausal women taking a combination of estrogen and a progestin had higher levels of PAI-i than women taking estrogen alone after adjustment for covariants such as age and other risk factors (204).

Information on the combination of estrogen and progesterone in women on the clinical consequences of atherosclerosis is scant but suggests a net beneficial effect. For example, in a study of 168 women taking an estrogen-progesterone combination, the relative risk of coronary artery disease was 0.3 (205). In a prospective cohort study from Sweden, women who received estradiol-levonorcrestin had a 50% reduction in the risk of myocardial infarction, whereas the risk in women taking estrogen alone was 0.74 (206). In view of the conflicting data on serum lipids and PAI-i on the one hand and the beneficial clinical results from relatively small trials on the other in women taking a combination of estrogen and a progestin compared to estrogen alone, further study is clearly needed.

Grady et al. (200) concluded on the basis of available data that women most likely to benefit from estrogen replacement therapy are those with a history of coronary artery disease and those with multiple risk factors for coronary artery disease. The net benefit of hormone replacement therapy is currently being explored in the women's health study, which is assessing the effect of estrogen, estrogen-progesterone, and placebo in a large cohort study which will determine the relative risk on coronary heart disease, breast cancer, and osteoporosis. These data and the data from other studies such as PEPI (203) and the heart estrogen replacement study should have an important public health impact (196). In the long run, however, women's use of hormone replacement therapy with estrogen or the combination of estrogen and a progestin may depend not so much on the magnitude of benefit shown in these trials but as on their perceived risk and attitudes concerning breast cancer. Thus it will be important to determine whether or not the results of these studies influence the clinical use of HRT even if they are statistically and clinically significant.

IX. ANTIPLATELET AGENTS

Aspirin has been shown to be effective in the secondary prevention of ischemic heart disease (207). Patients with a history of a prior myocardial infarction, acute myocardial infarction, unstable angina pectoris, and/or TIAs have a significant reduction in ischemic events when randomized to aspirin. These results can be explained by the effect of aspirin in inhibiting prostaglandin synthesis, platelet aggregation, and thrombosis. Inhibition of platelet aggregation may also have important effects on the development of atherosclerosis and its progression. Numaro et al. (208) have suggested that the release of thromboxane B_2 by platelets causes edema in the vascular wall and results in the release of adenine, suggesting that activated platelets could play a role in endothelial injury. Activated platelets also cause a decrease in cyclic AMP, an increase in intracellular calcium, and a decrease in nitric oxide in endothelial cells. These changes, due to platelet activation and the subsequent release of growth factors from the platelet such as PDGF, could play an important role in the initiation or acceleration of the atherosclerotic process. It has also been shown that intramural thrombosis formation is an important mechanism for the progression of the atherosclerotic plaque (209,210). Plaque rupture and subsequent thrombosis are relatively common but only occasionally lead to complete thrombosis and vascular occlusion causing infarction (211–213). In many instances of plaque rupture the thrombus may be incomplete or intramural and after organization becomes incorporated into the vascular wall contributing to the extent of the obstructive coronary artery disease. In other instances the thrombus after plaque rupture may be complete but infarction avoided because of collateral vessel formation. The platelet trialists (207) have summarized the data suggesting the effectiveness of aspirin and other antiplatelet agents in the secondary prevention of ischemic events.

There is also evidence suggesting that aspirin may play a role in the primary prevention of ischemic heart disease. The physicians' health study (214) demonstrated a 44% reduction in the risk of myocardial infarction among men taking 325 mg of aspirin every other day. The role of aspirin in the primary prevention of ischemic heart disease in women is currently under investigation in the women's health study (215). The availability of orally active glycoprotein IIb/IIIa platelet inhibitors and other antithrombotic drugs provides an opportunity for an exploration of the role of activated platelets and thrombosis in preventing atherosclerosis and its complications. Further studies exploring the effects of these strategies on the development of atherosclerosis and its progression by serial quantitative angiography and/or intravascular ultrasound (IVUS) will be important in our understanding of the pathophysiologic importance of these mechanisms. It is likely, if they can be shown to be safe in regard to the risk of bleeding, that one or more of these new antiplatelet or antithrombotic strategies will find an important role in the secondary prevention of ischemic heart disease both in those with and without concomitant hyperlipidemia. Other elements of the clotting and fibrinolytic systems may also be of importance, such as fibrinogen and plasminogen activator inhibitor PAI-i. Thus, interference with platelet activation, thrombosis, and/or fibrinolysis appear to be of importance in the development, progression, and the consequences of atherosclerosis and could therefore provide attractive therapeutic targets.

X. CONCLUSION

In conclusion, while lipid accumulation and oxidation of LDL cholesterol may play a critical role in the development of experimental and human atherosclerosis and lipid lowering, several strategies have been shown to be effective in preventing the development and progression of atherosclerosis along with its consequences, there remains a significant atherosclerotic burden and incidence of ischemic events despite current lipid-lowering strategies. A large percentage of patients with occlusive atherosclerotic vascular disease have serum LDL cholesterol levels < 125 to 130 mg/dl, a level at which lipid lowering is of uncertain benefit. Strategies designed to prevent monocyte adhesion, oxidation of LDL cholesterol, angiotensin II and endothelin formation, endothelial dysfunction, intracellular calcium accumulation, increase in wall stress, and thrombosis are all attractive and deserve further intensive clinical investigation alone and/or in combination with lipid-lowering strategies.

In view of the complex nature of the human atherosclerotic process, plaque rupture, and thrombosis, it will be necessary to demonstrate that the net effect of any adjunctive strategy on the clinical consequences of atherosclerosis and, most importantly, total mortality, are beneficial before recommending them for clinical use, regardless of their effect on endothelial dysfunction or angiographic evidence of effectiveness in preventing the development or progression of atherosclerosis. This caution is exemplified by the experience with calcium channel blocking agents referred to above. It should also be recognized that to be clinically applicable in today's health care environment, any adjunctive or alternative strategy will not only have to be proven to reduce ischemic events and total mortality but also to be cost-effective. The economic implications for society of new and effective pharmacologic approaches to the development of atherosclerosis and its consequences are of great concern. While adjunctive approaches hold great promise and may be cost-effective for the secondary prevention of ischemic heart disease, we must be cautious in applying these strategies to the problem of primary prevention without a clear vision as to their financial impact. Life-style modification, exercise, more effective diets (such as the Mediterranean diet), and avoidance of smoking, although as yet difficult to achieve for large populations, hold the most promise for a cost-effective approach to the primary prevention of atherosclerosis and its complications.

REFERENCES

1. Waters D, Higginson L, Gladstone P, et al. Effects of monotherapy with an HMG-CoA reductase inhibitor on the progression of coronary atherosclerosis as assessed by serial quantitative arteriography. Circulation 1994; 89:959–968.
2. Blankenhom DH, Azen SP, Kramsch DM, et al. Coronary angiographic changes with lovastatin therapy. Ann Intern Med 1993; 119:969–976.
3. Zhao XQ, Brown BG, Hillger L, et al. Effects of intensive lipid lowering therapy on the coronary arteries of asymptomatic subjects with elevated apolipoprotein B. Circulation 1993; 88:2744–2753.
4. MAAS Investigators. Effect of simvastatin on coronary atheroma: the Multicentre Anti-Atheroma study (MAAS). Lancet 1994; 344:633–638.
5. Pitt B, Mancini GBJ, Ellis SG, et al. Pravastatin limitation of atherosclerosis in the coronary arteries (PLAC 1): reduction in atherosclerosis progression and clinical events. JACC 1995; 26(5):1133–1139.

6. Scandinavian Simvastatin Survival Study Group. Randomised trial of cholesterol lowering in 4444 patients with coronary heart disease: the Scandinavian Simvastatin Survival Study (4S). Lancet 1994; 344:1383–1389.

7. Campos CT, Nguyen PO, Buchwald, PSCH Group. Effect of cholesterol lowering on PTCA, CABG, and heart transplantation rates: POSCH long-term follow-up study. Circulation 1993; 88:1–386.

8. Watts GF, Mandalia S, Brunt JN, Slavin BM, Coltart DJ, Lewis B. Independent associations between plasma lipoprotein subtraction levels and the course of coronary artery disease in the St. Thomas' Atherosclerosis Regression Study (STARS). Metabolism 1993; 42:1461–1467.

9. Cashin-Hemphill L, Mack W, LaBree L, et al. Coronary progression predicts future cardiac events. Circulation 1993; 88:1–363.

10. Haskell WL, Alderman EL, Fair JM, et al. Beneficial angiographic and clinical response to multifactor modification in the Stanford Coronary Risk Intervention Project (SCRIP). Circulation 1994; 89:975–990.

11. Byington RP, Jukema W, Salonen JT, et al. Reduction in cardiovascular events during pravastatin therapy. Circulation 1995; 92:2419–2425.

12. Stewart BF, Brown G, Zhao XQ, et al. Coronary atherosclerosis regression is less pronounced during a second course of comparably effective lipid lowering therapy. Circulation 1993; 88:1–363.

13. Jukema JW, Bruschke VG, Vanboven AJ, et al. Effects of lipid lowering by pravastatin on progression and regression of coronary artery disease in symptomatic men with normal to moderatly elevated serum cholesterol levels. (REGRESS.) Circulation 1995; 91:2528–2540.

14. Shepherd J, Cobbe SM, Ford I, et al. Prevention of coronary heart disease with pravastatin in men with hypercholesterolemia. N Eng] J Med 1995; 333:1301–1307.

15. Anderson TJ, Meredith IT, Yeung AC, Frei B, Selwyn AP, Ganz P. The effect of cholesterol-lowering and antioxidant therapy on endothelium-dependent coronary vasomotion. N Engl J Med 1995; 332:488–493.

16. Braunwald E, Pfeffer M, Sacks F. CARE Trial Results. Reported at the American College of Cardiology 45th Annual Scientific Session, Orlando, FL: March 24–26, 1996.

17. National Cholesterol Education Program. Second Report of the Expert Panel on Detection, Evaluation, and Treatment of High Blood Cholesterol in Adutls. NIH Publ. No. 88–2925. Bethesda, MD: National Heart, Lung and Blood Institute; 1988.

18. Kannel WB, Castelli WP, Gordon T. Cholesterol in the prediction of atherosclerotic disease. New perspectives based on the Framingham study. Ann Intern Med 1979; 90:85–91.

19. Hunninghake DB, Stein EA, Dujovne CA, et al. The efficacy of intensive dietary therapy alone or combined with lovistatin in outpatients with hypercholesterolemia. N Engl J Med 1993; 328:1213–1219.

20. Law MR, Wald NJ, Thompson SG. By how much and how quickly does reduction in serum cholesterol concentration lower risk of ischemic heart disease? BMJ 1994; 308:367–373.

21. Kaplan JR, Manuck SB. Antiatherogenic effects of b–adrenergic blocking agents: theoretical, experimental, and epidemiologic considerations. Am Heart J 1994; 128:1316–1328.
22. Bondjers G. Anti-atherosclerotic effects of beta-blockers. Eur Heart J 1994; 15:8–15.
23. Cruickshank JM. Beta-blockers, plasma lipids, and coronary heart disease. Circulation 1990; 82(suppl II):1160–1165.
24. Winther K, Willich SN. Beta1 blockade and acute coronary ischemia: possible role of platelets. Circulation 1991; 84(suppl VI):68–71.
25. Pettersson K, Hansson G, Bjorkman J-A, Ablad B. Prostacyclin synthesis in relation to sympathoadrenal action: effects of beta-blockade. Circulation 1991; 84(suppl VI):38–43.
26. Willis AL, Smith DL, Vigo C. Suppression of principal atherosclerotic mechanisms by prostacyclins and other eicosanoids. Prog Lipid Res 1986; 25:645–666.
27. Spence JD, Perkins DG, Klein RL, Adams MR, Haust MD. Hemodynamic modifications of aortic atherosclerosis: effects of propranolol versus hydralazine in hypertensive hyperlipidemic rabbits. Atherosclerosis 1984; 50:325–333.
28. Orekhov AN, Andrianovia IV, Rekhter Md, et al. Beta-blockers: propranolol, metoprolol, atenolol, pindolol, alprenolol and timolol, manifest atherogenicity on in vitro, ex vivo and in vivo models. Elmination of propranolol atherogenic effects by papaverine. Atherosclerosis 1992; 95:77–85.
29. Kaplan JR, Manuck SB, Adams MR, Weingand KW, Clarkson TB. Inhibition of coronary atherosclerosis by propranolol in behaviorally predisposed monkeys fed an atherogenic diet. Circulation 1987; 76:1364–1372.
30. Pettersson K, Ablad B. Metoprolol inhibits platelet deposition at arterial bifurcations in rabbits with sympathetic activation. FASEB J 1988; 2:1580. Abstract.
31. Yue TL, McKenna PJ, Gu JL, Cheng HY, Ruffolo RR, Feuerstein GZ. Carvedilol, a new antihypertensive agents, prevents lipid peroxidation and oxidative injury to endothelial cells. Hypertension 1993; 22:922–928.
32. Lopez BL, Christopher TA, Yue-TL, Ruffolo R, Feuerstein GZ, Ma XL. Carvedilol, a new beta-adrenoreceptor blocker antihypertensive drug, protects against free-radical-induced endothelial dysfunction. Pharmacology 1995; 51:165–173.
33. Yusuf S, Peto R, Lewis J, Collins R, Sleight P. b-blockade during and after myocardial infarction: An overview of the randomized trials. Prog Cardiovasc Dis 1985; 27:335–371.
34. Kennedy HL, Brooks MM, Barker AH, et al. Beta-blocker therapy in the Cardiac Arrythmia Suppression Trial. Am J Cardiol 1994; 74:674–680.
35. Cruickshank JM. b-blockers, plasma lipids, and coronary heart disease. Circulation 1990; 82(suppl 2):60–65.
36. MacMahon S, Peto R, Cutler J, et al. Blood pressure, stroke, and coronary heart disease, part 1: prolonged differences in blood pressure-prospective observational studies corrected for the regression dilution bias. Lancet 1990; 335:765–774.
37. Furberg CD, Cutler JA. Diuretic agents versus beta-blockers: comparison of effects of mortality, stroke, and coronary events. Hypertension 1989; 13(suppl I):157–161.

38. Wikstrand J, Wamold 1, Olsson G, et al. Primary prevention with metoprolol in patients with hypertension: mortality results from the MAPHY Study. JAMA 1988; 259:1976–1982.

39. Wilhelmsen L, Berglund G, Elmfeldt D, et al. Beta-blockers versus diuretics in hypertensive men: main results from the HAPPHY trial. J Hypertens 1987; 5:561–572.

40. Tuomilehto J, Wikstrand J, Olsson G, et al. Decreased coronary heart disease in hypertensive smokers: mortality results from the MAPHY Study. Hypertension 1989; 13:773–780.

41. Waters D, Lesperance J, Francetich M, et al. A controlled clinical trial to assess the effect of a calcium channel blocker on the progression of coronary athero-sclerosis. Circulation 1990; 82:1940–1953.

42. Lam JYT, Latour JG, Lesperance J, Waters D. Platelet aggregation, coronary arthery disease progression, and future coronary events. Am J Cardiol 1994; 73:333–338.

43. Habib JB, Bossaller C, Wells S, Williams C, Morrisett JD, Henry PD. Preserva-tion of endothelium-dependent vascular relaxation in cholesterol-fed rabbit by treatment with the calcium blocker PN 200110. Circ Res 1986; 58:305–309.

44. Kramsch DM, Sharma RC, Hodis HN. Amlodipine suppresses in vivo lowdensity lipoprotein oxidation, hyperinsulinemia and atherosclerosis in primates. Circula-tion 1993; 88(suppl I):562. Abstract.

45. Etingin OR, Hajjar DP. Nifedipine increases cholesteryl ester hydrolytic activity in lipid-laden rabbit arterial smooth muscle cells. J Clin Invest 1985; 75:1554–1558.

46. Jackson LJ, Bush RC, Bowyer DE. Inhibitory effect of calcium antagonists on balloon catheter-induced arterial smooth muscle cell proliferation and lesion size. Atherosclerosis 1988; 69:115–122.

47. Nakao J, Ito H, Ooyama T, Change WC, Murota S. Calcium dependency of aortic smooth muscle cell migration induced by 12–L-hydroxy-5,8,10, 14–eicosatetra-enoic acid. Atherosclerosis 1983; 46:309–319.

48. Schmitz G, Robenek H, Bejck M. Ca++ antagonists and ACAT inhibitors promote cholesterol efflux from macrophages by different mechanicms. Arteriosclerosis 1988; 8:46–56.

49. Daugherty A, Rateri DL, Schonfeld G, Sobel BE. Inhibition of cholesteryl ester deposition in macrophages by calcium entry blockers: an effect dissociable from calcium entry blockade. Br J Pharmacol 1987; 91:113–118.

50. Lacoste LL, Lam JYT, Hung J, Waters D. Oral verapamil inhibits platelet throm-bus formation in men. Circulation 1994; 89:630–634.

51. Kramsch DM, Aspen AJ, Rozler LJ. Atherosclerosis: prevention by agents not affecting abnormal levels of blood lipids. Science 1981; 213:1511–1512.

52. Henry PD, Bentley KI. Suppression of atherogenesis in cholesterol-fed rabbit treated with nifedipine. J Clin Invest 1981; 68:1366–1369.

53. Loaldi A, Polese A, Montorsi P, et al. Comparison of nifedipine, propranolol and isosorbide dinitrate on angiographic progression and regression of coronary ar-terial narrowing in angina pectoris. Am J Cardiol 1989; 64:433–439.

54. Gottlieb SO, Brinker JA, Mellits ED, et al. Effect of nifedipine on the development of coronary bypass graft stenoses in high-risk patients: A randomized, double-blind, placebo-controlled trial. Circulation 1989; 80: II228. Abstract.

55. Lichtlen PR, Hugenholtz PG, Raffienbeul W, et al. Retardation of angiographic progression of coronary artery disease by nifedipine. Lancet 1990; 335:1109–1113.

56. Waters D, Lesperance J, Francetich M, et al. A controlled clinical trial to assess the effect of a calcium channel blocker on the progression of coronary atherosclerosis. Circulation 1990; 82:1940–1953.

57. Furberg CD for the MIDAS Research Group. Effect of isradipine and diuretic on early carotid atherosclerosis in hypertension. J Hypertens 1994; 12(suppl 3):S67. Abstract.

58. Schroeder JS, Gao SZ. Calcium blockers and atherosclerosis: Lessons from the Stanford Transplant Coronary Artery Disease/Diltiazem Trial. Can J Cardiol 1995; 11:710–715.

59. Hansson L, Zanchetti A. The antiatherosclerotic effect of calcium antagonists in man—What did MIDAS actually show? Blood Pressure 1995; 4:133–136.

60. Psaty BM, Koepsell TD, Yanex ND, et al. Temporal patterns of antlhypertensive medication use among older adults, 1989 through 1992. An effect of the major clinical trials on clinical practice? JAMA 1995; 273:1436–1438.

61. Furberg CD, Psaty BM, Meyer JV. Nifedipine. Dose-related increase in mortality in patients with coronary heart disease. Circulation 1995; 92:1326–1331.

62. Kramsch DM, Sharma RC. Limits of lipid-lowering therapy: the benefits of amlodipine as anti-atherosclerotic agent. J Human Hypertens 1995; 9(suppl I):53–59.

63. Packer M, Nicod P, Khandheria BR, et al. Randomized multicenter, double-blind, placebo-controlled evaluation of amlodipine in patients with mild-to-moderate heart failure. J Am Coll Cardiol 1991; 17:274a. Abstract.

64. Packer M. Personal communication, 1996.

65. Pitt B. Role of calcium channel blocking agents in the prevention of atherosclerosis. Cardiovasc Drugs Ther 1995; 9:313–316.

66. Pepine CJ. Ongoing clinical trial sof angiotensin-converting enzyme inhibitors for treatment of coronary artery disease in patients with preserved left ventricular function. J Am Coll Cardiol 1996; 27:1048–1052.

67. Pahor M, Guralnik JM, Salive ME, Corti MC, Carbonin P, Havlik RJ. Do calcium channel blockers increase the risk of cancer? Am J Hypertens 1996; 9:695–699.

67. Schultz KD, Schultz K, Schultz G. Sodium nitroprusside and other smooth muscle relaxants increase cyclic GMP levels in rat ductus deferens. Nature 1977; 265: 750–751.

68. Feelisch M, Noack E. Correlation between nitric oxide formation during degradation of organic nitrates and activation of guanylate cyclase. Eur J Pharmacol 1987; 139:19–30.

69. Chung SJ, Fung HL. Identification of the subcellular site for nitroglycerin metabolism to nitric oxide in bovine coronary smooth muscle cells. J Pharmacol Exp Ther 1990; 243:614–619.

70. Ludmer PL, Selwyn AP, Shook TL, et al. Paradoxical vasoconstriction induced by acetylcholine in atherosclerotic coronary arteries. N Engl J Med 1986; 315: 1046–1051.

71. Reddy KG, Nair RN, Sheeran HM, Hodgson JM. Evidence that selective endothelial dysfunction may occur in the absence of angiographic or ultrasound atherosclerosis in patients with risk factors for atherosclerosis. J Am Coll Cardiol 1994; 23:833–843.

72. Nakaki T, Nakayama M, Kato R. Inhibition by nitric oxide and nitric oxide-producing vasodilators of DNA-synthesis in vascular smooth muscle cells. Eur J Pharrnacol Mol Pharmacol 1990; 189:347–353.

73. Bruckdorfer KR, Jacobs M, Rice-Evans C. Endothelium-derived relaxing factor (nitric oxide), lipoprotein oxidation and atherosclerosis. Biochem Soc Trans 1990; 18:1061–1063.

74. Kojda G, Stein D, Kottenberg E, Schnalth EM, Noack E. In vivo effects of pentaerythrityl-tetranitrate and isosorbide-5–mononitrate on the development of atherosclerosis and endothelial dysfunction in cholesterol-fed rabbits. J Cardiovasc Pharmacol 1995; 25:763–773.

75. Fink B, Utepbergenov D, Skatchkov M, Stalleicken D, Bassenge E. Pentaerithrityletetranitrate in contrast to other nitrovasodialtors circumvents tolerance and enhances plasma and platelet thiol contents. Eur Heart J 1996. In press.

76. Yusuf S, Collins R, MacMahon S, Peto R. Effect of intravenous nitrates on mortality in acute myocardial infarction: an overview of the randomised trials. Lancet 1988; 1:1088–1092.

77. Gruppo Italiano per lo Studio della Sopravvivenza nell'Infarto Miocardico. GISSI-3: effects of lisinopril and transdermal glyceryl trinitrate singly and together on 6–week mortality and ventricular function after acute myocardial infarction. Lancet 1994; 343:1115–1122.

78. ISIS-4 (Fourth International Study on Infarct Survival) Collaborative group. ISIS-4: a randomised factorial trial assessing early oral captopril, oral mononitrate and intravenous magnesium in 58,000 patients with suspected acute myocardial infarction. Lancet 1995; 345:669–685.

79. Alderman MH, Madhavan S, Ooi WL, Cohen H, Sealey JE, Laragh Ja. Association of renin-sodium profile with risk of myocardial infarction in patients with hypertension. N Engl J Med 1991; 324:1098–1104.

80. Pitt B. Angiotensin-converting enzyme inhibitors in patients with coronary atherosclerosis. Am Heart J 1994; 128:1328–1332.

81. Lonn Em, Yusuf S, Jha P, et al. Emerging role of angiotensin-converting enzyme inhibitors in cardiac and vascular protection. Circulation 1994; 90:2056–2069.

82. Farber HW, Center DM, Rounds S, Danilov SM. Components of the angiotensin system cause release of a neutrophil chemoattractant from cultured bovine and human endothelial cells. Eur Heart J 1990; 11 (suppl B):100–107.

83. Keidar S, Kaplan M, Aviram M. Angiotensin II. Modified LDL is taken up by macrophages via the scavenger receptor, leading to cellular cholesterol accumulation. Arterioscler Thromb Vasc Biol 1996; 16:97–105.

84. Griendling KK, Minieri CA, Ollerenshaw JD, Alexander RW. Angiotensin II stimulates NADH and NADPH oxidase activity in cultured vascular smooth muscle cells. Circ Res 1994; 74:1141–1148.

85. Keidar S, Brook JG, Aviram M. Angiotensin II enhanced lipid peroxidation of low-density lipoprotein. J Am Physiol Soc 1993; 8:245–248.

86. Dohi Y, Hahn AWA, Boulanger CM, Buhler FR, Luscher TF. Endothelin stimulated by angiotensin II augments contractility of spontaneously hypertensive rat resistance arteries. Hypertension 1992; 19:131–137.

87. Ridker PRM, Gaboury CL, Conlin PR, Seely EW, Williams GH, Vaughan DE. Stimulation of plasminogen activator inhibitor in vivo by infusion of angiotensin II: evidence of a potential interaction between the renin-angiotensin system and fibrinolytic function. Circulation 1993; 87:1969–1973.

88. Linz W, Wiemer G, Gohlke P, Unger T, Scholkens BA. Contribution of kinins to the cardiovascular actions of angiotensin-converting enzyme inhibitors. Pharmacol Rev 1995; 47:25–49.

89. Finta KM, Fischer MJ, Lee L, Gordon D, Pitt B, Webb RC. Ramipril prevents impaired endothelium-dependent relaxation in arteries from rabbits fed an atherogenic diet. Atherosclerosis 1993; 100:149–156.

90. Chobanian AV, Haudenschild CC, Nickerson C, Drago R. Antiatherogenic effect of captopril in the Watanabe heritable hyperlipidemic rabbit. Hypertension 1990; 15:327–331.

91. deCavanagh EMV, Inserra F, Ferder L, Romano L, Ercole L, Fraga CG. Superoxide dismutase and glutathione peroxidase activates are increased by enalapril and captopril in mouse liver. FEBS Lett 1995; 361:22–24.

92. Zhang X, Xie YW, Nasjletti A, Wolin MS, Hintze TH. Role of local coronary vascular kinin formation in the control of myocardial oxygen consumption in the canine heart. Circulation 1995; 92:I–110.

93. Ridker PM, GHaboury CL, Conlin PR, Seely EW, Williams GH, Vaughan DE. Stimulation of plasminogen activator inhibitor in vivo by infusion of angiotensin evidence of a potential interaction between the renin angiotensin system and fibrinolytic function. Circulation 1993; 87:1969–1973.

94. Yusuf S, Pepine CJ, Garces C, et al. Effect of enalapril on myocardial infarction and unstable angina pectoris in patients with low ejection fractions. Lancet 1992; 340:1173–1178.

95. Pfeffer MA, Braunwald E, Moye LA, et al. Effect of captopril on mortality and morbidity in patients with left ventricular dysfunction after acute myocardial infarction: results of the Survival and Ventricular Enlargement trial. N Engl J Med 1992; 327:669–677.

96. Mancini GBJ, Henry GC, Macaya C, et al. Angiotensin converting enzyme inhibition with Quinapril improves endotehlial vasomotor dysfunction in patients with coronary artery disease: the TREND Study (Trial on Reversing Endothelial Dysfunction). Circulation 1996. In press.

97. Creager MA, Roddy MA. Effect of captopril and enalapril on endothelial function in hypertensive patients. Hypertension 1994; 24:499–505.

98. Kiowski W, Linder L, Nuesch R, Martina B. Effects of cilazapril on vascular structure and function in essential hypertension. Hypertension 1996; 27:371–376.

99. Seruys P. Personal communication. 1996
100. Johnston Cl, Fabris B, Yamada H, et al. Comparative studies of tissue inhibition by angiotensin converting enzyme inhibitors. J Hypertens 1989; 7:11S–16S.
101. Texter M, Lees RS, Pitt B, Dinsmore RE, Uprichard ACG. The Quinapril Ischemic Event Trial (QUIET) design and methods: evaluation of chronic ACE inhibitor therapy after coronary artery intervention. Cardiovasc Drugs Ther 1993–7:273–282.
102. Timmermans PBMWM, Smight RD. A new class of therapeutic agents: the angiotensin II receptor antagonists. Cardiologia 1994; 39:397–400.
103. Azuma H, Niimi Y, Hamasaki H. Prevention of intimal thickening after endothelial removal by a nonpeptide angiotensin II receptor antagonist, losartan. Br J Pharmacol 1992; 106(3):665–671.
104. Yanagiwsawa M, Kurihara H, Kimura S, et al. A novel potent vasocontrictor peptide produced by vascular endothelial cells. Nature 1988; 332:411–415.
105. Achmad TH, Rao GS. Chemotaxis of human blood monocytes toward endothelin-1 and the influence of calcium channel blockers. Biochem Biophys Res Commun 1992; 189:994–1000.
106. Ohlstein EH, Arleth A, Bryan H, Elliott JD, Sung CP. The selective ETA receptor antagonist BQ 123 antagonizes endothelin-1-mediated mitogenesis. Eur J Pharmacol 1992; 225:347–350.
107. Lerman A, Edwards BS, Hallett JW, Heublein DM, Sandberg SM, Burnett JC Jr. Circulating and tissue endothelin immunoreactivity in advanced atherosclerosis. N Engl J Med 1991; 325:997–1001.
108. Winkles JA, Alberts GF, Brogi E, Libby P. Endothelin and endothelin receptor MRNA expression in normal and atherosclerotic artiers. Biochem Biophys Res Commun 1993; 191:1081–1088.
109. Boulanger CM, Tanner FC, Bea ML, Hahn AWA, Wemer A, Luscher TF. Oxidized low density lipoproteins induce MRNA expression and release of endothelin from human and porcine endothelium. Circ Res 1992; 70:1191–1197.
110. Kowala MC, Rose PM, Stein PD, et al. Selective blockade of the endothelin subtype A receptor decreases early atherosclerosis in hamsters fed cholesterol. Am J Pathol 1995; 146:819–826.
111. Steinberg D, Parthasarathy S, Carew TE, Khoo JC, Witztum JL. Beyond cholesterol. Modifications of low density lipoprotein that increase its atherogenicity. N Engl J Med 1989; 32:915–924.
112. Witztum JL, Steinberg D. Role of oxidized low density lipoprotein in atherogenesis. J Clin Invest 1991; 88:1785–1792.
113. Goldstein JL, Ho YK, Basu SK, Brown MS. Binding site of macrophages that mediates uptake and degradation of acetylate low density lipoprotein, producing massive cholesterol deposition. Proc Natl Acad Sci USA 1979; 76:333–337.
114. Morel DW, Hcsslcr JR, Chisolm GM. Low density lipoprotein cytotoxicity induced by free radical peroxidation of lipid. J Lipid Res 1983; 24:1070–1076.
115. Parthasarathy S, Rankin SM. Role of oxidized low density lipoprotein in atherogenesis. Prog Lipid Res 1992; 31:127–143.

116. Jialal I, Fuller CJ. Effect of vitamin E, vitamin C and beta-carotene on LDL oxidation and atherosclerosis. Can J Cardiol 1995; 11(suppl G): 97G–103G.
117. Steinberg D. Role of oxidized LDL and antioxidants in atherosclerosis. In: Longenecker J.B., ed. Nutrition and Biotechnology in Heart Disease and Cancer. New York: Plenum Press, 1995.
118. Daugherty A, Roselaar SE. Lipoprotein oxidation as a mediator of atherogenesis: insights from pharmacological studies. Cardiovasc Res 1994; 29:297–311.
119. Latron Y, Chautan M, Anfosso F, et al. Stimulating effect of oxidized low density lipoproteins on plasminogen activator inhibitor-I synthesis by endothelial cells. Arterioscler Thromb 1991; 11:1821–1829.
120. Tanner FC, Noll G, Boulanger CM, Luscher TF. Oxidized density lipoproteins inhibit relaxations of porcine coronary arteries: role of scavenger receptor and endothelium-derived nitric oxide. Circulation 1991; 83:2012–2020.
121. Chin JH, Azhar S, Hoffman BB. Inactivation of endothelial derived relaxing factor by oxidized lipoproteins. J Clin Invest 1992; 89:10–18.
122. Thomas CE, Jackson RL, Dhlweiler DF, Ku G. Multiple lipid oxidation products in low density lipoproteins induce interleukin-I beta release from human blood mononuclear cells. J Lipid Res 1994; 35:417–427.
123. Drake TA, Hannani K, Fei HH, Lavi S, Berliner JA. Minimally oxidized low-density lipoprotein induces tissue factor expression in cultured human endothelial cells. Am J Pathol 1991; 138:601–607.
124. Leung WH, Lau CP, Wong CK. Beneficial effects of cholesterol-lowering therapy on coronary endothelium-dependent relaxation in hypercholesterolemic patients. Lancet 1993; 341:1496–1500.
125. Egashira K, Hirooka Y, Kai H, et al. Reduction in serum cholesterol with pravastatin improves endothelium-dependent coronary vasomotion in patients with hypercholesterolemia. Circulation 1994; 89:2519–2524.
126. Treasure CB, Klein JL, Weintraub WS, et al. Beneficial effects of cholesterol-lowering therapy on the coronary endothelium in patients with coronary artery disease. N Engl J Med 1995; 332:481–487.
127. Anderson TJ, Meredith IT, Yeung AC, Frei B, Selwyn AP, Ganz P. The effect of cholesterol-lowering and antioxidant therapy on endothelium-dependent coronary vasomotion. N Engl J Med 1995; 332:488–493.
128. Ting HH, Timimi FK, Boles KS, Creager SJ, Ganz P, Creager MA. Vitamin C improves endothelium-dependent vasodilation in patients with non-insulin-dependent diabetes mellitus. J Clin Invest 1996; 97:22–28.
129. Keaney JF Jr, Xu A, Cunningham D, Jackson T, Frei B, Vita JA. Dietary probucol preserves endothelial function in cholesterol-fed rabbits by limiting vascular oxidative stress and superoxide generation. J Clin Invest 1995; 95:2520–2529.
130. Simon BC, Haudenschild CC, Cohen RA. Preservation of endothelium-dependent relaxation in atherosclerotic rabbit aorta by probucol. J Cardiovasc Pharmacol 1993; 21:893–901.
131. Bjorkhem I, Henriksson-Freyschuss A, Breuer 0, Diezfalusy U, Berglund L, Henriksson P. The antioxidant butylated hydroxytoluene protects against atherosclerosis. Arterioscler Thromb 1991; 11:15–22.

132. Sparrow CP, Doebber TW, Olsezewski J, et al. Low density lipoprotein is protected from oxidation and the progression of atherosclerosis is slowed in cholesterol-fed rabbits by the antioxidant N,N'-diphenylphenylenediamine. J Clin Invest 1992; 89:1885–1891.

133. Shaish A, Daughtery A, O'Sullivan F, Schonfeld G, Heinecke JW. Beta-carotene inhibits atherosclerosis in hypercholesterolemic rabbits. J Clin Invest 1995; 96: 2075–2082.

134. Mahley RW. Development of accelerate datherosclcrosis: concepts derived from cell biology and animal models. Arch Pathol Lab Med 1983; 107:393–399.

135. Yla-Herttuala S, Palinski W, Rosenfeld ME, et al. Evidence for the presence of oxidatively modified low density lipoprotein in atherosclerotic lesions of rabbit and man. J Clin Invest 1989; 84:1086–1095.

136. Salonen JT, Yla-Herttuala S, Yamamoto R, et al. Auto-antibody against oxidized LDL and progression of carotid atherosclerosis. Lancet 1992; 339:883–887.

137. Blann AD, Maxwell SRJ, Barrows G, Miller JP. Antioxidants, Von Willebrand factor and endothelial cell injury in hypercholesterolaemia and vascular disease. Atherosclerosis 1995; 116:191–198.

138. Regnstrom J, Nilsson J, Tomvall P, Landou C, Hamsten A. Susceptibility to low-density lipoprotein oxidation and coronary atherosclerosis in man. Lancet 1992; 339:1183–1186.

139. Gey KF, Puska P, Jordan P, Moser UK. Inverse correlation between plasma vitamin E and mortality from ischemic heart diseae in cross-cultural epidemiology. Am J Clin Nutr 1991; 53:326–334.

140. Riemersma RA, Oliver MF, Elton RA, et al. Plasma antioxidants and coronary heart disease: vitamins C and E and selenium. Eur J Clin Nur 1990; 44:143–150.

141. Office of Population and Censuses and Surveys. Dietary Nutrional Study of British Adults. London: HMSO, 1990.

142. Fulton M, Thomson M, Elton RA, et al. Cigarette smoking, social class and nutrient intake: relevance to coronary heart disease. Eur J Clin Nutr 1988; 42: 797–803.

143. Hertog MGL, Feskens EJM, Hollman PCH, et al. Dietary antioxidant flavonoids and risk of coronary heart disease: the Zutphen Elderly Study. Lancet 1993; 342:1007–1011.

144. Frankel EN, Kanner J, German GB, et al. Inhibition of oxidation of human lowdensity lipoprotein by phenolic substances in red wine. Lancet 1993; 341: 454–457.

145. Kalra J, Chaudhary AK, Prasad K. Increased production of oxygen free radicals in cigarette smokers. Int J Exp Path 1991; 72:1–71.

146. Mancini M, Parfitt VJ, Rubba P. Antioxidants in teh Mediterranean diet. Can J Cardiol 1995; 11 (suppl G) 105G–109G.

147. Riemersma RA, Wood DA, Macintyre CAA, et al. Risk of angina pectoris and plasma concentrations of vitamins A, C, and E and carotene. Lancet 1991; 337:1–5.

148. Stampfer MJ, Hennekens CH, Manson JE, et al. Vitamin E consumption and the risk of comary heart disease in women. N Engl J Med 1993; 328:1444–1449.

149. Kritchevsky SB, Shimakawa T, Tell GS, et al. Dietary antioxidants and carotid artery wall thickness. The ARIC Study. Circulation 1995; 92:2142–2150.
150. Hodis HN, Mack WJ, LaBree L, et al. Serial coronary angiographic evidence that antioxidant vitamin intake reduces progression of coronary artery atherosclerosis. JAMA 1995; 273:1849–1854.
151. Alpha-Tocopherol, Beta Carotene Cancer Prevention Study Group. The effect of vitamin E and beta carotene on the incidence of lung cancer and the other cancers in male smokers. N Engl J Med 1994; 330:1029–1035.
152. Walldius G, Erikson U, Olsson AG, et al. The effect of probucol on femoral atherosclerosis: the Probucol Quantitative Regression Swedish Trial (PQRST). Am J Cardiol 1994; 74:875–883.
153. Carew T, Schwenke DC, Steinberg D. Antiatherogenic effect of probucol unrelated to its hypocholesterolemic effect: evidence that antioxidants in vivo can selectively inhibit low density lipoprotein degradation in macrophagerich fatty streaks and slow the progression of atherosclerosis in the Watanabe heritable hyperlipidemic rabbit. Proc Natl Acad Sci USA 1987; 84:7725–7729.
154. Bagdade JD, Kaufmann D, Ritter MC, Subbaiah PV. Probucol treatment in hypercholeserolemic patients: effects of lipoprotein composition, HDL partical size, cholesteryl ester transfer. Atherosclerosis 1990; 84:145–154.
155. Schaefer-Elinder L, Hadell K, Johansson J, et al. Probucol treatment decreases serum concentrations of diet-derived antioxidants. Arterloscler Thromb Vasc Biol 1995; 15:1057–1063.
156. Stephesn NG, Parsons A, Schofield PM, et al. Randomised controlled trial of vitamin E in patients with coronary disease: Cambridge Heart Antioxidant Study (CHAOS). Lancet 1996; 347:781–786.
157. Steinberg D. Clinical trials of antioxidants in atherosclerosis: are we doing the right thing? Lancet 1995; 346:36–38.
158. Oliver MF. Antioxidant nutrients, atherosclerosis, and coronary heart disease. Br Heart J 1995; 73:299–301.
159. Jialal I, Fuller CJ. Effect of vitamin E, vitamin C and beta-carotene on LDL oxidation and atherosclerosis. Can J Cardiol 1995; 11(suppl G): 97G–103G.
160. Daugherty A, Roselaar SE. Lipoprotein oxidation as a mediator of atherogenesis: insights from pharmacological studies. Cardiovasc Res 1995; 29:297–311.
161. Tikkanen MJ, Nikkila EA, Vartianen E. Natural oestrogen as an effective treatment for type-II hyperlipoproteinemia in postmenopausal women. Lancet 1978; 2:490–491.
162. Granfone A, Campos H, McNamara JR, et al. Effects of estrogen replacement on plasma lipoproteins and apolipoproteins in postmenopausal, dyslipidemic women. Metabolism 1992; 41:1193–1198.
163. Lobo RA. Effects of hormonal replacement on lipids and lipoproteins in postmenopausal women. J Clin Endocrinol Metab 1991; 73:925–930.
164. Walsh BW, Schiff 1, Rosner B, Greenberg L, Ravnikar V, Sacks FM. Effects of postmenopausal estrogen replacement on the concentrations and metabolism of plasma lipoproteins. N Engl J Med 1991; 325:1196–1204.

165. The Writing Group for the PEPI Trial. Effects of estrogen or estrogen/progestin regimens on heart disease risk factors in postmenopausal women: the Postmenopausal Estrogen/Progestin Interventions (PEPI) trial. JAMA 1995; 273:199–208.
166. Bush TL, Barrett-Connor E, Cowan LD, et al. Cardiovascular mortality and noncontraceptive use of estrogen in women: results from the Lipid Research Clinics Program follow-up study. Circulation 1987; 75:1102–1109.
167. Williams JK, Adams MR, Klopfenstein HB. Estrogen modulates responses of atherosclerotic coronary arteries. Circulation 1990; 81:1680–1687.
168. Gisclard V, Miller VM, Vanlioutte PM. Effect of 17-b estradiol on endothelium-dependent responses in the rabbit. J Pharmacol Exp Ther 1988; 244:19–22.
169. Miller VM, Gisclard V, Vanhoutte PM. Modulation of endothelium-dependent and vascular smooth muscle responses by oestrogens. Phlebology 1988; 3:63–69.
170. Gilligan DM, Quyyumi AA, Cannon RO. Effects of physiological levels of estrogen on coronary vasomotor function in postmenopausal women. Circulation 1994; 89:2545–2551.
171. Reis SE, Gloth ST, Blumenthal RS, et al. Ethinyl estradiol acutely attenuates abnormal coronary vasomotor responses to acetylcholine in postmenopausal women. Circulation 1994; 89:52–60.
172. Lieberman EH, Gerhard M, Yeung AC, et al. Estrogen improves coronary vasomotor responses to acetylcholine in postmenopausal women. Circulation 1993; 88(suppl 1):1–79. Abstract.
173. Williams JK, Adams MR, Herrington DM, Clarkson TB. Short-term administration of estrogen and vascular responses of atherosclerotic coronary arteries. J Am Coll Cardiol 1992; 20:452–457.
174. Lieberman EH, Gerhard MD, Uehata A, et al. Estrogen improves endothelium-dependent flow-mediated vasodilation in postmenopausal women. Ann Intem Med 1994; 121:936–941.
175. Gerhard M, Ganz P. How do we explain the clinical benefits of estrogen? From bedside to bench. Circulation 1995; 92:5–8.
176. Hayashi T, Yamada K, Esaki T, et al. Estrogen increases endothelial nitric oxide by a receptor-mediated system. Biochem Biophys Res Comm 1995; 214:847–855.
177. Hayashi T, Fukoto JM, Ignarro LJ, Chaudhuri C. Basal release of NO from aortic rings is greater in female rabbits than in male rabbits: implications for atherosclerosis. Proc Natl Acad Sci USA 1992; 89:11259–11263.
178. Sugioka JM, Shimosegawa Y, Nakano MM. Estrogens as natural antioxidants of membrane lipid peroxidation. FEBS Lett 1987; 210:37–39.
179. Miller VM, Gisclard V, Vanhoutte PM. Alpha adrenergic responses of blood vessels of rabbits after ovariectomy and administration of estrogen. J Pharmacol Exp Ther 1987; 240:466–470.
180. Chang WC, Nakao J, Orimo H, Murota SI. Stimulation of prostacyclin activity in rat aorta smooth muscle cells in culture. Biochim Biophys Acta 1980; 619:107–118.
181. Gisclard V, Miller VM, Vanhoutte PM. Effect of estrogen on endothelium-dependent responses in the rabbit. J Pharmacol Exp Ther 1988; 244:19–22.

182. Miller VM, Vanhoutte PM. Progesterone and modulation of endothelium-dependent responses in canine coronary arteries. Am J Physiol 1991; 261:1022–1027.
183. Gisclard V, Flavahan NA, Vanhoutte PM. Alpha adrenergic responses, of blood vessels of rabbits after ovariectomy and administration of estrogen. J Pharmacol Exp Ther 1987; 240:466–470.
184. Jiang C, Sarrel PM, Poole-Wilson PA, Collins P. Acute effect of 17b-estradiol on rabbit coronary artery contractile responses to endothelin-1. Am J Physiol 1992; 263:H271–H275.
185. Zhang F, Ram JL, Standley PR, Sowers JR. 17b-estradiol attenuates voltage-dependent Ca2l currents in vascular smooth muscle. Am J Physiol 1994; 193: C975–C980.
186. Proudler AJ, Ahmed AIH, Crook D, Fogelman I, Rymer JM, Stevenson JC. Hormone replaement therapy and serum angiotensin-converting-enzyme activity in postmenopausal women. Lancet 1995; 346:89–90.
187. Morales DE, McGowan KA, Grant DS, et al. Estrogen promotes angiogenic activity in human umbilical vein endothelial cells in vitro and in a murine model. Circulation 1995; 91:755–763.
188. Little WC, Constantinescu M, Applegate RJ, et al. Can coronary angiography predict the site of a subsequent myocardial infarction in patients with mild to moderate coronary artery disease? Circulation 1988; 78:1157–1166.
189. Beldekas JC, Smith B, Gerstenfeld LC, Sonenshein GE, Franzblau C. Effects of estrogen on the biosynthesis of collagen in cultured bovine aortic smooth muscle cells. Biochemistry 1981; 20:2162–2167.
190. Fischer GM, Swain ML. Effects of estradiol and progesterone on the increased synthesis of collagen in atherosclerotic rabbit aortas. Atherosclerosis 1985; 54: 1770–1785.
191. Fischer GM, Cherian K, Swain ML. Increased synthesis of aortic collagen and elastin in experimental atherosclerosis. Atherosclerosis 1981; 39:463–467.
192. Shahar E, Folsom AR, Salomaa VV, et al. Relation of hormone-replacement therapy to measure sof plasma fibrinolytic activity. Circulation 1996; 93:1970–1975.
193. Nabulshi AA, Folsom AR, White A, et al. Association of hormone-replacement therapy with various cardiovascular risk factors in postmenopausal women. N Engl J Med 1993; 328:1069–1075.
194. Meade TW. Clotting factors and ischamic heart disease: the epidemiologic evidence. In: Meade TW, ed. Anticoagulants and Myocardial Infarction: A Reappraisal. New York: John Wiley, 1984:91–111.
195. Ylikorkala O, Kuusi T, Tikkanen MJ, Viinikka L. Desogestrel- and levonorgestrel-containing oral contraceptives have different effects on urinary excretion of prostacyclin metabolites and serum high density lipoproteins. J Clinc Endocrinol Metab 1987; 65:1238–1242.
196. Manson JE. Postmenopausal hormone therapy and atherosclerotic disease. Am Heart J 1994; 128:1337–1343.

197. Eaker ED, Chesebro JK, Sacks FM, Wenger NK, Whisnant JP, Winston M. Cardiovascular disease in women. Circulation 1993; 88:1999–2009.

198. Kannel WB, Hjortland MC, McNamara PM, Gordon T. Menopause and the risk of cardiovascular disease: the Framingham Study. Ann Intern Med 1976; 85:447–452.

199. Stampfer MJ, Colditz GA, Willett WC, et al. Postmenopausal estrogen therapy and cardiovascular disease: ten-year follow-up from the Nurses' Health Study. N Engl J Med 1991; 325:756–762.

200. Grady D, Rubin SM, Petitti DB, et al. Hormone therapy to prevent disease and prolong life in postmenopausal women. Ann Intern Med 1992; 117:1016–1037.

201. Miller VM, Vanhoutte PM. Progesterone and modulation of endothelium-dependent responses in canine coronary arteries. Am J Physiol 1991; 261:R1022–1027.

202. Williams JK, Honore EK, Washburn SA, Clarkson TB. Effects of hormone replacement therapy on reactivity of atherosclerotic coronary arteries in cynomolgus monkeys. J Am Coll Cardiol 1994; 24:1757–1761.

203. Writing Group for the PEPI Trial. Effects of estrogen or estrogen/progestin regimens on heart disease risk factors in postmenopausal women: the Postmenopausal Estrogen/Progestin Interventions (PEPI) trial. JAMA 1995; 273:199–208.

204. Gebara OCE, Mittleman MA, Sutherland P, Lipinska I, Matheney. Association between increased estrogen status and increased fibrinolytic potential in the Framingham Offspring Study. Circulation 1995; 91:1952–1958.

205. Nachtigall LE, Nachtigall RH, Nachtigall RD, Beckman EM. Estrogen replacement therapy. II. A prospective study in the relationship to carcinoma and cardiovascular and metabolic problems. Obstet Gynecol 1979; 54:74–79.

206. Falkebom M, Persson I, Adami HO, et al. The risk of acute myocardial infarction after oestrogen and oestrogen-progestogen replacement. Br J Obstet Gynaecol 1992; 99:821–828.

207. Hennekens CH, Buring JE, Sandercock P, Collins R, Peto R. Aspirin and other antiplatelet agents in the secondary and primary prevention of cardiovascular disease. Circulation 1989; 80:746–756.

208. Numano F, Kishi Y, Ashikaga T, Hata A, Makita T, Watanabe R. What effect does controlling platelets have on atherosclerosis?

209. Davies MJ, Thomas AC. Plaque fissuring: the cause of acute myocardial infarction, sudden ischemic death and crescendo angina. Br Heart J 1985; 53:363–373.

210. Fuster V, Badimon L, Badimon JJ, Chesebro JH. The pathogensis of comary artery disease and the acute coronary syndromes. N Engl J Med 1992; 326:242–250.

211. Fuster V, Badimon L, Badimon JJ, Chesebro JH. Pathogenesis of coronary artery disease and the acute coronary syndromes, 2. N Engl J Med 1992; 326:310–318.

212. Davies MJ, Bland JM, Haiigartner JWR, Angelini A, Thomas AC. Factors influencing the presence or absence of acute coronary artery thrombi in sudden ischaemic death. Eur Heart J 1989; 10:203–208.

213. Wilcox JN. Thrombotic mechanisms in atherosclerosis. Coron Artery Dis 1994; 5:223–229.

214. Steering Committee of the Physicians' Health Study Research Group. Final report on the aspirin component of the onging Physicians' Health Study. N Engl J Med 1989; 321:129–135.
215. Buring JE, Hennekens CH, Women's Health Study Research Group. The Women's Health Study: rationale and background. J Myocard Ischemia 1992; 4:30–40.

8
Prevention of Atherosclerosis in Clinical Practice

Robert A. Vogel
University of Maryland School of Medicine, Baltimore, Maryland

I. INTRODUCTION

Coronary heart disease is both highly prevalent and preventable. As is detailed in prior chapters, coronary risk factors play key roles in the genesis of atherosclerosis and the occurrence of cardiovascular events (1–8). Lipid accumulation and modification, endothelial dysfunction, vasoactivity, local plaque inflammation, and thrombogenicity are major pathophysiological factors in plaque accumulation and disruption. The presence of established coronary heart disease increases the risks of an additional event approximately sixfold at any given risk factor burden (9). Risk factor modification and the use of vasoprotective drugs have been shown to extend overall survival, improve the quality of life, decrease the need for coronary revascularization procedures, and reduce the incidence of subsequent myocardial infarctions in patients with established coronary heart disease (secondary prevention) (10–21). Despite considerable evidence supporting a substantial effect for risk factor modification, many patients are not counseled regarding risk factors and do not receive vasoprotective medications (22–25). This "treatment gap" adversely affects the outcome of patients with established coronary heart disease (26,27). The treatment gap is due to several complex factors, including physician misperceptions, difficulty in changing lifestyles, long-term patient compliance, and economics (28,29). This chapter summarizes the current secondary prevention standards for patient counseling, risk factor modification, and administration of vasoprotective drugs, and provides clinical treatment algorithms and suggestions for real-world implementation.

Guide to Comprehensive Risk Reduction
for Patients With Coronary and Other Vascular Disease

Risk Intervention	Recommendations
Smoking: Goal complete cessation	Strongly encourage patient and family to stop smoking. Provide counseling, nicotine replacement, and formal cessation programs as appropriate.
Lipid management: Primary goal LDL<100 mg/dL Secondary goals HDL>35 mg/dL; TG<200 mg/dL	Start AHA Step II Diet in all patients: ≤30% fat, <7% saturated fat, <200 mg/d cholesterol. Assess fasting lipid profile. In post-MI patients, lipid profile may take 4 to 6 weeks to stabilize. Add drug therapy according to the following guide:

LDL<100 mg/dL	LDL 100 to 130 mg/dL	LDL>130 mg/dL	HDL<35 mg/dL
No drug therapy	Consider adding drug therapy to diet, as follows:	Add drug therapy to diet, as follows:	Emphasize weight management and physical activity. Advise smoking cessation. If needed to achieve LDL goals, consider niacin, statin, fibrate.

	↘		↙	
		Suggested drug therapy		

TG <200 mg/dL	TG 200 to 400 mg/dL	TG >400 mg/dL
Statin Resin Niacin	Statin Niacin	Consider combined drug therapy (niacin, fibrate, statin)

If LDL goal not achieved, consider combination therapy.

Risk Intervention	Recommendations
Physical activity: Minimum goal 30 minutes 3 to 4 times per week	Assess risk, preferably with exercise test, to guide prescription. Encourage minimum of 30 to 60 minutes of moderate-intensity activity 3 or 4 times weekly (walking, jogging, cycling, or other aerobic activity) supplemented by an increase in daily lifestyle activities (eg, walking breaks at work, using stairs, gardening, household work). Maximum benefit 5 to 6 hours a week. Advise medically supervised programs for moderate- to high-risk patients.
Weight management:	Start intensive diet and appropriate physical activity intervention, as outlined above, in patients >120% of ideal weight for height. Particularly emphasize need for weight loss in patients with hypertension, elevated triglycerides, or elevated glucose levels.
Antiplatelet agents/ **anticoagulants:**	Start aspirin 80 to 325 mg/d if not contraindicated. Manage warfarin to international normalized ratio=2 to 3.5 for post-MI patients not able to take aspirin.
ACE inhibitors **post-MI:**	Start early post-MI in stable high-risk patients (anterior MI, previous MI, Killip class II [S₃ gallop, rales, radiographic CHF]). Continue indefinitely for all with LV dysfunction (ejection fraction≤40%) or symptoms of failure. Use as needed to manage blood pressure or symptoms in all other patients.
Beta-blockers:	Start in high-risk post-MI patients (arrhythmia, LV dysfunction, inducible ischemia) at 5 to 28 days. Continue 6 months minimum. Observe usual contraindications. Use as needed to manage angina rhythm or blood pressure in all other patients.
Estrogens:	Consider estrogen replacement in all postmenopausal women. Individualize recommendation consistent with other health risks.
Blood pressure **control:** Goal ≤140/90 mm Hg	Initiate lifestyle modification—weight control, physical activity, alcohol moderation, and moderate sodium restriction—in all patients with blood pressure>140 mm Hg systolic or 90 mm Hg diastolic. Add blood pressure medication, individualized to other patient requirements and characteristics (ie, age, race, need for drugs with specific benefits) if blood pressure is not less than 140 mm Hg systolic or 90 mm Hg diastolic in 3 months or if *initial* blood pressure is >160 mm Hg systolic or 100 mm Hg diastolic.

ACE indicates angiotensin-converting enzyme; MI, myocardial infarction; TG, triglycerides; and LV, left ventricular.

Figure 1   Overall preventive cardiology recommendations of the American Heart Association (30).

II. SECONDARY PREVENTION TREATMENT GOALS

Ten treatment goals are recommended for secondary prevention of coronary heart disease by the American Heart Association (30) (Figure 1). The recommendations for lipid management follow the guidelines of the National Cholesterol Education Program (NCEP) (31). Additionally, the control of diabetes mellitus and moderation in the use of alcohol in patients with hypertension or congestive heart failure are helpful measures (30,32–34). Together, these 12 goals should be integrated into the management of all coronary heart disease patients:

A. Patient Counseling Measures

1. Smoking cessation
2. Weight reduction to a body mass index < 25 kg/m^2
   Total fat intake < 60 g/day
   Saturated fat intake < 15 g/day
   Cholesterol intake < 200 mg/day
3. Physical exercise for at least 30 min three to five times per week
4. Limitation of alcohol intake to < 1 oz/day for patients with hypertension or hypertriglyceridemia
   Alcohol abstinence for patients with congestive heart failure

B. Risk Factor Modification

5. Reduction of low-density lipoprotein cholesterol (LDL-C) to < 100 mg/dl
6. Increase in high-density lipoprotein cholesterol (HDL-C) to > 35 mg/dl
7. Control of blood pressure to $< 140/90$ mm Hg
8. Control of diabetes by reducing hemoglobin-A$_{1c}$ to $< 7\%$

C. Vasoprotective Drugs

9. Aspirin 80 to 325 mg/day
10. Beta blocker for patients within 2 years of a Q-wave myocardial infarction
11. ACE-inhibitor for patients with left ventricular ejection fraction (LVEF) $< 40\%$
12. Hormone replacement therapy for postmenopausal women

Hypertension, hypercholesterolemia, and cigarette smoking are the three major modifiable risk factors for coronary heart disease (35,36). The recent decline in age-adjusted mortality from coronary heart disease is substantially due to decreases in these factors (37–40). A 1% decline in mean blood pressure and serum cholesterol results in a 2% to 4% and 1% to 1.5% decrease in subsequent cardiovascular events, respectively (41–44). For every 1% decrease in cigarette smoking prevalence, a 0.5% reduction in clinical events results (45–47). The strongest evidence that total cholesterol and LDL-C are causally related to the development of coronary heart disease is derived from randomized, controlled primary and secondary prevention clinical trials. The Lipid Research Clinic Coronary Primary Prevention Trial (LRC-CPPT) and the Helsinki Heart Study, also a primary prevention trial, demonstrated significant decreases in nonfatal cardiovascular events in hypercholesterolemic healthy men using cholestyramine and gemfibrozil, respectively (41,42).

During the past 10 years, 16 randomized trials have investigated whether cholesterol lowering was associated with reduced rates of angiographic progression of coronary atherosclerosis (13,48–57). Fifteen of the 16 trials demonstrated angiographic improvement in those randomized to lipid lowering in the form of less disease progression, more stability of lesions, and/or more disease regression than in the control group. An unexpected observation in these angiographic trials was a 40% to 50% reduction in clinical cardiovascular events, despite modest although statistically significant decreases in coronary heart disease progression. These preliminary findings set the stage for three major clinical trials: the Scandinavian Simvastatin Survival Study (4S) (16) (secondary prevention, markedly hypercholesterolemic population); West of Scotland Coronary Prevention Study (WOSCOPS) (17) (primary prevention, markedly hypercholesterolemic population); and Cholesterol and Recurrent Events Study (CARE) (58) (secondary prevention, mildly hypercholesterolemic population). Importantly, the 4S trial demonstrated a 30% reduction in all-cause mortality (182 and 256 deaths, treatment and control groups, respectively) in subjects with established coronary heart disease (80% prior myocardial infarction) randomized to simvastatin. Mean cholesterol was reduced from 260 to 189 mg/dl in this 5.4-year trial. Cholesterol reduction was also associated with an approximately 40% reduction in myocardial infarction, need for coronary revascularization, stroke or transient ischemic attack, and episodes of unstable angina. No increases were observed in noncardiovascular morbidity or mortality. Estimates of cost-effectiveness for translating the 4S trial results into an American population suggests an expense of $3800 per year of life saved (59). Treating less hypercholesterolemic individuals would cost an approximately $10,000 per year of life saved (60–62). (See chapter on cost-effectiveness.)

Unlike the population studied in the 4S trial, the mean cholesterol of coronary heart disease patients in the United States is 224 mg/dl. The CARE (58) trial assessed the effect of pravastatin 40 mg/day in patients with prior myocardial infarction and serum cholesterol < 240 mg/dl. Mean baseline total and LDL-cholesterol in this study were 209 mg/dl and 139 mg/dl, respectively. A 32% reduction in LDL-cholesterol was observed in the treatment group. Two hundred six and 269 coronary heart disease deaths plus nonfatal myocardial infarctions were observed in the pravastatin and control groups, respectively (24% risk reduction). Significant reductions in total myocardial infarctions and need for coronary revascularization were also observed. Similar benefit was observed for subjects above and below 60 years of age, men and women, ejection greater or < 40%, as well as in smoking, diabetic, and hypertensive patients.

The WOSCOPS trial assessed the effect of pravastatin 40 mg/day in middle-aged men without known coronary heart disease with a mean cholesterol of 272 mg/dl (17). In this high-risk primary prevention population, 20% and 26% reductions in total and LDL-cholesterol were associated with 248 definite coronary events (coronary heart disease, death plus nonfatal myocardial infarction) in the control group and 174 in the pravastatin group (31% risk reduction). Taken together, the 4S, CARE, and WOSCOPS trials demonstrated conclusive reductions in cardiovascular mortality and morbidity in patients with established coronary heart disease and in high-risk primary prevention populations. Justification for the NCEP recommendation to lower LDL-cholesterol to < 100 mg/dl comes from the post-CABG trial. (63) This angiographic progression study of 1351 men and women who had previously undergone coronary artery bypass surgery compared moderate versus aggressive cholesterol reduction and low-dose warfarin versus placebo administration in a 2 × 2 factorial design trial. The mean LDL-cholesterol levels in the moderate and aggressive cholesterol reduction groups were 135 and 95 mg/dl, respectively. Preliminary data suggest reduced progression of bypass graft atherosclerosis in the aggressive versus moderate cholesterol reduction group. No benefit was observed in the use of low-dose warfarin. An 18% reduction in cardiovascular events ($P = .09$) was observed in the aggressive cholesterol reduction group. This trial strongly supports the use of aggressive dietary and drug means for lowering cholesterol in coronary heart disease (CHD) patients.

As is detailed in the following management algorithms, NCEP/AHA step II diets should be employed in all CHD patients (30,31,64). Whereas encouragement of dietary modification should be undertaken for a protracted period of time in primary prevention populations, diet and drug therapy should be initiated simultaneously in patients with CHD and LDL-cholesterol > 130 mg/dl with a goal of reducing LDL-cholesterol to < 100 mg/dl. Justification for the simultaneous institution of drug and dietary therapy comes from both the 4S and WOSCOPS trials, which demonstrated significant reductions in cardiovascular events within 1 to 2 years of institution of drug therapy. The demonstrated early benefit supports the practice of aggressively lowering cholesterol as soon as the diagnosis of CHD is made. Aggressive diet modification (< 10% of calories from fat) has also been demonstrated to slow the progression of angiographic coronary artery disease (Lifestyle Heart Trial) without need for additional drugs (51). Improvements in myocardial perfusion have also been shown with aggressive diet modification and are probably related to improvements in small vessel endothelial function (65). Aggressive diet modification beyond a step II diet should be instituted in all patients willing to undertake this lifestyle change.

As with cholesterol, there is a large body of data relating both diastolic and systolic blood pressure to cardiovascular disease risk. Although significant diastolic hypertension (> 105 mm Hg) is associated with a fourfold increase in risk of CHD relative to the lowest quartile of risk, there appears to be a continuous, graded relationship between blood pressure and risks, with no evidence of a "threshold" (44). The importance of systolic blood pressure was emphasized in the MRFIT trial, which demonstrated that the risk of CHD, stroke, and all-cause mortality was more correlated with systolic than with diastolic pressure (66). This was confirmed in the Systolic Hypertension in the Elderly Program (SHEP), which demonstrated a 25% reduction in CHD events and a 36% reduction in stroke in subjects > 60 years of age with control of systolic hypertension (67). In general, randomized controlled trials of blood pressure reduction have demonstrated greater decreases in cerebrovascular events than in CHD events.

Cigarette smoking ranks as the largest preventable cause of CHD and is responsible for 400,000 premature deaths in the United States annually (45,46). Observational studies have consistently shown that nonsmokers and former smokers have significantly lower rates of CHD events than current smokers. Three randomized smoking cessation trials in primary prevention populations have demonstrated 7% to 47% reductions in CHD event rates. After acute myocardial infarction (AMI), smoking cessation is associated with an approximately 50% reduction in mortality (47). Despite this evident benefit, only 28% of patients with AMI are counseled to stop smoking (Cooperative Cardiovascular Project; see below) (23). As part of a comprehensive risk factor management program, smoking cessation counseling cost-effectiveness has been estimated at $200/year of life saved (47).

In addition to reductions in cholesterol, hypertension, and smoking, antiplatelet therapy in all patients with established CHD and beta-blocking therapy in medium- and high-risk coronary disease patients are clearly beneficial (14,68,69,70). Other data from the Cooperative Cardiovascular Project suggests that patients with AMI prescribed aspirin at discharge have 50% less mortality at 6 months (8.4% versus 17%) compared with those not receiving aspirin (26,27). The value of aspirin in primary prevention is less clear. Whereas the 22,000 male subjects United States Physician Health Study found a 44% reduction in the incidence of myocardial infarction (0.4% to 0.2% per year), limited to those > 50 years, the 5000 male-subjects British Doctors' Trial found no benefit (71,72). Other interventions demonstrated to lower the risk of CHD include rehabilitation and increased physical activity, control of diabetes mellitus, ACE inhibitor administration with reduced LVEF and hormone replacement therapy (HRT) (10,15,20,73–85).

The following pages present management algorithms or "clinical pathways" for achieving these 12 goals.

D. Management Algorithm for Smoking

1. Determine past and present tobacco use.
2. Assess motivation for smoking cessation (major determinant for likelihood of success and approach).
3. Provide detailed patient (and family) education.
4. Present options (counseling, smoking cessation programs, hypnosis, nicotine substitution drugs).
5. Utilize organized long-term counseling and cessation programs.
6. Provide long-term encouragement and reinforcement.
7. Consider nicotine substitution drugs (nicotine gum 2 mg, initial dose approximately 10/day; nicotine patch, initial dose 21 mg/day) with gradually decreasing dosage. These are effective only when used with organized behavioral modification program. Patients must not smoke when using nicotine gum/patch.

E. Management Algorithm for Diet

1. Assess current diet, height, weight, activity level, and lipid profile.
2. Reduce caloric intake (and increase activity) to reduce BMI < 25 kg/m^2. [body mass index = weight in kg/(height in m^2)]
3. If LDL-cholesterol > 100 mg/dl (CAD), initiate following diet:
    Total fat intake < 60 g/day
    Saturated fat intake < 15 g/day
    Cholesterol intake < 200 mg/day
    Encourage monounsaturated (olive oil) over polyunsaturated fat intake
    Increase complex carbohydrate and soluble fiber intake
    No alcohol (LVEF < 40%)
    ≤ 1 oz alcohol/day (HTN, hypertriglyceridemia)

$Na^+ < 2.3$ g/day (HTN, CHF)
4. Utilize dietician and nurse counseling.
5. Recommend educational cookbooks (examples):
   AHA Cookbook (David McKay Co.)
   New American Diet (Simon and Schuster)
   Eater's Choice: A Food Lovers Guide to Lower Cholesterol
   (Houghton Mifflin Co.)
   Dean Ornish's Program for Reversing Heart Disease
   (Random House)
   Beyond Cholesterol (Johns Hopkins University Press)
6. Provide long-term follow-up and reinforcement.

F. Management Algorithm for Exercise

1. Assess activity level, anginal status, LVEF.
2. Manage angina/ischemia maximally including consideration of revascularization.
3. Perform symptom limited stress test (treadmill ECG or thallium preferred).
4. Determine safe METS level for exercise, $\geq$ 30 min, 3–5/week as maximum exercise level without angina, evidence ischemia, arrhythmias, hypotension, excessive fatigue, or exercise SOB up to 75% APMHR (APMHR = 220 − age)

Modified Bruce Protocol

MPH	% Grade	METS	Equivalent exercise
1.7	0	2	Walking (2 MPH)
1.7	5	3.5	Dancing or calisthenics (slow)
1.7	10	5	Brisk walking (4 MPH)
2.5	12	7	Bicycling (10 MPH)
3.4	14	10	Running (12 min/mile)

5. Consider supervised exercise (rehabilitation program) for all heart patients and recommend strongly for postmyocardial infarction and revascularization patients

G. Management Algorithm for Alcohol

1. Determine alcohol intake through patient history, family discussions, and signs of alcohol abuse.

2. Alcohol intake is contraindicated in CHF (LVEF < 40%) and should be limited (< 1 oz/day) in hypertension or hypertriglyceridemia.
3. Educate and counsel patients with these conditions.
4. Refer patients/families unable/unwilling to comply to alcohol/substance abuse programs.
5. Provide long-term follow-up and reinforcement.

H. Management Algorithm for LDL-C > 100 mg/dl

1. Measure fasting lipid profile (TC, LDL-C, HDL-C, Trig).
2. Exclude secondary causes (e.g., hypothyroidism, nephrotic syndrome, DM).
3. Initiate diet:
   Weight reduction if BMI > 25 kg/m^2
   Total fat intake < 60 g/day
   Saturated fat intake < 15 g/day
   Cholesterol intake < 200 mg/day
4. Start low-dose HMG CoA (simvastatin 10 mg/day, atorvastatin 10 mg/day, lovastatin 20 mg/day, pravastatin 20 mg/day, fluvastatin 40 mg/day) at the same time initiation if LDL > 130 mg/dl. Monitor liver function tests and symptoms of myositis.
5. Repeat lipid profile in 6 weeks. If LDL > 100 mg/dl:
6. Progressively increase HMG CoA reductase inhibitor
7. Repeat lipid profile in 6 weeks. If LDL > 100 mg/dl:
8. Add bile acid sequestrant (cholestyramine 8 to 16 g/day, colestipol 10–20 g/day) if necessary
9. Repeat lipid profile in 6 weeks. If LDL > 100 mg/dl:
10. Refer to lipidologist or cardiologist if unsuccessful in lowering LDL-C < 100 mg/dl.

I. Management Algorithm for HDL-C < 35 mg/dl

1. Obtain fasting lipid profile (TC, LDL-C, HDL-C, Trig).
2. Exclude secondary causes (smoking, anabolic steroids, beta-blockers [do not discontinue latter]).
3. Increase aerobic exercise (goal 75% APMHR 30 min, 3–5/week)
4. Substitute mono-unsaturated dietary fat (olive oil) for polyunsaturated fat
5. Start nicotinic acid (niacin) 50 mg t.i.d., increase slowly to 500 mg t.i.d. Monitor liver function tests, uric acid, glucose. HMG CoA reductase inhibitors result in increased incidence (1% to 5%) of myositis (and rhabdomyolysis) if combined with nicotinic acid or

gemfibrozil. HMG CoA drug dosage should be kept low if combined with these agents.

6. Repeat lipid profile in 6 weeks.
7. If patient intolerant or nicotinic acid ineffective, replace with gemfibrozil 600 mg b.i.d.
8. If unable to raise HDL-C > 35 mg/dl, lower LDL-C (see LDL-C algorithm).
9. Refer to lipidologist or cardiologist if unable to increase HDL-C > 35 mg/dl and lower LDL-C < 100 mg/dl

J. Management Algorithm for Hypertension

1. Obtain repeated resting, seated BP determinations (both arms). If average > 140/90 manage as follows:
2. Assess fundoscopic changes, carotid bruits, cardiac heave, S_3 or S_4, abdominal bruits, peripheral pulses, neurological status.
3. Obtain urine analysis, electrolytes, creatinine, ECG, echocardiogram (for LVH, segmental dyskinesis)
4. Evidence for cardiac, cerebrovascular, or renal end-organ disease warrants more aggressive management.
5. Initiate lifestyle modifications: Weight reduction < 25 kg/m^2, increased aerobic exercise, Na$^+$ intake < 2.3 g/day (salt < 6 g/day), maintain normal K$^+$ (especially from food sources), ≤ 1 oz alcohol/day.
6. If BP response is inadequate, initiate diuretic or beta-blocker (Fifth Report of the Joint National Committee on Detection, Evaluation, and Treatment of High Blood Pressure).
7. If BP response is inadequate, increase dose and substitute or combine with ACE inhibitor or calcium antagonist.
8. If BP response is inadequate, combine with diuretic therapy or add another class of drug.
   Representative Drugs and Dosages:
   Diuretic: hydrochlorothiazide 12.5–25 mg/day
   Beta blocker: atenolol 25–100 mg/day
   Beta blocker with ISA: acebutalol 100–600 mg BID
   Alpha-beta blocker: labetolol 100–600 mg b.i.d.
   Alpha$_1$–blocker: doxazosin 1–16 mg/day
   ACE-inhibitor: lisinopril 5–40 mg/day
   Calcium antagonist: amlodipine 2.5–10 mg/day
   Central-acting alpha$_2$–agonist: clonidine 0.1–0.6 mg b.i.d.
   Peripheral acting adrenergic antagonist: guanethidine 10–100 mg/day

Direct vasodilator: minoxidil 2.5 mg/daily–40 mg b.i.d. (use with diuretic).

9. Clinical considerations:

African-Americans: beta blockers and ACE inhibitors less effective

CAD: beta blockers recommended (without ISA)

CHF: ACE inhibitors recommended

Elderly patients: treat systolic HTN

LVH: maintain effective BP control

Renal disease: often requires high-dose diuretic

10. Refer to hypertension specialist if unable to control BP < 140/90.

K. Management Algorithm for Diabetes Mellitus

1. Obtain fasting glucose in all heart patients.
2. Aggressive insulin-dependent diabetic glucose management lessens retinopathy, neuropathy, and nephropathy; may lessen cardiovascular events.
3. Institute ADA diet and exercise program to achieve BMI < 25 kg/m^2
4. Administer insulin $\geq$ 3 times/day using self-monitored glucose $\geq$ 4 times/day to achieve:

preprandial glucose: 70–120 mg/dl

postprandial glucose: < 180 mg/dl

3:00 AM glucose: > 65 mg/dl

average hemoglobin A$_{1c}$: $\leq$ 7%

5. Avoid hypoglycemia, especially in CAD and arrhythmic patients.

L. Management Algorithm for ASA

1. Identify patients with suspected or proven CAD.
2. ASA (80–325) mg/day) recommended for all CAD patients without absolute contraindications (hypersensitivity, active bleeding, high risk of bleeding)
3. Full dose warfarin (INR 2.5–3.5) or ticlopidine (250 mg b.i.d.) may be substituted, but there have not yet been established to be of equivalent efficacy.

M. Management Algorithm for Beta Blockers

1. Obtain history of myocardial infarction: obtain ECG, echocardiogram.
2. Beta blocker therapy should be administered for 2 years to patients with Q-wave myocardial infarction other than those at low risk

(asymptomatic, negative stress test, LVEF > 50%) or with absolute contraindications (bronchial asthma, symptomatic bradycardia (usually < 50 beats/min), symptomatic hypotension, 2° or 3° heart block, cardiogenic pulmonary edema, or cardiogenic shock). Dose: metoprolol 100 mg b.i.d., atenolol 100 mg/day, or equivalent.
3. Beta blocker therapy should be administered acutely after diagnosis of Q-wave myocardial infarction beginning with intravenous therapy.

N. Management Algorithm for ACE Inhibitors

1. Obtain LVEF in all heart disease or HTN patients.
2. ACE inhibitors are recommended for all patients with LVEF < 40% (also DM).
3. Obtain baseline BP, creatinine, K^+.
4. Avoid initiation in hypovolemic patients.
5. Single test dose: captopril 6.25 mg, enalapril 2.5 mg, lisinopril 5 mg or equivalent.
6. Begin captopril 12.5 mg t.i.d., enalapril 5 mg b.i.d., lisinopril 10 mg/day or equivalent.
7. Follow BP, creatinine and K^+.
8. Increase to captopril 50 mg t.i.d., enalapril 10 mg b.i.d. (maximum dose 20 mg b.i.d.), lisinopril 20 mg/day (maximum dose 40 mg/day) unless symptomatic hypotension, increased creatinine (consider decreasing diuretic if creatinine increases), or hyperkalemia occurs.

O. Management Algorithm for Hormone Replacement Therapy

1. Determine menopausal status in women with CAD.
2. HRT is recommended in postmenopausal women with CAD unless breast or uterine cancer risk outweighs benefit.
3. Breast and uterine cancer screenings must be provided for women on HRT.
4. Frequently used regimens:
    A. Conjugated estrogens 0.625 mg/day and medroxyprogesterone 10 mg/day for 10 out of 30 days
    B. Conjugated estrogens 0.625 mg/day and medroxyprogesterone 2.5 mg/day
5. HRT initiation in older women not previously on therapy needs to be individualized.

III. RISK FACTOR TREATMENT GAP

Most patients with coronary heart disease do not receive adequate risk factor modification. At the time of diagnosis, 91% and 56% of CHD patients have elevated LDL-cholesterol and low HDL-cholesterol, respectively, using the NCEP and the American Heart Association guidelines detailed above (86). In 1993, only 18% of United States and Canadian patients received lipid-lowering drugs after myocardial infarction (87). Currently, less than 10% of CHD patients are treated to NCEP lipid goals. At present, drug treatment rates for CHD patients are 78%, 41%, and 13% for patients with cholesterol levels > 300 mg/dl, between 240 and 300 mg/dl, and between 200 and 240 mg/dl, respectively (88).

The Cooperative Cardiovascular Project studied treatment rates for Medicare patients experiencing acute myocardial infarction during 1994 (23). As with cholesterol management, many patients did not receive appropriate medical therapy for which they were ideal candidates (see Table 2). As an example, smoking cessation counseling was documented in only 28% of actively smoking patients experiencing myocardial infarction. Only 50% of the patients evaluated received aspirin within 2 days of the diagnosis of AMI (26). As would be predicted from the randomized trials, follow-up data showed significantly poorer prognoses in patients not discharged on long-term aspirin therapy (27).

Roberts has summarized the reasons for lack of cardiologists' interest in secondary prevention focusing on cholesterol management (28). Explanations include a lack of belief in the cholesterol hypothesis, the routine nature of cholesterol management, lack of lifestyle and drug management knowledge,

Table 2 Cooperative Cardiovascular Pilot Project Data

	Ideal patients	Use in ideal patients	Use in excl. patients
Early interventions			
ASA	61%	83%	64%
Thrombolytics	10%	70%	12%
Late interventions			
ASA	58%	77%	51%
B blockers	30%	45%	27%
ACE I (low EF)	72%	59%	64%
Smoking cessation advice	100%	28%	N/A

Source: Ref. 23.

Table 3 Beliefs of 1211 Physicians in NY and TX that Treatment
Definitely Improves Survival in Acute MI

	Cardiologists	Internists	Family practitioners
Thrombolytics within 6 hr	93%	85%	81%
ASA within 24 hr	76%	52%	45%
ASA long-term	71%	55%	50%
Beta-blocker long-term	75%	54%	52%
Prophylactic lidocaine	2%	7%	9%

Source: Ref. 88.

guideline confusion, drug treatment expense, adverse effects, and poor reim-
bursement for instituting preventive measures. Despite numerous trials demonstrating the efficacy of secondary preventive measures, many physicians remain
unconvinced of the value of risk factor modification and vasoprotection. About
a quarter of cardiologists and half of family practitioners surveyed do not
believe that aspirin and beta blockers improve survival following AMI (Table
3) (89). Physicians in managed care networks exhibit similar practices (90).

IV. ORGANIZED APPROACH TO SECONDARY PREVENTION

A formal, organized approach to secondary prevention integrating the efforts
of physicians, nurses, dietitians, and rehabilitation therapists has proven highly
effective in several settings (91–93). Programs dependent on nurses and nurse
clinicians have been especially successful (91, 92). Organized programs have
been shown to improve the management of risk factors (92) as well as patient
outcomes (91). Whether centralized or community-based, essential ingredients
of an organized approach include:

1. Acquisition of a comprehensive patient data base on risk factors
   and medication in patients with cardiovascular disease (94).
2. Patient and family member education covering the value of risk
   factor modification and secondary preventive measures.
3. Physician and nurse counseling and early institution of therapeutic
   measures as is covered in the above management algorithms.
4. Both short- and long-term follow-up and reinforcement of patient
   compliance (95,96).

Table 4 Effect of Instituting a Preventive Cardiology Practice Index (Report Card) on Resident (MD) Treatment of Cardiac Patients

	Baseline Sept. 1994 (n = 83)	Postnotification April 1995 (n = 81)
Counseling		
Smoking	11/33	11/30
Alcohol (CHF)	0/1	2/5
Activity	23/79	50/77
Management		
LDL	11/20	21/26
HDL	9/11	13/15
HTN	36/72	45/58
DM	24/69	26/44
Vasoprotection		
ASA (CAD)	46/47	42/52
BB (Post-MI)	38/50	38/46
ACE-I (CHF)	23/36	30/38
HRT (Postmenop)	0/34	4/24
Total	221/452	282/415
($P < .001$)	(49%)	(68%)

5. Coordination of primary physician and specialist care.
6. Evaluation of physician practice and documentation of practice patterns.

Our institution has initiated a comprehensive cardiovascular diseases secondary prevention program incorporating several of these measures (92). A risk factor profile and summary of cardioprotective medication is obtained by the admitting nurse on all patients hospitalized on the cardiology and cardiothoracic surgery services. Teaching modules are given to all patients covering their specific risk factors, goals of therapy, and community resources available. Two risk factor nurse coordinators provide specialized patient education and program monitoring. A preventive cardiology physician is available for consultation on patients with nonroutine management issues. A letter is sent to referring physicians documenting the presence and management of risk factors. Predischarge exercise prescriptions and a phase II rehabilitation program are employed. House staff and cardiology fellows receive formal training in preventive measure and rehabilitation. Periodic surveys of patient management are used to document program quality.

Table 5 Potential Improvement in 1-Year Survival Following Myocardial
Infarction

Treatment	Treatment effect	Candidates	Not treated	Potential value
Smoking cessation	3%	40%	72%	0.9%
ASA	4%	90%	23%	0.8%
HMG CoA	1%	90%	75%	0.7%
B-blockers	2%	50%	55%	0.6%
ACE inhibitors	2%	50%	41%	0.4%
Thrombolytics	5%	25%	18%	0.2%

An important component of a high-quality preventive cardiology program is documentation of physician practice. We have used formal physician "report cards" covering preventive measures undertaken by our house staff on our coronary care unit and telemetry services. Providing physician feedback from chart reviews has been demonstrated to lead to an improvement in attention to patient counseling, management of risk factors, and provision of vasoprotective medications (Table 4).

V. CLINICAL VALUE OF PREVENTIVE CARDIOLOGY PROGRAM

Organized preventive programs have been shown to increase risk factor documentation and management, reduce the progression of coronary artery disease, and decrease cardiovascular events (91,92). Aggressive risk factor modification is competitive with coronary revascularization for improving long-term outcome (97).

The potential value of instituting an organized secondary prevention program with near universal adoption of proven measures can be estimated from trials demonstrating the treatment effect, the proportion of patients who are appropriate candidates for intervention, and the frequency of patients not currently receiving therapeutic measures (Table 5). Available data suggest that preventive measures could increase the absolute 1-year survival of patients experiencing an acute myocardial infarction from 0.4% to 0.9%. Substantial medical and economic benefit would also be obtained from decreased nonfatal cardiovascular events and need for coronary revascularization procedures.

REFERENCES

1. Steinberg D, Parthasarathy S, Carew TE, et al. Beyond cholesterol: modifications of low-density lipoprotein that increase its atherogenicity. N Engl J Med 1989; 320:915–924.
2. Davies MJ. A macro and micro view of coronary vascular insult in ischemic heart disease. Circulation 1990; 82(suppl II):II-38–II-46.
3. Ip JH, Fuster V, Badimon L, et al. Syndromes of accelerated atherosclerosis: Role of vascular injury and smooth muscle cell proliferation. J Am Coll Cardiol 1990; 15:1667–1687.
4. Fuster V, Badimon L, Badimon JJ, et al. The pathogenesis of coronary artery disease and the acute coronary syndromes. N Engl J Med 1992; 326:242–250.
5. Fuster V, Badimon L, Badimon JJ, et al. The pathogenesis of coronary artery disease and the acute coronary syndromes (second of two parts). N Engl J Med 1992; 326:310–318.
6. Brown BG, Zhao X-Q, Sacco DE, et al. Lipid lowering and plaque regression. New insights into prevention of plaque disruption and clinical events in coronary disease. Circulation 1993; 87:1781–1791.
7. Falk E, Shah PK, Fuster V. Coronary plaque disruption. Circulation 1995; 92: 657–671.
8. Libby P. Molecular bases of the acute coronary syndromes. Circulation 1995; 91:2844–2850.
9. Pekkanen J, Linn S, Heiss G, et al. Ten-year mortality from cardiovascular disease in relation to cholesterol levels among men with and without pre-existing cardiovascular disease. N Engl J Med 1990; 322: 1700–1707.
10. O'Connor GT, Buring JE, Yusuf S, et al. An overview of randomized trials of rehabilitation with exercise after myocardial infarction. Circulation 1989; 80:234–244.
11. Tsevat J, Weinstein MC, Williams LW, et al. Expected gains in life expectancy from various coronary heart disease risk factor modifications. Circulation 1991; 83:1194–1201.
12. Pfeffer MA, Braunwald E, Moye LA. Effect of captopril on mortality and morbidity in patients with left ventricular dysfunction after myocardial infarction. N Engl J Med 1992; 327:669–677.
13. LaRosa JC. Cholesterol lowering, low cholesterol, and mortality. Am J Cardiol 1993; 72:776–786.
14. Antiplatelet Trialists' Collaboration. Collaborative overview of randomised trials of antiplatelet therapy. I. Prevention of death, myocardial infarction, and stroke by prolonged antiplatelet therapy in various categories of patients. Br Med J 1994; 308:81–106.
15. Belchetz, PE. Hormonal treatment of postmenopausal women. N Engl J Med 1994; 330:1062–1071.
16. Scandinavian Simvastatin Survival Study Group. Randomised trial of cholesterol lowering in 4444 patients with coronary heart disease: the Scandinavian Simvastatin Survival Study (4S). Lancet 1944; 344:1383–1389.

17. Shepherd J, Cobbe SM, Ford I, et al. Prevention of coronary heart disease with provastatin in men with hypercholesterolemia. N Engl J Med 1995; 333:1301–1307.
18. Kendall MJ, Lynch KP, Hjalmarson A, et al. β-Blockers and sudden cardiac death. Ann Intern Med 1995; 123:358–367.
19. Gotto AM Jr. Lipid lowering, regression, and coronary events. Circulation 1995; 92:646–656.
20. The Diabetes Control and Complications Trial (DCCT) Research Group. Effect of intensive diabetes management on macrovascular events and risk factors in the diabetes control and complications trial. Am J Cardiol 1995; 75:894–903.
21. Fuster V, Pearson TA. Matching the intensity of risk factor management with the hazard for coronary disease events. J Am Coll Cardiol 1996; 27:957–1047.
22. Cohen MV, Byrne MJ, Levine B, et al. Low rate of treatment of hypercholesterolemia by cardiologists in patients with suspected and proven coronary artery disease. Circulation 1991; 83:1294–1304.
23. Ellerbeck EF, Jencks SF, Radford MJ, et al. Quality of care for medicare patients with acute myocardial infarction. JAMA 1995; 273:1509–1514.
24. Clinical Quality Improvement Network (CQIN) Investigators. Low incidence of assessment and modification of risk factors in acute care patients at high risk for cardiovascular events, particularly among females and the elderly. Am J Cardiol 1995; 76:570–573.
25. Shahar E, Folsom AR, Romm FJ, et al. Patterns of aspirin use in middle-aged adults: The Atherosclerosis Risk in Communities (ARIC) study. Am Heart J 1996; 131:915–922.
26. Krumholz HM, Radford MJ, Ellerbeck EF, et al. Aspirin in the treatment of acute myocardial infarction in elderly medicine beneficiaries. Patterns of use and outcome. Circulation 1995; 92:2841–2847.
27. Krumholz HM, Radford MJ, Ellerbeck EF, et al. Aspirin for secondary prevention after acute myocardial infarction in the elderly: prescribed use and outcomes. Arch Intern Med 1996; 124:292–298.
28. Roberts WC. Getting cardiologists interested in lipids. Am J Cardiol 1993; 72:744–745.
29. Vogel RA. Risk factors intervention and coronary artery disease: clinical strategies. Coronary Art Dis 1995; 6:466–471.
30. Smith SC JR, Blair SN, Criqui MH, et al. Preventing heart attack and death in patients with coronary disease. Circulation 1995; 92:2–4.
31. Summary of the second report of the National Cholesterol Education Program (NCEP): Expert panel on detection, evaluation and treatment of high blood cholesterol in adults (adult treatment panel II). JAMA 1993; 269:3015–3023.
32. The fifth report of the Joint National Committee on Detection, Evaluation, and Treatment of High Blood Pressure (JNCV). Arch Intern Med 1993; 153:154–183.
33. Steinberg D, Pearson TA, Juller LH: Alcohol and atherosclerosis. Ann Intern Med 1991; 114:967–976.

34. Klatsky AL, Armstrong MA, Friedman GD. Alcohol and mortality. Ann Intern Med 1992; 117:646–654.
35. Wong ND, Cupples LA, Ostefeld, Levy D, Kannel WB. Risk factors for long-term coronary prognosis after initial myocardial infarction: the Framingham Study. Am J Epidemiol 1989; 130:469–480.
36. Wong ND, Wilson PWF, Kannel WB. Sterum cholesterol as a prognostic factor after myocardial infarction: the Framingham Study. Ann Intern Med 1991; 115: 687–693.
37. Goldman L, Cook EF. The decline in ischemic heart disease mortality rates: an analysis of the comparative effects of medical interventions and changes in lifestyle. Ann Intern Med 1984; 101:825–836.
38. Sytowski PA, Kannel WB, D'Agostino RB. Changes in risk factors and the decline in mortality from cardiovascular disease. The Framingham Heart Study. N Engl J Med 1990; 322:1635–1641.
39. Gillum RF. Trends in acute myocardial infarction and coronary heart disease death in the United States. J Am Coll Cardiol 1993; 23:1273–1277.
40. McGovern PG, Pankow JS, Shahar E, et al. Recent trends in acute coronary heart disease. N Engl J Med 1996; 334:884–890
41. Lipid Research Clinics Program. The Lipid Research Clinics Coronary Primary Prevention Trial results. I. Reduction in incidence of coronary heart disease. JAMA 1984; 251:351–364.
42. Frick MH, Elo O, Haapa K, et al. Helsinki Heart Study: primary prevention trial with gemfibrozil in middle-aged men with dyslipidemia: safety of treatment, changes in risk-factors, and incidence of coronary heart disease. N Engl J Med 1987; 317:1237–1245.
43. Stamler J, Wentworth D, Neaton JD, MRFIT Research Group. Is relationship between serum cholesterol and risk of premature death from coronary heart disease continuous and graded? Findings in 356,222 primary screenees of the Multiple Risk Factor Intervention Trial (MRFIT). JAMA 1986; 256:2823–2828.
44. Colins R, Peto R, MacMahon S, et al. Blood pressure, stroke and coronary heart disease. Part 2. Short-term reductions in blood pressure: an overview of randomized drug trials in their epidemiological context. Lancet 1990; 335:827–838.
45. Bartecchi CE, MacKenzie TD, Schrier RW. The human cost of tobacco. N Engl J Med 1994; 330:907–912.
46. MacKenzie TD, Bartecchi CE, Schrier RW. The human cost of tobacco. N Engl J Med 1994; 330:975–980.
47. Krumholz HM, Cohen BJ, Tsevat J, et al. Cost-effectiveness of a smoking cessation program after myocardial infarction. J Am Coll Cardiol 1993; 22:1697–1702.
48. Cashin-Hemphill L, Mack WJ, Pogoda JM, et al. Beneficial effects of colestipol-niacin on coronary atherosclerosis. JAMA 1990; 264:3013–3017.
49. Buchwald H, Varco RL, Matts JP, et al. Effect of partial ileal bypass surgery on mortality from coronary heart disease in patients with hypercholesterolemia: report of the Program on the Surgical Control of the Hyperlipidemias (POSCH). N Engl J Med 1990; 323:946–955.

50. Brown G, Albers JJ, Fisher LD, et al. Regression of coronary artery disease as a result of intensive lipid-lowering therapy in men with high levels of apolipoprotein B. N Engl J Med 1990; 323:1289–1298.

51. Ornish D, Brown SE, Scherwitz LW, et al. Can lifestyle changes reverse coronary heart disease? The Lifestyle Heart Trial. Lancet 1990; 336:129–133.

52. Kane JP, Malloy MJ, Ports TA, et al. Regression of coronary atherosclerosis during treatment of familial hypercholesterolemia with combined drug regimens. JAMA 1990; 264:3007 3012.

53. MAAS Investigators. Effect of simvastatin on coronary atheroma: the multicentre antiatheroma study (MAAS). Lancet 1994; 344:633–638.

54. Jukema JW, Bruschke AUG, van Boven AJ, et al. Effects of lipid lowering by provastatin on progression and regression of coronary artery disease in symptomatic men with normal to moderately elevated serum cholesterol levels. The regression growth evaluation study (REGRESS). Circulation 1995; 91:2528–2540.

55. Ericsson C-G, Hamsten A, Nilsson J, et al. Angiographic assessment of effects of bezafibrate on progression of coronary artery disease in young male post infarction patients. Lancet 1996; 347:849–853.

56. Brown BG, Maher VMG. Reversal of coronary heart disease by lipid-lowering therapy. Observations and pathological mechanisms circulation 1994; 89:2928–2933.

57. Waters D, Craven TE, Lesperance J. Prognostic significance of progression of coronary atherosclerosis. Circulation 1993; 87:1067–1075.

58. Sacks FM, Pfeffer MA, Moye LA, et al. The effect of provastatin on coronary events after myocardial infarction in patients with average cholesterol levels. N Engl J Med 1996; 335:1001–1009.

59. Pedersen TR, Kjekshus J, Berg K, et al. Cholesterol lowering and the use of healthcare resources. Circulation 1996; 93:1796–1802.

60. Goldman L, Weinstein M, Goldman P, Williams L. Cost-effectiveness of HMG CoA reductase inhibition for primary and secondary prevention of coronary heart disease. JAMA 1991; 265:1145–1151.

61. Hay JW, Wittels EH, Gotto AM. An economic evaluation of lovastatin for cholesterol lowering and coronary artery disease reduction. Am J Cardiol 1991; 67:789–796.

62. Gaspoz J-M, Kennedy JW, Orav EJ, Goldman L. Cost-effectiveness of prescription recommendations for cholesterol-lowering drugs. A survey of a representative sample of American cardiologists. J Am Coll Cardiol 1996; 27:1232–1237.

63. Post Coronary Artery Bypass Graft Trial Investigators. The effect of aggressive lowering of low-density lipoprotein cholesterol levels and low-dose anticoagulation on obstructive changes in saphenous-vein coronary-artery bypass grafts. N Engl J Med 1996; 336:153 162.

64. Katzel LI, Bleecker ER, Colman EG, et al. Effects of weight loss vs aerobic exercise training on risk factors for coronary disease in healthy, obese, middle-aged and older men. JAMA 1995; 274:1915–1921.

65. Gould KL, Martucci JP, Goldberg DI, et al. Short-term cholesterol lowering decreases size and severity of perfusion abnormalities by positron emission tomography after dipyridamole in patients with coronary artery disease. A potential non-invasive marker for healing coronary endothelium. Circulation 1994; 89: 1530–1538.

66. Neaton JD, Kuller LH, Wentworth D, Borhani NO. Total and cardiovascular mortality in relation to cigarette smoking, serum cholesterol concentration, and diastolic blood pressure among black and white males followed up for five years. Am Heart J 1984; 108:759–769.

67. SHEP Cooperative Research Group. Prevention of stroke by antihypertensive drug treatment in older persons with isolated systolic hypertension: final results of the systolic hypertension in the elderly program (SHEP) JAMA 1991; 265: 3255–3264.

68. Fuster V, Cohen M, Halperin J. Aspirin in the prevention of coronary disease. N Engl J Med 1989; 321:183–185.

69. Yusuf S, Sleight P, Held P, McMahon S. Routine medical management of acute myocardial infarction: Lessons from overviews of recent randomized controlled trials. Circulation 1990; 82(suppl II):11117–11134.

70. Roberts R, Rogers WJ, Mueller IIS, et al. Immediate versus deferred B-blockade following thrombolytic therapy in patients with acute myocardial infarction. Results of the Thrombolysis in Myocardial Infarction (TIMI)II-B study. Circulation 1991; 83:422–437.

71. Steering Committee of the Physicians Health Study Research Group. Final report on the aspirin component of the ongoing Physicians Health Study. N Engl J Med 1989; 321:129–135.

72. Peto R, Gray R, Collins R, et al. Randomized trial of prophylactic daily aspirin in British male doctors. Br Med J 1988; 296:313–316.

73. Bierman EL. Atherogenesis in diabetes. Arterio and Thromb 1992; 12:647–656.

75. Schuler G, Hambrecht R, Schlierf G, et al. Regular physical exercise and low-fat diet: effects on progression of coronary artery disease. Circulation 1992; 86:1–11.

75. Lakka TA, Venalainen JM, Raurmaa R, et al. Relation of leisure-time physical activity and cardiorespiratory fitness to the risk of acute myocardial infarction in men. N Engl J Med 1994; 330:1549–1554.

76. Wenger NK, Froelicher ES, Smith LK, et al. Cardiac Rehabilitation. AHCPR Publication No. 96–0672. October 1995.

77. SOLVD Investigators: Effect of enalapril on the mortality and the development of heart failure in asymptomatic patients with reduced left ventricular ejection fractions. N Engl J Med 1992; 327:685–691.

78. Pfeffer MA, Braunwald E, Moye LA, et al. Effect of captopril on mortality and morbidity in patients with left ventricular dysfunction after myocardial infarction. Results of the Survival and Ventricular Enlargement Trial. N Engl J Med 1992; 327:669–677.

79. Eaker ED, Chesebro JH, Sacks FM, et al. Cardiovascular disease in women. Circulation 1993; 88:1999–2009.

80. Bush TL, Barrett-Connor E, Cowan LD, et al. Cardiovascular mortality and non-contraceptive use of estrogen in women: results from the Lipid Research Clinics Program Follow-up Study. Circulation 1987; 75:1102–1109.

81. Sulllivan JM, Vander Zwaag R, Hughes JP, et al. Estrogen replacement and coronary artery disease: effect on survival in post-menopausal women. Arch Intern Med 1990; 150:2557–2562.

82. Samaan SA, Crawford MH. Estrogen and cardiovascular function after menopause. J Am Coll Cardiol 1995; 26:1403–1410.

83. Walsh JME, Grady D. Treatment of hyperlipidemia in women. JAMA 1995; 274:1152–1158.

84. Guetta V, Cannon RO. Cardiovascular effects of estrogen and lipid-lowering therapies in post-menopausal women. Circulation 1996; 93:1928–1937.

85. Writing Group for the PEPI Trial. Effects of estrogen or estrogen/progestin regimens on heart disease risk factors in post-menopausal women. JAMA 1995; 273:199–208.

86. Pearson TA. Personal communication, 1994.

87. Rouleau JL, Mayé LA, Pfeffer MA, et al. A comparison of management patterns after acute myocardial infarction in Canada and the United States. N Engl J Med 1993; 328:779–784.

88. Shepherd J. Cholesterol monitor survey, 1994.

89. Ayanian JZ, Hauptman PJ, Guadagnoli E, et al. Knowledge and practices of generalist and specialist physicians regarding drug therapy for acute myocardial infarction. N Engl J Med 1994; 331:1138–1142.

90. Brana DA, Newcomer LE, Freibuerger A, Tian H. Cardiologists' practices compared with practice guidelines: use of beta-blockade after acute myocardial infarctions. J Am Coll Cardiol 1995; 26:1432–1436.

91. Haskell WL, Alderman EL, Fair JM, et al. Effects of intensive multiple risk factor reduction on coronary atherosclerosis and clinical cardiac events in men and women with coronary artery disease. The Stanford Coronary Risk Intervention Project (SCRIP). Circulation 1994; 89:975–990.

92. Vogel RA. The effect of a risk factor modification program on the management of hypercholesterolemia: the University of Maryland experience. Lipid Rev 1994; 1:1–4.

93. Cupples ME, McKnight A. Randomized controlled trial of health promotion in general practice for patients at high cardiovascular risk. Br Med J 1994; 309:993–996.

94. Miller M, Kankel K, Fitzpatrick D, et al. Divergent reporting of coronary risk factors before coronary bypass surgery. Am J Cardiol 1995; 75:736–737.

95. Rigotti NA, McKoul KM, Shiffman S. Predictors of smoking cessation after coronary artery bypass survey. Results of a randomized trial with 5–year follow-up. Ann Intern Med 1994; 120:287–293.

96. Jorenby DE, Smith SS, Fiore MC, et al. Varying nicotine patch dose and type of smoking cessation counseling. JAMA 1995; 274:1347–1352.

97. Vogel RA. Comparative clinical consequences of aggressive lipid management, coronary angioplasty and bypass surgery in coronary artery disease. Am J Cardiol 1992; 69:1229–1233.

9

Economics of Medical Management of Atherogenesis: Cost-Effectiveness Analyses of Medical Interventions

Orlando Rodríguez and David J. Cohen
Beth Israel-Deaconess Medical Center, and
Harvard Medical School, Boston, Massachusetts

I. INTRODUCTION

The preceding chapters have reviewed much of the data regarding medical interventions to prevent or retard the development of atherosclerosis and its various clinical manifestations. While the appeal of such preventive strategies is undeniable, such interventions frequently have unanticipated economic consequences. Since clinical studies to evaluate the efficacy of medical interventions are generally performed on relatively high-risk populations, extrapolation of these findings to a much broader treatment group is tenuous at best and is likely to be associated with a much lower degree of absolute clinical benefit. Moreover, medical interventions to prevent the development of atherosclerosis often involve considerable "hidden" costs such as the screening program, itself, and additional unnecessary costs that may be induced as indirect consequences of the screening process (1,2). Consequently, economic evaluation can play a critical role in demonstrating the magnitude of the benefit of such preventive strategies when applied to specific populations and whether these strategies represent a wise use of health care dollars.

In this chapter, we will review the economic implications of many of these interventions. First, we will review the principles of economic analysis as it applies to health care interventions, with particular emphasis on cost-effectiveness analysis. We will then review the available data on the cost-effectiveness of a wide variety of treatments to prevent the development of atherosclerosis or to limit cardiovascular events in patients with established coronary heart disease (CHD). Our goal in this overview is to provide the reader with a basic understanding of both the strengths and limitations of cost-effectiveness analysis and the implications of the available data for both clinical decision making and the development of public policy for the prevention and management of atherosclerosis.

II. PRINCIPLES OF COST-EFFECTIVENESS ANALYSIS

Three major types of economic analyses can be used to evaluate medical programs: cost-identification analysis, benefit-cost analysis, and cost-effectiveness analysis. Cost-identification (or cost-minimization) analysis simply determines the net cost of a health care intervention, expressed as the cost per unit of service provided (3). While such analyses may provide certain insights into the appropriateness of alternative forms of care, these findings are limited by the implicit underlying assumption that the outcomes of the alternative treatments are equivalent. If this assumption is incorrect, however, cost-minimization analysis cannot be used to determine the relative appropriateness of alternative treatment programs.

Benefit-cost analysis compares the costs and benefits of a medical program by expressing both in monetary terms (3). The *net benefit* of the program is then calculated as the difference between its benefits and its costs. Although this method has the advantage of being able to compare medical programs with different outcomes, the technical and ethical challenges of assigning monetary value to health outcomes have limited the acceptance of such studies by the medical community.

Cost-effectiveness analysis is the most commonly used form of medical economic analysis. It is a technique for identifying (and thus maximizing) the net health benefits that can be derived by allocating a fixed amount of scarce health care resources (4), By explicitly quantifying the tradeoffs between health care costs and health benefits, cost-effectiveness analysis allows physicians to compare the health benefits gained by use of a new treatment program to those benefits that could be achieved by alternative uses for the same health care resources. In contrast to benefit-cost analysis, cost-effectiveness analysis has the advantage of measuring health benefits in natural units. For comparisons among programs to treat a single condition, disease-specific intermediate outcomes can be used as effectiveness measures. For example, in an analysis of alternative treatments for hypertension, a natural unit of effectiveness would be the change in diastolic blood pressure; similarly, for lipid-lowering interventions, the change in total cholesterol (or low-density cholesterol; LDL) might be an appropriate measure. Similarly, for comparisons among alternative programs to prevent coronary heart disease, effectiveness might be measured in terms of myocardial infarctions avoided or incident cases of CHD prevented.

While such endpoints would be useful for prioritizing among a variety of preventive strategies, determining which (if any) of these strategies are worthy of funding requires comparison with other programs that compete for the same health care dollars. Since many of these programs are designed to treat noncardiovascular disease, generic measures of overall health benefit are required to make appropriate comparisons. In general, health benefits may include extensions of life or improvements in quality of life and are measured as years of life or "quality-adjusted life years" (QALYs). Quality-adjusted life years are derived by multiplying the time spent in a given health state by a "utility weight" that represents the individual's preference for the specific health state relative to death (utility = 0) and perfect health (utility = 1) (3,4).

Once a program's overall cost and quality-adjusted life expectancy have been estimated, an incremental cost-effectiveness ratio is derived by dividing the program's incremental cost relative to the next most effective alternative by its incremental effectiveness. Programs that both reduce costs and improve clinical outcomes are favored on both grounds and should clearly be adopted, but most medical interventions (including preventive strategies) improve health outcomes only by increasing costs (5,6). In theory, the remaining programs should be selected for funding in order of increasing cost-effectiveness ratios until the available budget is exhausted. By this method, a decision maker can allocate the available health care resources so as to maximize the total health benefits that can be achieved.

In practice, however, an exhaustive analysis of all potential health care programs is rarely practical. As a result, cost-effectiveness analysis cannot determine definitively whether a specific program or treatment under evaluation is "cost-effective." Although programs with lower cost-effectiveness ratios are clearly more cost-effective than programs with higher ratios, the threshold cost-effectiveness ratio above which a program should not be funded depends on both the alternative uses available for the same resources and the overall size of the health care budget. Nonetheless, at least within the U.S. health care system, there is an emerging consensus about the desirability of cost-effectiveness ratios (7). In general, incremental cost-effectiveness ratios < $20,000 per quality-adjusted year of life gained—such as those for coronary artery bypass grafting for left main disease (5) or for treatment of severe hypertension (8)—are viewed as quite favorable. Cost-effectiveness ratios between $20,000 and $40,000 per quality-adjusted year of life gained are also consistent with many other accepted practices including hemodialysis (9), use of tissue plasminogen activator for treatment of suspected acute myocardial infarction (MI), and implantable defibrillator placement for survivors of out-of hospital cardiac arrest (11–13). On the other hand, cost-effectiveness ratios greater than $60,000 to $100,0000/QALY are higher than those of most accepted treatments and are generally regarded as unattractive (7).

A.   Incremental Cost-Effectiveness

Several specific principles of cost-effectiveness analysis are particularly relevant to the evaluation of interventions to treat and prevent atherosclerosis. First, the importance of incremental cost-effectiveness analysis cannot be overemphasized. As in general economics, the principle of diminishing marginal returns also applies to medical economics, and thus the incremental benefits of any medical treatment generally decline as the scope of the program is broadened. In the context of medical economics, this implies that any intervention must be evaluated in comparison to the next most intensive (and presumably next most effective) alternative. For example, in the case of cholesterol lowering, both the overall costs and benefits of a program that treats all patients with serum cholesterol > 240 mg/dl will be greater than those of a program that treats only those individuals whose cholesterol is > 300 mg/dl. Thus, it is important to calculate the costs and effectiveness of cholesterol-lowering treatment for individuals with cholesterol levels between 240 and 300 mg/dl as *incremental* to the costs and effectiveness of treating just those individuals with cholesterol levels above 300 mg/dl. In an analogous fashion, the cost-effectiveness of a primary prevention program for hypercholesterolemic individuals should be calculated relative to the less intensive strategy of restricting cholesterol lowering to individuals with proven CHD (i.e., secondary prevention).

B.   Discounting

The concept of discounting is also critical to the economic evaluation of preventive interventions. A general principle of economics is that the value of both money and goods may vary with time. Future costs are generally less onerous than present costs, while future health benefits are less desirable than current health benefits. Cost-effectiveness analyses generally incorporate these principles by discounting both future costs and future benefits (4). Although there is no universally accepted discount rate, most analysts currently recommend a rate of 3% to 5% and explore the sensitivity of their results to modest variations in this rate (14). In the case of cholesterol lowering and other preventive interventions, costs are generally incurred long before any expected benefits, Thus, discounting tends to reduce benefits more than costs and results in less favorable cost-effectiveness ratios than would have been obtained by analyses that do not incorporate discounting.

C. Sensitivity Analysis

In general, data for cost-effectiveness analyses are incomplete for a variety of reasons. Clinical trials usually evaluate an intervention in highly selected patient populations and under tightly controlled circumstances. In contrast, cost-effectiveness analyses often address the "real-world" application of these treatments to a much broader target population, and thus extrapolation from trial data is frequently necessary. Moreover, no single trial can address all of the possible clinical scenarios and therapeutic options that should be examined in a meaningful economic evaluation. Accordingly, synthesis of data from a variety of sources is frequently required. Finally, the true costs of any medical treatment are impossible to measure and will vary with the scope of the intervention and the time frame to be considered (15).

Because of the inherent uncertainties and gaps in the medical data, cost-effectiveness analyses generally employ simulation models built from a set of assumptions and based on empirical evidence from multiple sources. Obviously, such models are no more or less accurate than the assumptions on which they are based. Thus, *sensitivity analyses*, in which the effect of varying one or more of the model's assumptions are examined, are critical to the interpretation of any cost-effectiveness analysis. If the results of the analysis are stable, even in the face of plausible variations in the underlying assumptions, the conclusions of the analysis may be viewed with a fair degree of confidence. On the other hand, if the results are highly sensitive to plausible variations in one or more assumptions, any conclusions of the analysis should be viewed with caution and further empirical studies would be needed to reduce the uncertainty regarding the specific assumptions.

III. COST-EFFECTIVENESS OF LIPID-LOWERING THERAPY

Over the past decade, at least 11 studies have examined the cost-effectiveness of lipid-lowering therapy in adults (16–26). Although a comprehensive discussion of each study is beyond the scope of this chapter, we will attempt to review a number of general findings in these analyses. Given the limitations of the existing data, each of these studies involves a simulation model, most of which share a number of similar features. Most analyses have assumed that the effect of cholesterol reduction for primary prevention of CHD can be modeled using the logistic risk equations developed by the Framingham Heart Study to describe the relationship between serum cholesterol level and the incidence of CHD (27). The use of the Framingham risk equations to extrapolate the benefits of lipid lowering to patients who have generally been excluded from clinical trials (i.e., women, low-risk men, the elderly) is based on the finding that the relationship between the degree of cholesterol reduction and the observed reduction in CHD risk in the major intervention studies is similar to that predicted by the Framingham equations (28). Another important similarity is the assumption of a 2-year delay between initiation of treatment and any risk reduction. This assumption is based on the observed divergence of coronary event and survival curves in many of the major lipid-lowering trials (29–31).

A.   Cholesterol Reduction for Secondary Prevention of CHD

The most cost-effective indication for cholesterol-lowering therapy is for the secondary prevention of coronary events in patients with established CHD. Goldman and colleagues used the Coronary Heart Disease Policy Model—a simulation of the incidence and outcomes of CHD within the overall U.S. population between the ages of 35 and 85 (32)—to study the cost-effectiveness of HMG-CoA reductase inhibition with lovastatin for secondary coronary prevention (22). In general, they found that the use of lovastatin in individuals with known CHD had highly favorable cost-effectiveness ratios. For example, among both men and women with total cholesterol > 250 mg/dl, the cost-effectiveness ratio for lovastatin 20 mg/day was < $25,000 per year of life saved (in 1989 dollars). Moreover, among men ages 35–54, lovastatin was estimated to *save both money and lives.* Even with serum cholesterol levels < 250 mg/dl, the estimated cost-effectiveness ratios for secondary prevention with lovastatin 20 mg/day were less than $40,000 per year of life saved except in young women.

More recently, data from two large-scale clinical trials—the Scandinavian Simvastatin Survival Trial (4S) (30), and the Cholesterol and Recurrent Events (CARE) trial (31)—have provided further support for these findings. In the 4S trial, treatment with simvastatin 20 mg/day in patients with established CHD and total cholesterol levels of 212 to 309 mg/dl resulted in a 25% reduction in total serum cholesterol and a 30% reduction in all-cause mortality over a 5-year follow-up period (30). Pedersen and colleagues collected medical resource utilization data in conjunction with the 4S trial and converted these data into direct medical care costs based on 1994 U.S. DRG weights (33). Thus, their analysis represents a cost-minimization analysis from the perspective of a third-party payer (i.e., Medicare). They found that treatment

Table 1 Costs per Patient According to Principal Diagnosis During Follow-Up in the 4S Trial

Hospitalization category	Average cost per patient[a]	
	Placebo	Simvastatin
Acute MI	3100	1955
Angina	1038	825
LV failure	153	77
Any acute CHD	4291	2857
Arrhythmia	234	374
Other acute cardiac	664	516
Stroke	419	320
TIA	83	54
Any revascularization procedure	6608	4305
CABG	6087	3874
PTCA	450	431
Total cardiovascular		
Discounted	12,300	8,428
Undiscounted	13,670	9,285

Source: Adapted with permission from Ref. 33.
[a] Costs are given in 1995 US dollars and discounted at an annual rate of 5%.

with simvastatin resulted in a 26% reduction in the number of acute hospitalizations for cardiovascular disease (primarily for revascularization procedures or acute myocardial infarction) and a 34% reduction in total days of hospitalization during follow-up. As a result, follow-up medical care costs were reduced by $3800 per patient, on average, in the simvastatin group compared with placebo treatment (Table 1). Although the cost of simvastatin treatment and monitoring over the 5-year follow-up period ($4625) was greater than the resulting cost savings, > 85% of the drug treatment costs were offset by savings in direct medical care costs; the net cost of simvastatin treatment was thus reduced to just $0.28/day.

Finally, a formal cost-effectiveness analysis of simvastatin for secondary coronary prevention has recently been published. Johannesson and colleagues developed a computer simulation model of overall survival and lifetime medical care costs based on statistical models derived from the 5-year results of the 4S trial (34). Costs were based on Swedish health care costs for the observed resource utilization of the trial participants, converted to U.S. dollars, and projected beyond the time-frame of the trial using a Markov model.

Table 2 Cost-Effectiveness Ratios for Secondary Coronary Prevention with Simvastatin Based on the Results of the 4S Trial (Dollars per Year of Life Saved)

Total cholesterol before treatment (mg/dl)	Age 35		Age 59		Age 70	
	Men	Women	Men	Women	Men	Women
Analysis of direct costs only						
213	$11,400	$27,400	$7,000	$16,400	$6,200	$13,300
261	8,800	18,800	5,500	10,300	4,700	4,700
309	6,700	13,200	4,200	7,100	3,800	6,200
Analysis of direct and indirect costs						
213	Savings	Savings	2,100	8,600	6,200	13,300
261	Savings	Savings	1,600	4,900	4,700	8,500
309	Savings	Savings	1,200	3,200	3,800	6,200

Source: Adapted with permission from Ref. 34.

They estimated that for a 59-year-old man with established CHD, treatment with simvastatin would increase life-expectancy by an average of 0.28 years and increase direct medical expenditures by $1500, with an resulting cost-effectiveness ratio of $5500 per year of life saved. For a 59-year-old woman, the gain in life expectancy was projected to be somewhat smaller (0.16 years), but the overall cost-effectiveness ratio remained favorable at $10,300 per year of life saved. In fact, over a wide range of ages (35 to 70 years) and serum cholesterol levels (213 to 309 mg/dl), they projected that simvastatin would be reasonably cost-effective with incremental cost-effectiveness ratios between $4000 and $27,000 per year of life saved (Table 2). When indirect costs (due to lost productivity) were also included in the analysis, the cost-effectiveness of simvastatin improved even further and was estimated to be cost saving for young men and women.

B. Cholesterol Reduction for Primary Prevention of CHD

Evaluating the cost-effectiveness of lipid-lowering therapy for the primary prevention of CHD is more complex than for secondary prevention. Numerous observational studies have demonstrated that the risk of developing CHD is a multiplicative function of serum cholesterol and other risk factors (e.g., sex, age, cigarette smoking, hypertension, glucose intolerance) (27,35–37). The multiplicative nature of this risk function implies that the effect of any degree of cholesterol reduction on overall CHD risk is greater for individuals whose baseline risk is higher. Most cost-effectiveness analyses have found that primary coronary prevention is highly cost-effective only for individuals with multiple additional coronary risk factors (17,20,22,23,25).

Hay and colleagues examined the cost-effectiveness of lovastatin for primary coronary prevention using a model of CHD incidence based on the Framingham risk equations and data regarding mortality after the onset of CHD derived from Framingham observations (23). Estimates of the costs of specific CHD events and procedures were based on expert consensus. They found that using lovastatin 20 mg/day to treat a 35-year-old man with serum cholesterol of 240 to 299 mg/dl and no other risk factors, had a cost-effectiveness ratio of $34,000 per year of life saved (in 1990 dollars). The cost-effectiveness ratio improved to $13,000 per year of life saved, however, when the same treatment was applied to a 35-year-old male smoker with hypertension. Using a similar model, Oster and Epstein found that for a 50-year-old man with a cholesterol level of 240 mg/dl but no other risk factors, the cost-effectiveness ratio for lifetime treatment with cholestyramine was $135,000 per year of life gained (19). The addition of three major coronary risk factors (smoking, hypertension, and diabetes mellitus) improved the cost-effectiveness ratio for the same intervention to $58,000 per year of life gained.

The higher absolute risk of CHD for men than that for women implies that if other risk factors are equal, interventions to lower serum cholesterol will be more effective on an absolute basis and thus more cost-effective in men than in women (20,22,23). Goldman and colleagues used the Coronary Heart Disease Policy Model to study the cost-effectiveness of lovastatin for primary coronary prevention (22). For women aged 35 to 64, cost-effectiveness ratios were generally three to five times higher than for men with equivalent risk profiles (Table 3). For women < 54 years or > 74 years, lovastatin was estimated to have a cost-effectiveness ratio above $60,000 per year of life saved regardless of the pretreatment cholesterol level or other risk factors. Even for women aged 55 to 74 (the most cost-effective age group), the cost-effectiveness of lifetime treatment with lovastatin was reasonable (< $60,000 per year of life saved) only in subgroups with multiple additional risk factors.

In addition to the population targeted for treatment, the choice of the lipid-lowering agent has an important effect on the cost-effectiveness of primary prevention. Martens and colleagues compared the cost-effectiveness of an HMG-CoA reductase inhibitor (simvastatin) with a bile-acid resin (cholestyramine) for the primary prevention of CHD in Dutchmen with serum cholesterol > 310 mg/dl (20). Given the slightly lower cost and much greater effectiveness of simvastatin in lowering serum cholesterol, they estimated simvastatin to be nearly five times more cost-effective than cholestyramine in most patient subgroups.

Table 3 Cost-Effectiveness Ratio[a] (Dollars per Year of Life Saved) of 20 mg/day Lovastatin for Primary Prevention of Coronary Heart Disease

	Age (yrs)				
	35–44	45–54	55–64	65–74	75–84
Men, pretreatment cholesterol > 300 mg/dl					
High risk[b]	24,000	13,000	15,000	23,000	66,000
Moderate risk[c]	130,000	49,000	29,000	32,000	92,000
Low risk[d]	330,000	110,000	58,000	58,000	150,000
Women, pretreatment cholesterol > 300 mg/dl					
High risk[b]	195,000	62,000	34,000	39,000	67,000
Moderate risk[c]	480,000	140,000	62,000	46,000	87,000
Low risk[d]	1,500,000	320,000	130,000	68,000	110,000

Source: Adapted with permission from Ref. 22.
[a] All cost-effectiveness ratios are in 1989 dollars.
[b] High risk = diastolic blood pressure >105 mmHg, smoker, weight > 130% of ideal.
[c] Moderate risk = diastolic blood pressure 90–104 mmHg, nonsmoker, weight 110%–129% of ideal.
[d] Low risk = diastolic blood pressure < 95 mmHg, nonsmoker, weight < 110% of ideal.

The cost of lipid-lowering drugs is a critical factor in determining the cost-effectiveness of lipid-lowering therapy as well. In one analysis, Kinosian and Eisenberg found that substituting bulk cholestyramine for individual patients decreased the cost-effectiveness ratio from $108,000 to $58,000 per year of life saved (18). Similarly, Goldman and colleagues found that cost-effectiveness ratios for lovastatin declined by approximately 30% if the cost of lovastatin decreased by 40% (22). Such cost reductions are likely to occur in the near future due to increasing competition among similar HMG-CoA reductase inhibitors as well as the potential availability of generic lovastatin in 1997.

Schulman and colleagues used a unique study design to compare the cost-effectiveness of multiple alternative drug regimens (21). By assuming that cholesterol-lowering medications are effective only to the extent that they alter serum lipid levels, they calculated a cost-effectiveness ratio for each specific agent in terms of net cost per unit change in serum cholesterol (or LDL, HDL, or a weighted average of LDL and HDL). Although their analysis is not directly comparable to any other study, it can nonetheless provide important insights into those treatment regimens that are "efficient" ways to treat hypercholesterolemia. For example, in their analysis of cost per unit decrement in overall coronary risk, Schulman and colleagues found that only nicotinic acid and lovastatin (20, 40, or 80 mg/day) were cost-effective treatment strategies (21). Nicotinic acid appeared to be relatively cost-effective because it produced modest decreases in LDL cholesterol and modest increases in HDL cholesterol at a comparatively low cost. Although lovastatin was among the most expensive agents, it was also potentially cost-effective because it lowered LDL levels to the greatest extent and thus produced the greatest expected reduction in overall coronary risk. The other drugs considered (cholestyramine, gemfibrozil, colestipol, and probucol) did not appear to be as cost-effective as either niacin or lovastatin in their model. If long-term compliance with niacin therapy was somewhat lower than their baseline estimates, however, gemfibrozil replaced niacin as a cost-effective alternative.

Overall, these studies suggest that cholesterol lowering for primary coronary prevention is less cost-effective than for secondary coronary prevention. This finding should not be surprising. Since the absolute risk of subsequent coronary events and CHD mortality is five to seven times higher for patients with established CHD than for individuals without known coronary disease (38–40), the potential for risk reduction for an individual is far greater in secondary than in primary prevention. Moreover, any potential adverse effects of cholesterol lowering on either quality of life or noncardiovascular mortality will be less important in patients with preexisting CHD. Since the overall benefit of any intervention represents the sum of its effects on cardiovascular and noncardiovascular mortality, to the extent that treatments to lower serum cholesterol might increase noncardiovascular mortality (41), cholesterol-lowering interventions will be most effective—and most cost-effective—in those individuals with the greatest absolute risk of mortality due to CHD. Thus, most analyses suggest that use of cholesterol-lowering medications for primary prevention of CHD is reasonably cost-effective only in young or middle-aged men with at least moderate hypercholesterolemia (> 240 mg/dl) and several additional risk factors.

C. Population-Based Interventions to Lower Cholesterol

Population-based interventions to lower serum cholesterol levels are attractive for several reasons. Most "individualized" treatments such as dietary counseling or drug therapy are targeted at high-risk individuals, but because CHD is so prevalent, most cases develop in individuals who are, in fact, "low risk" (42,43). For example, simulations based on the CHD Policy Model suggest that 50% to 70% of new cases of CHD will occur in individuals with serum cholesterol < 250 mg/dl (19). As a result, life expectancy gains for an ambitious policy of targeted intervention that reduced serum cholesterol to 250 mg/dl in all individuals with current cholesterol levels > 250 mg/dl could also be obtained by a more modest populationwide intervention that reduced serum cholesterol by an average of 10 mg/dl in men and 23 mg/dl in women (19). Moreover, population-based interventions are relatively inexpensive on a per-capita basis. Populationwide education programs in the Stanford Five-Community Study and the North Karelia (Finland) Study reduced serum cholesterol levels by 1% to 4% at an estimated annual cost of just $4 to $10 per person (44,45). Finally, populationwide interventions may affect multiple CHD risk factors simultaneously. In both the North Karelia and Stanford Five-City studies there were significant reductions in diastolic blood pressure as well as serum cholesterol levels (44,46). The Stanford project led to significant reductions in the smoking rate as well (44).

Based on these data, several analyses suggest that population-based interventions to lower serum cholesterol can be highly cost-effective. Kristiansen and colleagues examined the cost-effectiveness of a population-based strategy to promote healthier dietary habits in Norwegian men aged 40 to 49 compared with targeted individual dietary or combined diet and drug therapy (24). They found the population-based strategy to be highly cost-effective, with an estimated cost-effectiveness ratio of $20 per year of life saved. In contrast, the incremental cost-effectiveness ratios for individualized dietary or combined dietary and drug therapy were estimated to be $20,000 per year of life saved and $150,000 per year of life saved, respectively.

More recently, Tosteson and colleagues used the CHD Policy Model to analyze the cost-effectiveness of a populationwide educational program to improve dietary habits (47). Based on the costs and cholesterol-lowering effects observed in the Stanford Five-City project, they estimated that a 25-year program would save 624,000 life-years at a net cost of $2.1 billion, with an incremental cost-effectiveness ratio of $3200 per life-year gained. When the impact of this program on multiple risk factors (including blood pressure and smoking rates) was considered, such a populationwide intervention was projected to save both money and lives. These highly favorable cost-effectiveness ratios suggest that populationwide interventions should form a key element of any comprehensive national strategy to prevent coronary heart disease.

IV. ANTIHYPERTENSIVE THERAPY

The benefits of antihypertensive therapy in preventing the development of atherosclerosis and its consequences are well-known (48). Given the high prevalence of hypertension and the long duration of latent disease before the development of clinical complications, however, cost-effectiveness analyses are critical for understanding the public policy implications of widespread antihypertensive therapy. Two major studies have examined the overall cost-effectiveness of hypertension screening and treatment programs. In one of the first medical cost-effectiveness analyses, Weinstein and Stason evaluated the cost-effectiveness of antihypertensive therapy using a "stepped-care" approach involving diuretics, alpha-blockers, and centrally acting agents (8). Using a model of CHD and stroke incidence based on observations from the Framingham

Heart Study and incorporating adjustments to account for reduced quality of life due to adverse side effects, they estimated the cost-effectiveness of treatment for moderate diastolic hypertension (diastolic blood pressure > 105 mm Hg) to be $20,000 per quality-adjusted year of life gained (updated to 1984 dollars). For patients with mild hypertension (diastolic blood pressure 95 to 104 mm Hg), they estimated the cost-effectiveness ratio to be $42,000/ QALY. The cost-effectiveness ratio varied considerably with age, gender, and level of diastolic blood pressure. The most favorable ratios were for young men with severe hypertension, while young women had the least favorable ratios.

More recently, Littenberg and colleagues reexamined the cost-effectiveness of screening for and treating hypertension (49). Despite their use of more recent data and consideration of additional antihypertensive agents, their findings were similar to those of Weinstein and Stason. They found that hypertension screening and treatment was associated with generally favorable cost-effectiveness ratios (range: $12,000 to $43,000/QALY in 1990 dollars) for men aged 20 to 60 and for women aged 40 to 60. Similar to the earlier analysis, they found the cost-effectiveness of antihypertensive therapy to be somewhat less favorable for young women ($65,000/QALY).

With the recent introduction of several additional classes of antihypertensive medications, the choice of a specific agent has become increasingly complex and involves multiple considerations including drug efficacy, side effects, drug interactions, coexisting conditions, compliance, and cost. In an attempt to evaluate several of these tradeoffs explicitly, Edelson and colleagues used the CHD Policy Model to estimate the cost-effectiveness of various antihypertensive monotherapies in patients with diastolic blood pressures > 95 mm Hg (50). Their analysis took into account differences in drug efficacy, compliance, and effects on serum cholesterol, but they did not consider any potential impact of treatment on quality of life. In their analysis, propranolol was estimated to be both the least expensive and most effective agent in the long run, with a cost-effectiveness ratio of $17,000 per year of life saved (1987 dollars). For the other agents, the cost-effectiveness ratios (relative to no therapy) were projected to be $25,000/YOLS for hydrochlorothiazide; $49,000/YOLS for nifedipine; $96,000/YOLS for prazosin; and $112,000/YOLS for captopril. These findings suggest that for treatment of mild to moderate hypertension, a generic beta-blocker is the preferred option on the grounds of both overall effectiveness and cost-effectiveness. Sensitivity analyses demonstrated that differences in blood pressure effects far outweighed the impact of cholesterol effects among the available antihypertensive agents; a 1 mm Hg change in diastolic blood pressure was projected to be roughly equivalent to a 6 mg/dl change in serum cholesterol. On the other hand, the cost-effectiveness of treatment was sensitive to modest differences in quality of life across antihypertensive agents. For example, if 1 year of propranolol treatment were equivalent to 0.98 years without treatment (i.e., utility of propranolol treatment = 0.98), all of the improvement in life expectancy by antihypertensive therapy would be negated by the associated decrement in quality of life. Thus, even modest differences in quality of life with alternative treatments would be expected to have important effects on their relative cost-effectiveness.

V. SMOKING CESSATION INTERVENTIONS

Cost-effectiveness analyses of smoking cessation interventions, including physician counseling, nicotine gum, and nicotine patches in primary prevention as well as a nurse-managed program following myocardial infarction have all demonstrated highly favorable cost-effectiveness ratios (51–54). These findings reflect both the modest costs of these interventions and the sizable benefits of smoking cessation for those who quit, in spite of low overall cessation rates.

Cummings and colleagues estimated the cost-effectiveness of brief advice and counseling by a physician about quitting smoking during a routine office visit (51). Based on three randomized studies, they estimated a 1-year cessation rate of 2.7% as a result of physician counseling, and they assumed that 10% of those who quit would eventually relapse. In their analysis, the cost-effectiveness ratios for physician counseling ranged from $1300 to $1850 per year of life saved in men and $2300 to $3900 per year of life saved in women. Even in a "worst-case scenario," assuming a 1% 1-year cessation rate and a 50% relapse rate, the cost-effectiveness ratios remained < $15,000 per year of life saved for men and < $30,000 per year of life saved for women.

More recently, Oster and colleagues examined the cost-effectiveness of nicotine gum as an adjunct to physician advice in men and women aged 35 to 69 years (52). Based on the results of randomized trials, they estimated a smoking cessation rate of 6.1% in patients prescribed nicotine gum after physician advice compared to physician advice alone. In contrast to the analysis by Cummings et al., they assumed no relapse after successful smoking cessation at 1 year. Based on observational data, they projected undiscounted gains in life expectancy as a result of quitting ranging from 1 to 5 years, depending on gender and age. Based on these data, they estimated the incremental cost-effectiveness ratio for nicotine gum to range from $8000 to $18,000 per year of life saved. The cost-effectiveness ratios increased but remained favorable at $9000 to $20,000 per year of life saved when a 10% relapse rate was assumed in a sensitivity analysis.

Following the development of the transdermal nicotine patch, Fiscelia and Franks estimated the incremental cost-effectiveness of its use as an adjunct to physician counseling in men and women ages 25 to 69 (53). Based on effectiveness data from published meta-analyses (56,57), they assumed a 1-year cessation rate of 7.9% with nicotine patch as compared to 1.5% after counseling alone and projected gains in life expectancy after smoking cessation that ranged from 0.76 to 6.71 years, depending on age and gender. They estimated the benefits of smoking cessation using published mortality data for non-smokers, smokers, and quitters and adjusted for the impact of smoking on health-related quality of life. Additional assumptions included a 50% rate of patch prescription acceptance, a 95% rate of compliance with the patch, and a 35% relapse rate after 1 year of abstinence. In their analysis, the cost-effectiveness ratios for prescribing a nicotine patch as an adjunct to physician counseling ranged from $4390/QALY in men aged 35 to 39 years to $10,943/QALY in men aged 65 to 69 years. The cost-effectiveness ratios were slightly less favorable for women in the young age groups and slightly more favorable in women > 50 years old (due to their longer life expectancy than men of similar age). Sensitivity analyses showed that the cost-effectiveness ratios were most sensitive to changes in the probability of quitting smoking, but even using the lower bound of the 95% confidence intervals for this effect estimate yielded highly favorable cost-effectiveness ratios of < $8000/QALY for most patients.

Given the highly favorable cost-effectiveness ratios for smoking cessation interventions in primary prevention of atherosclerosis, it is not surprising that programs to promote smoking cessation in patients with established CHD are among the most cost-effective medical interventions. In the only such analysis to date, Krumholz and colleagues examined the cost-effectiveness of a nurse-managed smoking cessation program compared to physician advice alone soon after an acute myocardial infarction (54). Based on a published clinical trial (55), they assumed that an additional 26% of smokers would quit as a result of the nurse-managed program and estimated the mean gain in life expectancy as a result of smoking cessation among MI survivors to be 1.7 years. They also estimated the cost of such a program to be $ 100 per patient (mainly to cover nursing time and administrative expenses). Based on this assumption, they projected an incremental cost-effectiveness ratio of $250 per year of life saved, which remained < $1000 per year of life saved under a wide range of plausible alternative assumptions. These findings confirm that targeting a relatively labor-intensive smoking cessation program to survivors of myocardial infarction is highly cost-effective.

VI.   HORMONE REPLACEMENT THERAPY

Evaluating the cost-effectiveness of hormone replacement therapy for post-menopausal women is complicated by the lack of definitive data from randomized clinical trials and by the multiple effects of such treatment including a reduction in the risk of osteoporosis and related fractures, a potential reduction in the risk of CHD and cardiovascular death, and a potential increased risk of endometrial and breast cancers. Although several early studies on the cost-effectiveness of hormone replacement therapy estimated favorable cost-effectiveness ratios of < $40,000 per year of life saved, these may represent conservative estimates as they did not consider any cardiovascular benefits of such therapy (58–60).

Subsequently, two analyses have examined the cost-effectiveness of hormone replacement therapy while taking into consideration its cardiovascular benefits (61–62). Daly and colleagues examined the cost-effectiveness of three strategies: (a) treating women with estrogen after hysterectomy only, (b) treating women with an intact uterus with combined estrogen and progestin, and (c) treating women with an intact uterus with unopposed estrogen (61). Assuming a 50% decrease in the risk of developing coronary heart disease with unopposed estrogen and a 25% risk reduction with combination therapy, the authors projected gains in life expectancy of 0.11 to 0.25 years over a 10-year follow-up period with associated cost-effectiveness ratios of $4600, $13,000 and $23,000 per year of life saved (in 1990 dollars), respectively, for the three strategies. Tosteson and colleagues developed a state-transition model incorporating the impact of hormone replacement therapy on osteoporotic fractures, ischemic heart disease deaths, and quality of life (62). Based on reviews of the epidemiologic data, they assumed a 50% reduction in cardiovascular mortality in patients with a prior hysterectomy, a 36% increase in the risk of breast cancer among women receiving unopposed estrogen, and no cardiovascular benefit or breast cancer risk for women on combined therapy. Under these assumptions, they estimated a cost-effectiveness ratio of $12,620 per year of life saved (1990 dollars) for a 10-year course of unopposed estrogen in women with a prior hysterectomy and $88,500 per year of life saved for combined therapy. Although hormone replacement therapy was reasonably cost-effective under the baseline assumptions of these analyses, in both studies the cost-effectiveness ratios were highly sensitive to plausible variations in the effect of estrogen on cardiovascular morbidity and mortality. Thus, despite the unequivocal benefits of hormone replacement therapy on osteoporosis, further data are necessary to reliably estimate the cost-effectiveness of this intervention. Ongoing randomized clinical trials of hormone replacement such as the Women's Health Initiative should provide reliable effect estimates to better inform this decision.

VII. LIFESTYLE INTERVENTIONS

Epidemiologic evidence suggests that regular aerobic exercise is associated with lower rates of coronary events and improved survival (63–65). Based on these data, Hatziandreu and colleagues examined the cost-effectiveness of an exercise regimen as intervention for the primary prevention of CHD (66). They used a decision-analytic model to compare medical care costs and quality-adjusted life expectancies of two hypothetical cohorts of 35-year-old men who did or did not engage in regular aerobic exercise. This model was based on age-specific CHD event rates derived from the Framingham Heart Study, and they assumed that coronary events would be reduced by 50% as a result of regular exercise. They considered direct and indirect costs of exercise, including exercise-related injuries, and measured effectiveness in quality-adjusted life years assuming that each year following a CHD event was equivalent to 0.8 years without an event (utility = 0.8). Under their (relatively favorable) assumptions, the cost-effectiveness ratio for regular aerobic exercise was $22,400/QALY. Not surprisingly, the cost-effectiveness of routine exercise was highly dependent on the relative risk of coronary events with exercise. Varying this relative risk from 0.4 to 0.67 resulted in cost-effectiveness ratios between $11,700 and $33,200/QALY. Moreover, for any individual, the cost-effectiveness of exercise was very sensitive to the level of enjoyment that the individual derived from exercise itself. For example, the cost-effectiveness ratio ranged from $2500/ QALY for those who enjoy exercise, to $86,500/QALY for those who hate it. This study thus suggests that regular aerobic exercise is reasonably cost-effective as a health promotion activity except in individuals who dislike it.

Aerobic exercise in conjunction with formal cardiac rehabilitation appears to be reasonably cost-effective as secondary prevention in post-MI patients as well. Based on a meta-analysis of published clinical trials, Oldridge and colleagues estimated a 17% relative reduction in 3-year mortality with cardiac rehabilitation compared with routine care for post-MI patients (67,68). One-year cost data and additional quality-of-life benefits were based on a separate randomized clinical trial (69). Over a 3-year time horizon, they estimated that cardiac rehabilitation would improve quality-adjusted life expectancy by 0.071 years at a net cost of $480, with a resulting cost-effectiveness ratio of $6800/QALY (68). Even if the quality-of-life benefits were excluded, the cost-effectiveness ratio remained < $25,000 per year of life saved. Thus, cardiac rehabilitation appears to be reasonably cost-effective for myocardial infarction survivors, but much of the apparent effectiveness can be attributed to improved short-term quality of life.

VIII. ANTITHROMBOTIC THERAPY

Although the benefits of antithrombotic therapy in the primary and secondary prevention of coronary events in unequivocal, few studies have been performed to evaluate the cost-effectiveness of this practice. Only one study, published in abstract form, has examined the cost-effectiveness of aspirin in the secondary prevention of CHD (70). Gaspoz and colleagues used the CHD Policy Model and aspirin efficacy data pooled from the literature to estimate the incremental cost-effectiveness of 100 mg aspirin daily given for 25 years to patients with a prior myocardial infarction. They estimated that such therapy would save both money and lives in women but increased costs slightly in men. Nonetheless, aspirin as secondary prevention in men was highly cost-effective with a cost-effectiveness ratio of $500 to $1000 per year of life saved. Given its low cost and proven efficacy, it is not surprising that aspirin is highly cost-effective in the secondary prevention of CHD. Despite its proven benefit as primary prevention in men (71), no studies to date have examined the cost-effectiveness of aspirin for primary coronary prevention.

The data on the cost-effectiveness of oral anticoagulation is also very limited. Based on the data from the Anticoagulants in the Secondary Prevention of Events in Coronary Thrombosis (ASPECT) trial, van Bergen and colleagues examined the cost-effectiveness of oral anticoagulation in survivors of a myocardial infarction followed for a mean of 37 months (72). The authors concluded that oral anticoagulation would result in cost savings estimated at $519 per patient compared to placebo. Because the authors did not compare oral anticoagulation therapy with aspirin, however, interpretation of these findings for clinical practice is difficult. The results of ongoing clinical trials comparing warfarin and aspirin directly should provide the basis for more relevant comparisons in the future (73).

IX. SUMMARY

In the current health care climate, it is increasingly apparent that medical care resources are not without limit. Thus, there has been increased interest in evaluating the economic as well as clinical outcomes of modern medical practices. In this chapter, we have attempted to review and synthesize the available data regarding the cost-effectiveness of alternative strategies for the prevention and treatment of atherosclerosis. In general, these studies suggest that many of the available interventions are reasonably cost-effective when compared with alternative uses for the same health care dollars within the U.S. health care system.

For patients with *established coronary heart disease,* a wide variety of medical and nonmedical interventions including aggressive lipid-lowering therapy, long-term anticoagulation (with aspirin), and intensive programs to promote smoking cessation all appear to be highly cost-effective (Table 4). While other interventions such as antihypertensive therapy and hormone replacement

Table 4 Overview of the Cost-Effectiveness of Medical Interventions in the Secondary Prevention of Atherogenesis

Intervention (Ref.)	Condition	Patient group	C/E ratio
Lovastatin 20 mg/d (22)	Hyperlipidemia	TC ≥ 250 mg/dl, men age 45–54	Dominant
ASA 100 mg/d (70)	CHD	Women	Dominant
Nurse-managed program (54)	Smoking	Smokers post-MI	250
ASA 100 mg/d (70)	CHD	Men	563
Lovastatin 20 mg/d (22)	Hyperlipidemia	TC ≥ 250 mg/dl, women age 45–54	4,700
Cardiac rehabilitation (69)	CHD	Post-MI	8,000[a]
Simvastatin (34)	Hyperlipidemia	CHD, men, TC = 261	5,500[b]
Simvastatin (34)	Hyperlipidemia	CHD, women, TC = 261	10,300[b]
Lovastatin 20 mg/d (22)	Hyperlipidemia	TC < 250 mg/dl, men age 55–64	22,900
Lovastatin 20 mg/d (22)	Hyperlipidemia	TC < 250 mg/dl, women age 55–64	48,600

Source: Adapted with permission from Ref. 74.
All ratios are in 1993 $/YOLS discounted at 5%, except when noted.
[a] Cost-utility ratio in $/QALY.
[b] 1995 dollars.
TC = total cholesterol; CHD = coronary heart disease; MI = myocardial infarction; Dominant = saves money and lives; YOLS = year of life saved; C/E = cost-effectiveness.

therapy for postmenopausal women have not been studied directly as secondary prevention, the fact that these interventions are reasonably cost-effective as primary prevention suggests that they are likely to be even more cost-effective when applied to individuals with known CHD. Finally, by impacting multiple independent CHD risk factors simultaneously, population-based educational approaches appear to be highly cost-effective as well and thus should be a key element of any national policy to reduce coronary heart disease.

Although primary coronary prevention is generally less cost-effective than secondary prevention, in many cases these interventions are reasonably cost-effective as well (Table 5). For example, a variety of primary prevention therapies including antihypertensive therapy for patients with moderate diastolic hypertension and unopposed estrogen as hormone replacement therapy for postmenopausal women are associated with cost-effectiveness ratios < $40,000 per year of life saved—similar to federally funded programs such as hemodialysis and other widely practiced medical interventions. Moreover,

Table 5 Overview of the Cost-Effectiveness of Medical Interventions for the Primary Prevention of Atherogenesis

Intervention (Ref.)	Condition	Patient group	C/E ratio
Physician counseling (51)	Smoking	Men age 50–54 or women age 55–59	< 2500
Nicotine patch/ counseling (53)	Smoking	Men age 35–39 or women age 45–49	< 5,000[a,b]
Unopposed estrogen (62)	Prophylaxis	Women age > 50, hysterectomy	12,620[c]
Lovastatin 20 mg/d (23)	Hyperlipidemia	Men age 35, TC = 240–299 mg/dl, smoking and hypertension	13,000[c]
Propranolol (50)	Hypertension	DBP ≥ 95 mm Hg	17,000
Common regimen (8)	Hypertension	DBP ≥ 105	20,000[a]
Aerobic exercise (66)	Prophylaxis	Men age 35	22,400[a]
Hydrochlorothiazide (50)	Hypertension	DBP ≥ 95 mm Hg	25,000
Lovastatin 20 mg/d (23)	Hyperlipidemia	Men age 35, TC = 240–299 mg/dl, no other risk factors	34,000[c]
Simvastatin 20 mg/d (20)	Hyperlipidemia	TC = 3 10 mg/dl, men age 40	36,300
Common regimen (8)	Hypertension	DBP 95–104 mm Hg	42,000[a]
Nifedipine (50)	Hypertension	DBP ≥ 95 mm Hg	49,000
Combined BRT (62)	Prophylaxis	Women ≥ 50 years, intact uterus	88,500[c]
Captopril (50)	Hypertension	DBP ≥ 95 mm Hg	111,600
Cholestyramine 12 g/d (20)	Hyperlipidemia	TC = 3 10 mg/dl, men age 40	159,800

Source: Adapted with permission from Ref. 74.
All ratios are in 1993 $/YOLS discounted at 5%, except when noted.
[a]Cost-utility ratio in $/QALY.
[b] 1995 dollars.
[c] 1990 dollars.
TC = total cholesterol; CHD = coronary heart disease; MI = myocardial infarction; DBP = diastolic blood pressure; HRT = hormone replacement therapy; C/E = cost-effectiveness.

interventions to promote smoking cessation such as physician counseling, nicotine gum, and the nicotine patch are among the most cost-effective forms of primary coronary prevention, with cost-effectiveness ratios between $5000 and $10,000 per year of life saved. On the other hand, lipid-lowering therapy for primary prevention of CHD appears to be reasonably cost-effective only for middle-aged men with multiple additional risk factors. The appropriateness of cholesterol reduction for other populations, including young men, most women, and the elderly, is less certain, however. Even if cholesterol reduction in these populations reduces the risk of developing CHD to a similar extent as in middle-aged men, most studies suggest that the cost-effectiveness ratios for such treatment exceed $100,000 per year of life saved.

These studies also demonstrate the critical importance of the choice of a specific drug or treatment strategy in determining the cost-effectiveness of programs to treat or prevent CHD. In the case of lipid lowering, for example, several studies have shown that niacin or the HMG-CoA reductase inhibitors represent cost-effective initial therapies. Similarly, in treating hypertension, generic beta blockers and hydrochlorothiazide appear to have favorable cost-effectiveness ratios as initial monotherapy, while captopril and calcium channel blockers are several times more expensive for comparable projected survival benefits.

Although medical economics have often been ignored in traditional medical education, we contend that such ignorance is a luxury clinicians can no longer afford. Cost-effectiveness analysis provides the theoretical framework for evaluating the relationship between dollars expended on medical care and the benefits that may be achieved, and thus the tools for maximizing the health benefits for society despite constrained resources. While medical economics often provides a sobering look at medical science, in the case of management of atherosclerosis and coronary heart disease, the message is generally favorable. Through basic science and clinical research, the medical community now has many tools and approaches to prevent CHD, and cost-effectiveness analysis suggests that many of these interventions are reasonable investments for our limited health care dollars.

REFERENCES

1. Garber AM, Littenberg B, Sox, HC Jr, et al. Costs and health consequences of cholesterol screening for asymptomatic older Americans. Arch Intern Med 199 1; 151:1089–1095.
2. Grover SA, Coupal L, Fahkry R, et al. Screening for hypercholesterolemia among Canadians: how much will it cost? Can Med Assoc J 1991; 144:161–168.
3. Eisenberg JM. Clinical economics. A guide to the economic analysis of clinical practices. JAMA 1989; 262:2879–2886.

4. Weinstein MC, Stason WB. Foundations of cost-effectiveness analysis for health and medical practices. N Engl J Med 1977; 296:716–72 1.
5. Weinstein MC, Stason WB. Cost-effectiveness of coronary artery bypass surgery. Circulation 1982; 66(suppl III):56–66.
6. Krumholz HM, Pasternak RC, Weinstein MC, et al. Cost effectiveness of thrombolytic therapy with streptokinase in elderly patients with suspected acute myocardial infarction. N Engl J Med 1992; 327:7–13.
7. Goldman L, Gordon DJ, Rifkind BM, et al. Cost and health implications of cholesterol lowering. Circulation 1992; 85:1960–1968.
8. Stason WB, Weinstein MC. Allocation of resources to manage hypertension. N Engl J Med 1977; 296:732–739.
9. Drummond NE. Economic evaluation and the rational diffusion and use of health technology. Health Policy 1987; 7:309–324.
10. Mark DB, Hlatky MA, Califf M, et al. Cost effectiveness of thrombolytic therapy with tissue plasminogen activator as compared with streptokinase for acute myocardial infarction. N Engl J Med 1995; 332:1418–1424.
11. Kuppermann M, Luce BR, McGovern B, et al. An analysis of the cost effectiveness of the implantable defibrillator. Circulation 1990; 81:91–100.
12. Larsen GC, Manolis AS, Sonnenberg FA, et al. Cost-effectiveness of the implantable cardioverter-defibrillator: effect of improved battery life and comparison with amiodarone therapy. J Am Coll Cardiol 1992; 19:1323–1334.
13. Owens DK, Sanders GD, Harris RA, et al. Cost-effectiveness of implantable cardioverter defibrillators relative to aminodarone for prevention of sudden cardiac death. Ann Intern Med 1997; 126:1–12.
14. Lipscomb J, Weinstein MC, Torrance GW. Time preference. In: Gold MR, Siegel JE, Russell LB, Weinstein MC, eds. Cost Effectiveness in Health and Medicine. New York: Oxford University Press, 1996:214–246.
15. Finkler SA. The distribution between cost and charges. Ann Intern Med 1982; 96:102–109.
16. Weinstein MC, Stason WB. Cost-effectiveness of interventions to prevent or treat coronary heart disease. Annu Rev Public Health 1985; 6:41–63,
17. Oster G, Epstein AM. Cost-effectiveness of antihyperlipemic therapy in the prevention of coronary heart disease. JAMA 1987; 258:2381–2387.
18. Kinosian BP, Eisenberg JM. Cutting into cholesterol. Cost-effective alternatives for treating hypercholesterolemia. JAMA 1988; 259:2249–2254.
19. Goldman L, Weinstein MC, Williams LW. Relative impact of targeted versus populationwide cholesterol interventions on the incidence of coronary heart disease. Projections of the coronary heart disease policy model. Circulation 1989; 80:254–260.
20. Martens LL, Rutten FFH, Erkelens DW, et al. Cost effectiveness of cholesterol lowering therapy in the Netherlands. Simvastatin versus cholestyramine. Am J Med 1989; 87(suppl 4A):54S–58S.
21. Schulman KA, Kinosian B, Jacobson TA, et al. Reducing high blood cholesterol level with drugs. Cost-effectiveness of pharmacologic management. JAMA 1990; 264:3025–3033.

22. Goldman L, Weinstein MC, Goldman PA, et al. Cost-effectiveness of HMG-CoA reductase inhibition for primary and secondary prevention of coronary heart disease. JAMA 1991; 265: 1145–1151.

23. Hay JW, Wittels EH, Gotto AM. An economic evaluation of lovastatin for cholesterol lowering and coronary artery disease reduction. Am J Cardiol 1991; 67:789–796.

24. Kristiansen IS, Eggen AE, Thelle DS. Cost effectiveness of incremental programmes for lowering serum cholesterol concentration: is individual intervention worth while? Br Med J 1991; 302:1119–1122.

25. Goldman L, Goldman PA, Williams LW, et al. Cost-effectiveness considerations in the treatment of heterozygous familial hypercholesterolemia with medications. Am J Cardiol 1993; 72:75D–79D.

26. Hamilton VH, Racicot FE, Zowall H, et al. The cost-effectiveness of HMG-CoA reductase inhibitors to prevent coronary heart disease. Estimating the benefits of increasing HDL-C. JAMA 1995; 273:1032–1038.

27. McGee D, Gordon T. The results of the Framingham study applied to four other U.S.-based epidemiological studies of cardiovascular disease. In: Kannel VM, Gordon T, eds. The Framingham Study: An Epidemiologic Investigation of Cardiovascular Disease. NIH publication No. 76–1083. Bethesda, MD: U.S. Goverment Printing Office, 1976.

28. Tyroler HA. Review of lipid-lowering clinical trials in relation to observational epidemiologic studies. Circulation 1987; 76:515–522.

29. Lipid Research Clinics Program. The Lipid Research Clinics Coronary Primary Prevention Trial results 1. Reduction in incidence of coronary heart disease. JAMA 1984; 251:351–364.

30. Scandinavian Simvastatin Survival Study Group. Randomised trial of cholesterol lowering in 4444 patients with coronary heart disease: the Scandinavian Simvastatin Survival Study (4S). Lancet 1994; 344:1383–1389.

31. Sacks FM, Pfeffer MA, Moye LA, et al. The effect of pravastatin on coronary events after myocardial infarction in patients with average cholesterol levels. N Engl J Med 1996; 335:1001–1009.

32. Weinstein MC, Coxson PG, Williams LW, et al. Forecasting coronary heart disease incidence, mortality and cost: the coronary heart disease policy model. Am J Public Health 1987; 77:1417–1426.

33. Pedersen TR, Kjekshus J, Berg K, et al. Cholesterol lowering and the use of healthcare resources. Results of the Scandinavian Simvastatin Survival Study. Circulation 1996; 93:1796–1802.

34. Johannesson M, Jonsson B, Kjekshus J, et al. Cost effectiveness of simvastatin treatment to lower cholesterol levels in patients with coronary heart disease. N Engl J Med 1997; 336:332–336,

35. Gordon T, Kannel YM. Multiple risk functions for predicting coronary heart disease: the concept, accuracy, and application. Am Heart J 1982; 103:1031–1039.

36. Pooling Project Research Group. Relationship of blood pressure, serum cholesterol, smoking habit, relative weight, and ECG abnormalities to incidence of major coronary events: final report of the Pooling Project. J Chron Dis 1978; 31:201–306.

37. Brand JRI, Rosenman RK Sholtz RI, et al. Multivariate prediction of coronary heart disease in the Western Collaborative Group Study compared to the findings of the Framingham Study. Circulation 1976; 53: 348–355.
38. Roussouw JE, Lewis B, Rifkind BM. The value of lowering cholesterol after myocardial infarction. N Engl J Med 1990; 323:1112–1119.
39. Kannel WB, Wolf PA, Garrison RF, eds. The Framingham Study: An Epidemiologic Investigation of Cardiovascular Disease. Section 35. Survival Following Initial Cardiovascular Events: Thirty Year Follow-Up. NIH publication No. 88–2969. Washington, DC: Government Printing Office, 1988.
40. Shaper AG, Pocock SJ, Walker M, et al. Risk factors for ischaemic heart disease: the prospective phase of the British Regional Heart Study. J Epidemiol Commun Health 1985; 39:197–209.
41. Gould AL, Roussouw JE, Santanello NC, Heyse JF, Furberg CD. Cholesterol reduction yields clinical benefit. A new look at old data. Circulation 1995; 91:227482.
42. Wilson PWF, Christiansen JC, Anderson KM, et al. Impact of national guidelines for cholesterol risk screening: the Framingham Offspring Study. JAMA 1989; 262:41–44.
43. Sempos C, Fulwood R, Haines C, et al. The prevalence of high blood cholesterol levels in the United States. JAMA 1989; 262:45–52.
44. Farquhar JW, Fortmann SP, Flora JA, et al. Effects of communitywide education on cardiovascular disease risk factors. The Stanford Five-City Project. JAMA 1990; 264:359–365.
45. Puska P, Salonen JT, Nissinen A, et al. Change in risk factors for coronary heart disease during 10 years of a community intervention programme (North Karelia Project). Br Med J 1983; 287:1840–1844.
46. Fortmann SP, Williams PT, Hulley SB, et al. Effect of health education on dietary behavior: the Stanford Three Community Study. J Clin Nutr 1981; 34:2030–2038,
47. Tosteson ANA, Weinstein MC, Hunink MGM, et al. Cost-effectiveness of populationwide educational approaches to reduce serum cholesterol levels. Circulation 1997; 95:24–30.
48. MacMahon SW, Cutler JA, Furberg CD, et al. The effects of drug treatment for hypertension on morbidity and mortatlity from cardiovascular disease: a review of randomized controlled trials. Prog Cardiovasc Dis 1086; 29:99–118.
49. Littenberg B, Garber AM, Sox HC. Screening for hypertension. Ann Intern Med 1990; 112:192–202.
50. Edelson JT, Weinstein MC, Tosteson ANA, et al. Long-term cost-effectiveness of various initial monotherapies for mild to moderate hypertension. JAMA 1990; 263:408–413.
51. Cummings SR, Rubin SM, Oster G. The cost-effectiveness of counseling smokers to quit. JAMA 1989; 261:75–79.
52. Oster G, Huse DM, Delea TE, Colditz GA. Cost-effectiveness of nicotine gum as an adjunct to physician's advice against cigarette smoking. JAMA 1986; 256:1315–1318.

53. Fiscelia K, Franks P. Cost-effectiveness of the transdermal nicotine patch as an adjunct to physician's smoking cessation counseling. JAMA 1996; 275:1247–1251.

54. Krumholz HM, Cohen BJ, Tsevat J, et al. Cost-effectiveness of a smoking cessation program after myocardial infarction. J Am Coll Cardiol 1993; 22:1697–1702.

55. Taylor AB, Houston-Miller N, Yillen JD, DeBusk RF. Smoking cessation after acute myocardial infarction: effect of a nurse-managed intervention. Ann Intern Med 1990; 113:118–123.

56. Silagy C, Mant D, Fowler G, et al. Meta-analysis on efficacy of nicotine replacement therapy in smoking cessation. Lancet 1994; 343:139–142.

57. Law M, Tang JL. An analysis of the effectiveness of interventions intended to help people stop smoking. Arch Intern Med 1995; 155:1933–1941.

58. Weinstein MC. Estrogen use in postmenopausal women-costs, risks and benefits. N Engl J Med 1980; 303:308–316.

59. Weinstein MC, Schiff I. Cost-effectiveness of hormone replacement therapy in the menopause. Obstet Gynecol Surv 1982; 38:445–455.

60. Weinstein MC, Tosteson ANA. Cost-effectiveness of hormone replacement. Ann NY Acad Sci 1990; 592:162–172.

61. Daly E, Roche M, Barlow D, et al. HRT: an analysis of benefits, risks and costs. Br Med Bull 1992; 48:368–400.

62. Tosteson ANA, Weinstein MC. Cost-effectiveness of hormone replacement therapy after the menopause. Ballieres Clin Obstet Gynaecol 1991; 5:943–959.

63. Powell KE, Thompson PD, Caspersen CJ, Kendrick JS. Physical activity and the incidence of coronary heart disease. Annu Rev Public Health 1987; 8:253–287.

64. Berlin JA, Colditz GA. A meta-analysis of physical activity in the prevention of coronary heart disease. Am J Epidemiol 1990; 132:639–646.

65. Paffenbarger RS Jr, Hyde RT, Wing AL, et al. The association of changes in physical-activity level and other lifestyle characteristics with mortality among men. N Engl J Med 1993; 328:538–545.

66. Hatziandreu EI, Koplan JP, Weinstein MC, et al. A cost-effectiveness analysis of exercise as a health promotion activity. Am J Public Health 1988; 78:1417–1421.

67. O'Connor GT, Buring JE, Yusuf S, et al. An overview of randomized trials of rehabilitation with exercise after myocardial infarction. Circulation 1989; 80:234–244.

68. Oldridge N, Furlong W, Feeney D, et al. Economic evaluation of cardiac rehabilitation soon after acute myocardial infarction. Am J Cardiol 1993; 72:154–161.

69. Oldridge NB, Guyatt G, Jones N, et al. Effects on quality of life with comprehensive rehabilitation after acute myocardial infarction. Am J Cardiol 1991; 67:1084–1089.

70. Gaspoz JM, Goldman P, Williams L, et al. Cost-effectiveness of aspirin in secondary prevention of coronary heart disease. Circulation 1995; 92(suppl):1–47. Abstract.

71. Final report on the aspirin component of the ongoing Physicians' Health Study. Steering Committee of the Physicians' Health Study Research Group. N Engl J Med 1989; 321:129–135.

72. van Bergen PFMM, Jonker JJC, van Hout BA, et al. Costs and effects of long-term oral anticoagulant treatment after myocadial infarction. JAMA 1995; 273:925–928.

73. Cairns JA, Markham BA. Economics and efficacy in choosing oral anticoagulants or aspirin after myocardial infaretion. JAMA 1995; 273: 965–967.

74. Kupersmith J, Holmes-Rovner M, Hogan A, et al. Cost-effectiveness analysis in heart disease. Part III: ischemia, congestive heart failure, and arrhythmias. Prog Cardiovasc Dis 1995; 37:307–346.

10

Applied Genetics Now and Gene Therapy in the Future

Roger R. Williams, Paul N. Hopkins, Lily Wu, and Steven C. Hunt
University of Utah School of Medicine, Salt Lake City, Utah

I. PRACTICE THE MEDICINE OF THE FUTURE NOW!

In the past two decades we have witnessed a virtual explosion in the understanding of genetic factors promoting or preventing atherosclerosis (1). In the next two decades we should see dramatic changes in they way we practice medicine. We stand at the intersection of discovery and application. This chapter will help you learn to apply the growing knowledge of genetics so you can start now practicing medicine of the future!

II. TWO TYPES OF GENETIC FACTORS

Genetic factors can be classified as *major genes* or *polygenes*. Both can contribute to a person's susceptibility and resistance to atherosclerosis as illustrated in Figure 1.

Polygenic traits (like LDL cholesterol in all of us) show a *continuous blending effect. Offspring* generally have a polygenically determined cholesterol level approximately halfway between the levels of the two parents when values are measured at about the same age for both generations. Classic polygenic traits lead to *sibling similarity*. If we find a patient with a polygenically high cholesterol, *all* siblings will usually have a similarly elevated cholesterol, as shown for one sibship in Figure 2. This leads to a practical application: when we find a patient who meets criteria for treatment of a polygenically elevated LDL cholesterol level (the most common cause), we

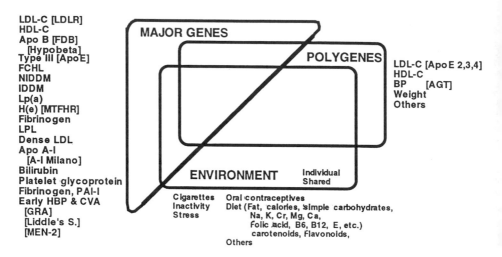

Figure 1   Multifactorial factors promoting atherosclerosis. Overlapping domains represent combined (additive or multiplicative) effects of major genes, polygenes, and environmental factors.

should routinely arrange for all siblings to be tested to find others with similar levels needing treatment (2). HDL cholesterol, blood pressure, and weight are examples of other common risk factors showing strong polygenic effects.

Major gene traits such as heterozygous familial hypercholesterolemia (FH) have Mendelian inheritance (dominant for FH heterozygotes). If one parent carries a dominant gene, on average half of the offspring will receive the gene and half will not, causing *segregation* or *bimodal separation* of the offspring into two groups: those with twice normal LDL cholesterol levels

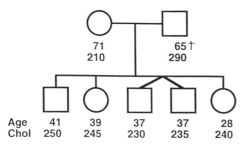

Figure 2   Sibship illustrating the common polygenic form of hypercholesterolemia.

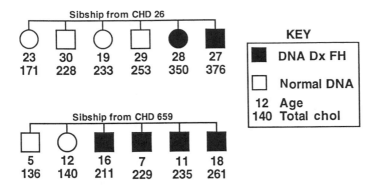

Figure 3   Two sibships with FH showing bimodality from presence of absence of the major gene (LDL receptor defect) and background polygenic effects shifting the entire sibship toward higher cholesterol levels in the upper sibship and toward lower levels in the bottom sibship.

and those with normal cholesterol levels (3). The separation is very evident in two sibships shown in Figure 3 from families with heterozygous FH. DNA markers for the LDL receptor locus on the short arm of chromosome 19 were used to genetically diagnose the presence or absence of FH in these two sibships as indicated. In Figure 3 the siblings were sorted in order of increasing cholesterol level. In the upper sibship there is a jump of almost 100 mg/dl (2.6 mmol/L) between the highest normal sibling and the lowest sib carrying the FH gene. In the second sibship on the bottom of Figure 3, a similar large "gap" is 71 mg or 1.8 mmol. Clear separation into two distinct groups (called *bimodality*) is characteristic of a major gene. These principles have been summarized into diagnostic criteria for FH (4) in Table 1.

The left side of Figure 1 lists other major gene risk factors for atherosclerosis. Other well-defined atherogenic major genes include familial defective apolipoprotein B (FDB), high Lp(a), dominant and recessive variants of Apo-E (type III hyperlipidemia), heterozygous lipoprotein lipase deficiency (LPL), and homozygous deficiency of methylene tetrahydrofolate reductase (hyperhomocysteinemia). There are three well-defined genetic variants that seem to be antiatherogenic including CETP deficiency with very high HDL (5), Apo-A-I Milano with apparent facilitated reverse cholesterol transport (6), and hypobetalipoproteinemia with very low apo-B and LDL cholesterol (7).

Diabetes, FCHL, and pure low HDL are clinical atherogenic syndromes that exhibit some of the characteristics of major gene traits (bimodality and vertical transmission in multigenerational pedigrees). Challenges encountered in some large genetic studies of these trait suggest that they are more complex

Table 1 Criteria for Diagnosing Heterozygous FH

Individual criteria	LDL-chol mg/dl (mmol/ml)[a]		
	Age	Index	Relative
1. Very high LDL-chol	40+	260 (6.7)	205 (5.3)
	30s	240 (6.2)	190 (4.9)
	20s	220 (5.4)	170 (4.4)
	< 18	200 (5.2)	160 (4.1)
2. No secondary cause (nephrosis, pregnancy, etc.)			
Family criteria			
3. Tendon xanthoma or youth > LDL criteria			
4. Bimodal LDL-chol (70–100 mg/dl gap)			

Source: From Ref. 4.
[a] Note: Because of higher a priori probability of having FH, relatives can be diagnosed with FH using lower LDL cholesterol criteria than persons evaluated as new index cases not known to be part of a family with FH.

than simple monogenic disorders. Two genes may work together to promote these disorders, and gene-environment interactions may play important roles yet to be defined in precise genetic models.

Causal mutations are also known for three dominant hypertension syndromes (GRA, Liddle's syndrome, and MEN-II) (8–10).

Table 2 presents a large number of "candidate gene loci" under investigation for their possible connections to atherogenesis. Some are known sequences with a physiological effect suspected of relating to atherogenesis. Others are loci suggested to be genetically linked or associated with either atherosclerosis or a risk factor.

Polygenic background influences phenotypic expression of a *major gene* as illustrated in Figure 3. In the upper sibship, polygenic influence has shifted the entire sibship toward higher background cholesterol, resulting in higher than average cholesterol for siblings without FH as well as higher than average levels for FH in the affected siblings. In the lower sibship of Figure 3, polygenic influence has shifted the entire sibship toward lower cholesterol, resulting in lower than average cholesterol (for their respective major gene status) in both the non-FH and FH siblings.

Recognizing *bimodality* in sibships establishes the "cut point" between gene carriers and noncarriers in families with traits like FH. Applying this

Table 2 Candidate Genes for Atherosclerosis and Its Risk Factor

Lipids and lipoproteins
  AI-CIII-AIV Apo group
  Apo-B (FDB, hypo-beta)
  Apo-E-2, 3, 4
  CETP chol ester transfer protein
  Cholesterol-7 alpha hydroxoylase
  CII Apo-C-II
  Fatty acid binding protein (FABP3)
  HMG-CoA reductase
  HTGL hepatic TGL lipase
  LCAT lecithin chol acetyl transferase
  LDL receptor
  Lp(a)/plasminogen
  LPL lipoprotein lipase
  Scavenger receptor (HDL receptor)
  VLDL receptor
Thrombogenic factors
  Antithrombin III
  Factor V Leiden (venous thrombosis) Factor VII
  Fibrinogen (FGA, FGG, FGB, HAEIII and Beta-854)
  PAI-1
  PDGF
  Platelet IIIa/IIb glycoprotein
  Platelet activating factor receptor (PTAFR)
  TGF-beta
  Thrombomodulin (THBD)
  Tromboxane A_2 receptor (TBXA$_2$R)
Obesity
  Leptin receptor
  OB/leptin
  TNF tumor necrosis factor
Diabetes and insulin resistance
  Glucagon receptor
  Glucokinase
  Glycogen synthase
  NIDDM1
  Sulfonurea receptor (SUR)
Adhesion molecules
  Endothelial leukocyte adhesion molecule (ELAM1)
  Vascular cell adhesion molecule-1 (VCAM-1)
  Intracellular adhesion molecule-1 (ICAM1)

Table 2   (Continued)

Antioxidants
  Piroxicam
  PAF hydrolase
Homocysteine
  MTHFR
  CBS
  Methionine synthase
Hypertension—renin angiotensin system
  AGT angiotensinogen
  ACE angiotensin converting enzyme
  REN structural gene for renin
  RBP renin binding protein
  AT2R1 angiotensin II receptor type-1
Hypertension—kallikrein system
  KALK1 kallikrein
  KIN kininogen
  KST kallistatin
  BDKRB2 bradykinin receptor B$_2$
Hypertension—nitric oxide system
  NOSe endothelial NO synthase
  NOSI inducible NO synthase
  NOSB NO synthase in brain
Hypertension—ion transport and ion channels
  Epithelial Na channel (Liddle's locus)/SA?
  NHE3 new Na-H antiporter
  Cl-HCO3 exchanger?
  Human anion exchanger isoform
  Glucocorticoid receptor
Hypertension—endothelin system
  Entothelins? (1, 2, 3 etc.)
  Endothelin receptor?
Hypertension—other candidates
  CYP11B1 11–beta hydroxylase/Aldo synthase
  Mineralocorticoid receptor
  ADRB3 beta-3 adrenergic receptor
  Atrionaturiuretic peptide receptor, type A
  Near LPL locus (8p22QTL)

practical knowledge to the two sibships in Figure 3 helps us correctly infer that the 29-year-old male in the top sibship with a cholesterol of 253 does not carry the gene for FH, while the 16-year-old male in the bottom sibship with a cholesterol of 211 does carry the gene for FH.

III. GENE-ENVIRONMENT INTERACTION

The relative impact of *environmental factors* depends on a patient's genetic resistance or susceptibility (11), as illustrated in Figure 4. Among persons ages 30 to 49, cigarette smoking shows a multiplicative interaction with genetic background identified in this case using family history of coronary heart disease (CHD). A CHD relative risk of 4 for smokers with a strong positive family history (+FHx) compares to the usual relative risk of 2 for ordinary smokers (–FHx). This translates into about 10 to 14 years of increased life for smoking cessation in patients with genes like FH, compared to about 2 to 4 years added longevity for smoking cessation in the general population. The practical application in this case leads to vigorous lifestyle modifications for genetically susceptible persons because they can benefit even more than average from risk reduction involving strongly interacting environmental factors such as smoking.

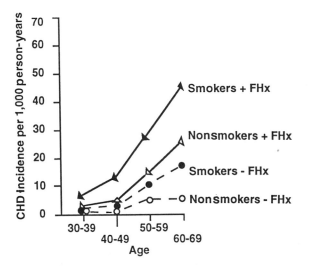

Figure 4 CHD incidence rates by family history and smoking status illustrates a multiplicative interaction, especially in the younger two age groups.

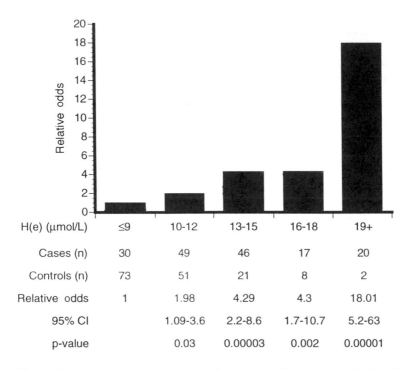

H(e) (μmol/L)	≤9	10-12	13-15	16-18	19+
Cases (n)	30	49	46	17	20
Controls (n)	73	51	21	8	2
Relative odds	1	1.98	4.29	4.3	18.01
95% CI		1.09-3.6	2.2-8.6	1.7-10.7	5.2-63
p-value		0.03	0.00003	0.002	0.00001

Figure 5   Relative odds of coronary disease according to plasma levels of homocysteine in 162 men and women with early coronary heart disease compared to 155 age- and sex-matched controls without coronary heart disease (12). Note substantially increased risk of CHD for persons with homocysteine levels above 13 μmol/L.

The relative impact of genetic factors may also depend on a patient's environmental exposure status. Homocysteine levels above 13 to 19 μmol/L seem to promote coronary atherosclerosis (12) (Figure 5). The level of homocysteine can be affected by a common "heat-labile" mutation of the gene for methylene tetrahydrofolate reductase (MTHFR) as well as by dietary intake of a common vitamin, folic acid. As illustrated in Figure 6, persons who developed the high homocysteine levels associated with high risk for coronary atherosclerosis generally required *both* genetic and environmental risk exposure. They were homozygous for the MTHFR heat labile mutation *and* had low folic acid intake (as reflected in serum levels) (13). These data suggest that neither low folate alone nor homozygous MTHFR mutation status would confer the strong risk of hyperhomocysteinemia and early CHD. *Both* genetic and environmental exposures are required for the strong risk CHD in this example.

Meaningful synergy has been suggested for selected environmental factors with specific genetic syndromes. Restricting saturated fat and cholesterol

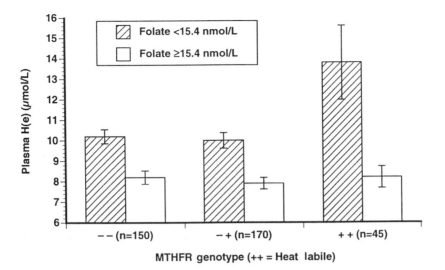

Figure 6   Plasma homocysteine levels (mean H(e) + SEM), according to presence (+) or absence (−) of the MTHFR mutation and folate intake levels (13). Note the degree of elevation associated with substantially increased risk for CHD [i.e., H(e) above 13 μmol/L] are limited mostly to those with *both* homozygous MTHFR deficiency *and* low folate intake.

helps lower cholesterol for persons with FH, while restricting calories or simple carbohydrates is not particularly helpful. Physical activity, weight reduction, and a diabetic type diet are beneficial for persons with familial combined hyperlipidemia (FCHL). Recent studies also indicate that the angiotensinogen gene variant promoting hypertension identifies a subset in whom sodium restriction may be especially beneficial (i.e., "salt-sensitive hypertension"). Generous intake of B vitamins and folate seem particularly important for persons carrying genes that promote hyperhomocysteinemia. Thus a proper genetic diagnosis can lead to very effective risk reduction by choosing interventions that focus on specific environmental factors found to have strong interaction with that particular genetic syndrome.

IV. RELATIVE MAGNITUDE OF GENES VERSUS ENVIRONMENT?

The maximal stable cholesterol lowering effect of diet seems to be about 20% to 30% based on good compliance with very strict diets like the Pritikin (14) and Dean Ornish (15). If we assume a "normal" cholesterol level to be about

200 mg/dl (about 5 mmol/L), then a 20% to 30% increase would be about 240 to 260 mg or about 6.0 to 6.5 mmol. Thus, it seems reasonable to assume that most persons who have a level > 240 to 260 mg or 6.0 to 6.5 mmol not only have a *cholesterol level needing treatment* but also must have one that is *genetically elevated*. This leads to several important conclusions. First, persons with cholesterol levels high enough to require therapy are not just reckless eaters; they are "genetically challenged" and deserve our sympathy and help. Second, whether their underlying genetic cause is major gene or polygenic, they all have siblings likely to share their need for screening and treatment. In other words, "every cholesterol patient is a proband" for family screening.

Obesity is another prominent factor in atherosclerosis. While diet and exercise obviously play an important role, genes likely play a very strong role especially for those who are extremely lean or extremely obese. Major research efforts are under way to map and understand genes for obesity. Future medications will likely include drugs to normalize weight for morbidly obese patients just as potent statins now help patients with FH normalize their cholesterol levels. This underscores another practical application of genetics. Discovering genes that promote or prevent disease also leads to new and better diagnostic and therapeutic approaches.

V.   APPLYING THE PRINCIPLES TO A LIPID CASE HISTORY

Assume you are caring for a 45–year-old man with a fasting total cholesterol of 310 mg/dl, normal triglycerides (125 mg/dl), low HDL cholesterol (33 mg/dl), and high calculated LDL cholesterol (252 mg/dl). He doesn't have any secondary causes such as hypothyroidism or nephrosis. His father and brother both had myocardial infarctions before age 55. The lipid levels in relatives are not known to the patient.

Practical questions:

1. Is this patient's high LDL-cholesterol most likely due to genes or environment or both?
2. What would be the differential diagnosis?
3. What would be required to determine the exact genetic diagnosis?
4. Will you likely prescribe medication for this patient's cholesterol regardless of the genetic causes?
5. If so, are there any important practical reasons to go to the trouble to make the genetic diagnosis?

6. His 43-year-old brother has about the same lipid levels and asks you what he should do about diet and exercise. What do you tell this brother?

Answers:

1. The magnitude of this cholesterol elevation (55% above the median for his age) strongly suggests an underlying genetic factor.
2. FH, FCHL, and polygenic hypercholesterolemia (PH) are all possibilities. It would be on the low-average end of the distribution for FH, high end of the distribution for PH, and high average for FCHL. PH and FH usually have normal triglycerides. Although 75% of affected persons in families with FCHL have high triglycerides, about 25% will have high LDL and normal triglycerides.
3. First examine the patient looking for tendon xanthoma that would establish the diagnosis of FH. In the absence of tendon xanthoma, obtaining lipid levels in siblings, children, aunts and uncles, nieces and nephews will help distinguish the diagnosis. Collecting a "lipid family history," as illustrated in Figure 7, is a key approach for diagnosing all familial lipid disorders as well as for finding affected relatives who need treatment. Finding high triglycerides as well as high cholesterol levels in siblings supports the diagnosis of familial combined (FCHL). Bimodal pure LDL-cholesterol elevations and very high LDL-cholesterol in children indicate FH. A blending effect producing similar levels in siblings and absence of severe pediatric hypercholesterolemia supports PH.
4. An *LDL-cholesterol* of 252 mg/dl will not drop below 200 mg/dl even with a superb diet. This 45–year-old male with low HDL and positive family history meets NCEP guidelines for medication. The goal should be to get the level down to about 130 mg/dl. Drug therapy will be indicated regardless of whether the diagnosis is FH, PH, or FCHL.
5. There are *several* practical reasons for making the proper genetic diagnosis. The treatment strategies are different for FH vs. PH or FCHL, thus justifying the effort required to make a specific genetic diagnosis. In addition the strategy for screening in relatives is also somewhat different:
    a. Screening relatives
        Screening lipids in relatives is necessary to help make the diagnosis. At the same time it will identify several other persons requiring treatment for FH, or PH, or FCHL. Extended relative screening is not recommended for PH but is for FH and FCHL. If this patient has FH, *screening should extend to third*

Medical Family History   This section is important. Please complete it as accurately as possible

List all relatives, not just those with problems. Please make an effort to obtain as much information as possible. **Give approximate age for first occurrence or diagnosis for each disease or problem listed.** See the example provided. You may need to call your relatives for missing information. **Circle either Bro / Sis, etc. for gender.**

BLOOD LEVELS: List the worst levels known (highest serum cholesterol, triglycerides, lowest HDL cholesterol). Approximate levels may be listed. Phone calls may be necessary to verify.

RELATIONSHIP	First Name	Living (L) or Dead (D)	AGE (now or at death)	CAUSE OF DEATH IF DECEASED	HEART ATTACK	CORONARY BYPASS SURGERY	CORONARY ANGIOPLASTY (PTCA)	STROKE	HIGH BLOOD PRESSURE (treated)	DIABETES	CIGARETTES (C)urrent (F)ormer (N)ever	WEIGHT (A)verage (O)verweight 50+ lbs	Total Cholesterol	Triglycerides	HDL Cholesterol
					AGE OF FIRST OCCURRENCE										
Example	John	D	70	Heart Attack	50	52			40		C	A	255	140	35
You															
Father															
Mother															
Bro / Sis															
Bro / Sis															
Bro / Sis															
Bro / Sis															
Bro / Sis															
Spouse															
Son / Dau															
Son / Dau															
Son / Dau															
Son / Dau															
Pat GF															
Pat GM															
Pat A / U															
Pat A / U															
Pat A / U															
Pat A / U															
Pat A / U															
Mat GF															
Mat GM															
Mat A / U															
Mat A / U															
Mat A / U															
Mat A / U															
Mat A / U															

Pat = paternal, Mat = maternal, GF = grandfather, GM = grandmother, A = aunt, U = uncle

Figure 7   A useful questionnaire for obtaining a detailed "Lipid Family History." It will often take about 6 months of letters and phone calls to collect all of this information from the relatives listed. Once collected it usually leads to a specific diagnosis and also identifies affected relatives needing treatment.

degree relatives including children because this major gene is easy to trace in extended relatives. For PH, only siblings and adult children need screening. In FCHL families extended adult relatives can be tested and found needing treatment.

b. Cardiology workup

FH experts recommend a treadmill and other tests for FH men in their 40s even in the absence of symptoms. They find a significant percentage will have lesions requiring bypass surgery or angioplasty. If you diagnose never-treated heterozygous FH in a 45-year-old male, you have identified a man with high risk of current silent coronary atherosclerosis and MI in the near future. Remember his very high cholesterol has been present for over four decades, in contrast to men the same age with PH or FCHL whose cholesterol may have only been this high for one or two decades.

c. Exercise prescription

Even with a normal treadmill, *jogging could be dangerous for this man with FH* as it has been the cause of death of many FH men in their 40s. Walking would be a safer form of exercise. The benefit of jogging is also limited for FH because exercise does not help LDL receptor defects or lower LDL cholesterol in persons with FH.

Exercise poses less risk and offers more benefit for FCHL men in their 40s than men with FH. Therefore jogging should be encouraged if this patient has FCHL and passes a treadmill ECG. Several common findings in FCHL patients often improve with regular aerobic exercise including hyperinsulinemia, obesity, high triglycerides, low HDL, and high blood pressure. In persons with PH, jogging is less dangerous and possibly more beneficial in those with FH but less dramatically beneficial than in those with FCHL.

d. Dietary prescription

Dietary prescriptions should be tailored to the specific genetic diagnosis. Patients with FCHL often need a diet like those prescribed for patients with NIDDM. *FH patients do not need to limit calories or simple carbohydrates*, as these have no effect on the LDL receptor defects that cause their high LDL cholesterol. The diet for an FH man will be pure low fat and low cholesterol. For patients with polygenic hypercholesterolemia, the diet is similar to that for FH.

6. The recommendation for an affected brother will be the same as for the patient and will depend on which genetic diagnosis is present in this family, FH, FCHL, or PH.

VI. DOMINANT HYPERTENSION SYNDROMES

Two severe dominant forms of hypertension (GRA and Liddle's syndrome) lead to early severe hypertension and strokes. Applying our new understanding of these disorders can lead to informative diagnostic tests and effective therapy tailored to the specific pathophysiology. Without this understanding many patients will die of early strokes in the fourth decade of life because they remain undiagnosed, severely hypertensive, and unresponsive to ineffective ordinary therapy.

Glucocorticoid remediable aldosteronism (GRA) results from a dominant "gain of function" mutation on chromosome 8, inducing high levels of abnormal adrenal steroids 18–hydroxy cortisol and 18–oxocortisol (8). This unusual chimeric mutation is derived from the combination of fragments of two genes—the aldosterone synthase gene, and the steroid 11–beta-hydroxylase gene. The DNA sequences of these two genes are 95% identical, they have identical intron-exon boundaries, and they are located next to each other on chromosome 8. During recombination, unequal crossing over has occurred, producing the mutant gene with sequences and functions of both genes combined into the variant. Administration of exogenous glucocorticoids (like dexamethasone) can often suppress aldosterone, abnormal steroids, and the severe blood pressure elevations. Persons with the gene for GRA often have early severe hypertension and close relatives dying of cerebral hemorrhage in their forties. GRA often fails to respond to ordinary antihypertensive medications but can respond to prednisone (suppress hormone production), spironolactone (competitively inhibit aldosterone receptor), or amiloride (inhibit distal renal epithelial sodium channel response to mineralocorticoid action).

Liddle's syndrome results from dominant mutations at a locus coding for the beta subunit of the epithelial sodium channel on chromosome 16p. A genetically activated channel cannot be maintained in a properly closed state (9). A low plasma renin activity and variable hypokalemia is seen in this syndrome as in GRA. However, Liddle's syndrome also causes suppressed aldosterone secretion in contrast to the hyperaldosteronism seen in GRA. Excessive reabsorption of sodium and exchange for potassium in the distal nephron probably account for the hypertension and hypokalemia. Both of these features of Liddle's syndrome are responsive to triamterine or amiloride, which specifically inhibit the epithelial sodium channel. Unlike GRA, this syndrome is not responsive to spironolactone, which inhibits the mineralocorticoid receptor. Kidney transplant also seems to eliminate the problem.

VII. ANGIOTENSINOGEN: A COMMON GENE FOR "SALT-SENSITIVE HYPERTENSION"?

Commonly occurring hypertension is also thought to result from the effects of milder effects of multiple genes in combination with environmental factors. Large studies under way in several countries are likely to produce a list of several common genes contributing to hypertension.

Variants of the gene for angiotensinogen (AGT) on chromosome 1 seem to promote hypertension, probably in a manner consistent with several theories of "salt-sensitive hypertension." Several different approaches have been taken. The AGT gene has been genetically linked to essential hypertension in several diverse populations (16–18), and genetically associated with both essential hypertension and pre-eclampsia in several populations(16,18,19). Higher levels by genotype suggest a pathophysiologic mechanism involving increased production of the substrate angiotensinogen. Homozygous carriers of this AGT variant show blunting of renal response to infusion of angiotensin II (thought be some to be a sign of salt-sensitive hypertension) (20).

VIII. APPLYING THE PRINCIPLES TO A HYPERTENSION CASE HISTORY

Assume you are caring for a 40-year-old man with a resting blood pressure of 210/135 mm Hg who has not responded to diuretics, beta blockers, ACE inhibitors, or calcium channel blockers. He has normal renal function and no evidence of renal artery stenosis. His older brother had a stroke when he was only 45. His 16-year-old daughter has a blood pressure of 160/95.

Practical questions:

1. What possible genetic diagnoses should be considered?
2. What could be done to establish or rule out one of the dominant hypertension syndromes?
3. How could screening relatives help prevent early strokes? Which relatives should be screened?
4. How specific should the medications be tailored to genetic diagnoses for these dominant hypertension syndromes?

Answers:

1. Glucocorticoid remediable aldosteronism (GRA) and Liddle's syndrome are both dominant hypertension syndromes leading to early severe hypertension and stroke. Both are unresponsive to the ordinary antihypertensive medications listed above.

2. GRA often responds to a trial with spironolactone or dexamethasone, which address the two problems of abnormal steroids causing hyperaldosteronism and severe hypertension. Severe hypertension with Liddle's syndrome responds to amelioride or triamterene. Once suspected on these clinical grounds, specific diagnoses may be made by testing blood and urine for endocrine abnormalities described above. DNA testing can often identify a specific causal mutation for these disorders.

3. All first- and second-degree relatives should be screened for hypertension or diagnostic endocrine abnormalities. If specific mutations are known for a given family, other relatives can be sequentially screened and given a definitive result (gene present or absent) from a single blood sample. It is important to make the diagnosis and institute effective treatment as early as possible. Once the hypertension has been present too long, it generates vessel and renal changes that cause irreversible hypertension even with proper medication. Tracing families with GRA and Liddle's syndrome can save relatives from early strokes and premature death. All easily found relatives should be traced on the affected side of the family. This should usually include siblings, offspring, parents, aunts and uncles, nieces and nephews, and first cousins and their offspring.

4. GRA and Liddle's syndrome are two excellent examples of clinical settings in which very specific medications can be chosen to match a specific genetic mechanism. Steroids or spironolactone are specific for GRA. Triamterene, amiloride, or renal transplantation are specific treatments for Liddle's syndrome.

IX. MAKE EARLY DIAGNOSES AND PREVENT EARLY DEATHS

Unfortunately, even well-understood and very treatable dominant disorders like FH are not diagnosed or treated in most gene carriers (21). For relatively uncommon gene traits like FH, FDB, GRA, and Liddle's syndrome, many cases can be found more efficiently by screening relatives than by screening the general population. If treatment can normalize levels and prevent or delay early CHD or stroke deaths, shouldn't there be a vigorous effort to find and help persons in these super high risk pedigrees? MED PED is a non-profit humanitarian project that attempts to answer that need. Currently organized in 21 collaborating countries, MED PED registries try to collect all known index cases with FH or FDB and then contact relatives for screening and treatment in both close and distant MEDical PEDigrees. From one index case 5 to 15 new FH cases can often be found among "close relatives" (siblings, parents, offspring, aunts, uncles, nieces, nephews, first cousins, and their offspring). In some cases hundreds of FH cases have been found by extending screening to "distant relatives" (second, third, and fourth cousins and their offspring).

The collection of detailed medical family histories together with contacting and helping relatives in high-risk pedigrees like these with FH, FDB, GRA, and Liddle's syndrome should become part of routinely supported medical care. At the present time the MED PED collaborators are setting an example of case detection through relative screening. The MED PED effort is supported by humanitarian funding to demonstrate the need and feasibility of this approach to justify future support by government and health insurance agencies. If you know of patients who seem to have FH (see criteria in Table 2), GRA, or Liddle's syndrome, you can obtain free help tracing relatives by calling this toll free number: 1-888-2HI-CHOL. MED PED staff will help you find undiagnosed or untreated relatives who have the same deadly gene.

MED PED collaborators in 21 countries have collectively identified over 16,000 patients with FH (22). By contacting relatives of known FH cases, many new cases are diagnosed every day. By educating patients and their personal physicians and by helping them get additional help from referral specialists, many FH patients are experiencing dramatic (40% to 50%) reductions in LDL cholesterol levels. Annual follow-up contacts and involvement in FH support groups and lay organizations help address the most important challenge to life long medication: *long-term compliance.*

X. MED PED PARADIGM FOR OTHER GENETIC DISEASES

This same approach could work for similar diseases as long as they meet these criteria:

1. A single dominant gene causes preventable serious illness.
2. Validated diagnostic tests are available (gene test or clinical test).
3. Some form of treatment or prevention is available and shown to be effective.

Several other single gene disorders fit these criteria (Table 3).

XI. SOCIAL ISSUES: COST AND CONFIDENTIALITY

The cost-effectiveness of drug therapy for FH has been rigorously analyzed and documented (23). Daily treatment with a low dose of lovastatin was

Table 3 Treatable Dominant Cardiovascular Diseases

Genetic trait	Description	Clinical diagnosis	Genetic diagnosis	Treatment or prevention
Familial hypercholester- olemia (FH)	High LDL cholesterol and very early heart attack deaths	LDL cholesterol and xanthoma; quite reliable	LDL receptor gene tests (> 200 caus- al mutations)	Drugs reduce cholesterol and likely extend life 10 to 30 years
Familial defective Apo-B (FDB)	High apolipoprotein-B and cholesterol with early heart attack deaths	High cholesterol can mimic FH, but some are lower	Two specific caus- al mutations.	Same as for FH for those with very high cholesterol
Dominant Type III hyperlipidemia	Very high beta VLDL cholesterol with early heart attack deaths	High triglyceride and abnormal TRIG/VLDL ratio	Several specific causal mutations	Specific medications can often normalize levels and prolong life
Long QT syndrome	High risk for sudden arrhythmic death in youth and young adults	Long duration of QT interval on ECG	Linkage found and mutations being sought	Medication can lower risk of sudden death and prolong life
GRA hypertension	Severe high blood pressure and early stroke	Abnormal steroid hor- mones; BP normal after dexamethasone	Several specific causal mutations	Suppress abnormal steroids with hormones like dexamethasone
Liddle's syndrome	Severe high blood pressure and early stroke	Selective BP response to ameloride and triamterene	Causal mutations	Ameloride or triamterene
MEN-II	Pheochromocytoma and other endocrine neoplasia	MRI and CT scans for tumors	Causal mutations	Surgical removal of endocrine tumors

projected *to save money as well as lives,* and higher-dose therapy was associated with an acceptable cost per year of life saved in this conservative
analysis (23).

Some social scientists raise concerns about projects like MED PED causing psychological stress by contacting relatives to talk about their family history.
MED PED collaborators in several countries report a *large preponderance of
positive reactions* from relatives contacted in FH families. The dramatic occurrence of very early heart attack deaths in FH families is usually well known
to relatives. Whether they know their cholesterol level or not, many relatives
in FH pedigrees already worry about having an early heart attack death long
before being contacted by MED PED. Because of MED PED, thousands of
relatives have been screened and found to have normal cholesterol and reas-
sured that their fear of early death was not warranted. Others found to have
very high cholesterol levels have learned something very few of them knew
before MED PED: their super high cholesterol levels can be dramatically
reduced and early heart attack deaths can be prevented! Similar observations
are likely to be found in the dominant hypertension families.

XII. GENE THERAPY—THE FRONTIER OF MOLECULAR MEDICINE!

The Wright brothers traveled a very short distance in a very crude airplane.
But it marked the beginning, and today air travel is a key part of our society
relied upon each day by many ordinary people. Gene therapy is already
beyond the historic first flight. For atherosclerotic diseases the first short flight
was launched in 1992 for a person with homozygous FH (24). To replace the
genetically absent LDL receptors, some of his liver cells were surgically
removed, infected with a virus containing the human gene sequence for normal LDL receptors, and "returned" to his liver. It required statin drug stimulation of the few newly acquired LDL receptors to produce a perceptible
drop in serum cholesterol from this procedure. The effect was much too small
to have meaningful clinical results. But like the first flight at Kitty Hawk,
the first gene therapy for FH in Michigan "got off the ground."

At this beginning stage, some probably view gene therapy as a last
chance hope for rare FH homozygotes. But it offers much more! For starters
it offers the potential for a *permanent* cure for 10 million FH *heterozygotes.*
Fully successful gene replacement will be a *cure,* not just a treatment. We
have drugs that help many FH heterozygotes now, but noncompliance deprives
many of them of the full benefit of therapy. Normal genes work night and
day without side effects, and a recipient of successful gene therapy won't
forget to take the next dose.

Basic technical challenges of gene therapy include: (a) obtaining a gene sequence with beneficial effects when expressed in the appropriate tissue; (b) attaching the therapeutic DNA to a vehicle like a virus; and (c) delivering it in large numbers to cells where its effect is needed. These are not trivial tasks, but solutions to technical challenges seem to take time until ingenious minds forge the path from first flight to jet flight.

Gene therapy has potential beyond replacing defective genes. It can override the effects of existing genes. It can carry the benefits of antiatherogenic genes from naturally protected humans to others born without this good fortune.

Citing some current gene therapy research projects illustrates progress well under way. In Rochester, Minnesota, the endothelial nitric oxide synthase gene (eNOs) is under study because nitric oxide is a potent vasodilator which may also inhibit platet aggregation and smooth muscle cell proliferation. An adenoviral vector encoding cDNA for eNOs was generated by homologous recombination and applied in vitro to porcine coronary smooth muscle cells achieving increased levels of nitrate and cGMP and diminished cell proliferation (25).

In Milan, Italy, apo-E-deficient mice were given intramuscular injections of naked supercoiled plasmids containing complete human apo-E cDNA. The injected DNA is maintained in an episomal, circular form and does not replicate. But transgene persistence has been demonstrated up to 19 months. In these apo-E-deficient mice, average total cholesterol levels were significantly decreased from the first week after plasmid injection and achieved a drop from 441 mg/dl to 273 mg/dl by the eighth week (26).

In Houston, Texas, synthetic DNA complexes have been constructed that are as efficient vectors as viruses but lack the immunological limitations. Furthermore, specific, high-level expression of these exogenous genes was achieved by receptor-mediated delivery of synthetic DNA vectors, coated, condensed, and targeted by lipophilic, nonexchangeable derivatives of apolipoprotein E-3 peptides, which are high-affinity ligands for the LDL and VLDL receptors. This method is being used to identify and modify the barriers to targeted delivery to hepatocytes in vivo (27).

In Parma, Italy, a molecular variant called Apo-A-I Milano, is under study because it seems to protect against coronary disease (despite causing a low HDL cholesterol). In transgenic mice it seems to promote more efficient cholesterol efflux from cells ("reverse cholesterol transport") (28). Within two decades, we may well be writing prescriptions for genes rather than medications. Compliance will be complete and automatic. High-risk genes causing tragedy in some families will be conquered, and protective genes that now prevent atherosclerosis in a few lucky families may be shared with everyone who needs them. The technology seems likely to succeed. The social and economic factors may be the rate-limiting step!

REFERENCES

1. Hopkins PN, Williams RR. Human genetics and coronary heart disease: a public health perspective. Ann Rev Nut 1989; 9:303–345.
2. Williams RR, Hopkins PN, Wu LL, Hunt SC. Guidelines for managing severe familial lipid disorders. Primary Cardiol 1995; 21:47–53.
3. Hobbes HH, Brown MS, Goldstein JL. Molecular genetics of the LDL receptor gene in familial hypercholesterolemia. Human Mutation 1992; 1:445–466.
4. Williams RR, Hunt SC, Schumacher MC, et al. Diagnosing heterozygous familial hypercholesterolemia using new practical criteria validated by molecular genetics. Am J Cardiol 1993; 72:171–176.
5. Inazu A, Brown ML, Hesler CB, et al. Increased high-density lipoprotein levels caused by a common cholesteryl-ester transfer protein gene mutation. N Engl J Med 1990; 323:1234–1238.
6. Sirtori CR, Franceschini G. Hypoalphalipoproteinemia: from a mutation to drug development. In: Woodford FP, Davignon, Sniderman A, eds. Atherosclerosis X. Amsterdam: Elsevier, 1995:50–55.
7. Pullinger CR, Hillas E, Hardman DA, et al. Two apolipoprotein B gene defects in a kindred with hypobetalipoproteinemia, one of which results in a truncated variant, apoB-61, in VLDL and LDL. J Lipid Res 1992; 33:699–710.
8. Lifton RP, et al. A chimaeric 11β-hydroxylase/aldosterone synthase gene causes glucocorticoid-remediable aldosteronism and human hypertension. Nature 1992; 355:262–265.
9. Shimkets RA, et al. Liddle's syndrome: heritable human hypertension caused by mutations in the β subunit of the epithelial sodium channel. Cell 1994; 79:1–8.
10. Neumann HPH, et al. Consequences of direct genetic testing for germline mutations in the clinical management of families with multiple endocrine neoplasia, type II. JAMA 1995; 274:1149–1151.
11. Hopkins PN, Williams RR, Hunt SC. Magnified risks from cigarette smoking for coronary prone families in Utah. Western J Med 1984; 141:196–202.
12. Hopkins PN, Wu LL, Wu J, et al. Higher plasma homocyst(e)ine and increased susceptibility to adverse effects of low folate in early familial coronary artery disease. Arterioscler Thrombos Vasc Biol 1995; 15: 1314–1320.
13. Jacques PF, Bostom AG, Williams RR, et al. Relation between folate status, a common mutation in methylenetetrahydrofolate reductase, and plasma homocysteine concentrations. Circulation 1996; 93:7–9.
14. Barnard RJ. Effects of life-style modification on serum lipids. Arch Intern Med 1991; 151:1389–1394.
15. Ornish D, Brown SE, Scherwitz LW, et al. Can Lifestyle changes reverse coronary heart disease? The Life Style Heart Trial. Lancet 1990; 336: 129–133.
16. Jeunemaitre X, et al. Molecular basis of human hypertension: role of angiotensinogen. Cell 1992; 71:169–180.
17. Caulfield M, et al. Linkage of the angiotensinogen gene to essential hypertension. N Engl J Med 1994; 330:1629–1633.
18. Hata A, et al. Angiotensinogen as a risk factor for essential hypertension in Japan. JCI 1993; 93:1285–1287.

19. Ward K, et al. A molecular variant of angiotensinogen associated with preeclampsia. Nature Genet 1993; 4:59–61.
20. Hopkins PN, et al. Blunted renal vascular response to angiotensin II is associated with a common variant of angiotensinogen gene and obesity. J Hypertens 1996; 14:199–207.
21. Williams RR, Schumacher MC, Barlow GK, et al 1993b Documented need for more effective diagnosis and treatment of familial hypercholesterolemia according to data from 502 heterozygotes in Utah. Am J Cardiol 72:18D–24D
22. Williams RR, Hamilton-Craig I, Kostner GM, et al. MED-PED: an integrated genetic strategy for preventing early deaths. In: Berg K, Boulyjenkov V, Christen Y, eds. Genetic Approaches to Noncommunicable Diseases. Heidelberg: Springer-Verlag, 1996:35–45.
23. Goldman L, Goldman PA, Williams LW, et al. Cost-effectiveness considerations in the treatment of heterozygous familial hypercholesterolemia with medications. Am J Cardiol 1993; 72:75D–79D.
24. Grossman M, Raper SE, Kozarsky K, et al. Successful ex vivo gene therapy directed to the liver in a patient with familial hypercholesterolemia. Nat Genet 1994; 6:335–341.
25. O'Brien TO, Kullo I, Chen A, Katusic Z. Adenoviral-mediated gene transfer of nitric oxide synthase (NOS) to the vascular wall yields functional enzymatic activity. Abstract Book, 66th Congress of the European Atherosclerosis Society, Florence, Italy, July 13–17, 1996. Milan, Italy: Giovanni Lorenzini Medical Foundation.
26. Vazio VM, Rinaldi M, Ciafre SA, et al. Functional chronic correction of dyslipidemia in apo E deficient mice by direct intramuscular injection of naked plasmid DNA. Abstract Book, 66th Congress of the European Atherosclerosis Society, Florence, Italy, July 13–17, 1996. Milan, Italy: Giovanni Lorenzini Medical Foundation.
27. Smith LC, Hauer J, Sparrow JT. Gene delivery by lipophilic apo E. Abstract Book, 66th Congress of the European Atherosclerosis Society, Florence, Italy, July 13–17, 1996, Milan, Italy: Giovanni Lorenzini Medical Foundation.
28. Chiesa G, Parolini C, Canavesi M, Rubin EM, Franceschini G, Bernini F. Cholesterol efflux potential in mice expressing human apolipoprotein A-I Milano. Abstract Book, 66th Congress of the European Atherosclerosis Society, Florence, Italy, July 13–17, 1996. Milan, Italy: Giovanni Lorenzini Medical Foundation.

11

Acute and Chronic Lesions in the Epicardial Coronary Arteries in Patients with Symptomatic and Fatal Myocardial Ischemia

William C. Roberts
Baylor University Medical Center, Dallas, Texas

This chapter describes the amounts of luminal narrowing in the three major epicardial coronary arteries in patients with fatal unstable angina pectoris (UAP), acute myocardial infarction (AMI), and sudden coronary death (SCD), and also the composition of atherosclerotic plaques in these 3 major epicardial arteries in patients with fatal coronary events. It also briefly summarizes the amounts of luminal narrowing and plaque composition in coronary endarterectomy specimens in patients having that procedure at the time of coronary artery bypass grafting because of myocardial ischemia, and it also describes acute lesions in the lumens and in atherosclerotic plaques of patients with fatal coronary events.

I. AMOUNTS OF CORONARY ARTERIAL LUMINAL NARROWING IN THE THREE CORONARY SUBSETS

The amount of coronary arterial narrowing observed at autopsy in patients with UAP, AMI, and SCD is generally enormous (1,2). As shown in Table 1, a study of 80 patients at autopsy with these 3 coronary events (SCD in 31, AMI in 27, and UAP in 22), an average of 2.9 of the 4 major (right, left main, left anterior descending, and left circumflex), coronary arteries were

Table 1 Number of Major (Right, Left Main, Left Anterior Descending, and Left Circumflex) Coronary Arteries Narrowed > 75% in Cross-Sectional Area by Atherosclerotic Plaques in Fatal Coronary Artery Disease

Coronary event	Patients (n)	Mean age (yr)	Number of 4 arteries/patient > 75% narrowed by CSA by plaque				
			4	3	2	1	Mean
Sudden coronary death	31	47	2	29	6	2	2.8
Acute myocardial infarction	27	59	3	14	10	0	2.7
Unstable angina pectoris	22	48	10	8	3	1	3.2
Total	80	51	16 (20%)	42 (52%)	19 (24%)	3 (4%)	2.9
Control	40	52	0 (0)	5 (5%)	12 (13%)	21 (23%)	0.7

CSA, Cross-sectional area.

severely (> 75% decrease in cross-sectional area) narrowed at some points, and no significant differences were observed among the 3 coronary subsets. (Cross-sectional area narrowing of 75% is roughly equivalent to diameter narrowing [the unit of angiography] of 50%.) Patients with UAP had a much higher frequency of severe narrowing of the left main coronary artery (10 of 22 patients [45%]) compared with those with AMI (3 of 27 patients [11%]) and SCD (3 of 31 patients [10%]).

A more sophisticated approach to determining narrowing is to examine the entire lengths of the major epicardial coronary arteries. One technique involves incising each of the 4 major coronary arteries transversely at 5-mm intervals and then preparing a histologic section from each 5–mm segment. Normally, the total length of the 4 major arteries is approximately 27 cm (right = 10 cm, left main = 1 cm, left anterior descending = 10 cm, and left circumflex = 6 cm), and thus approximately 55 5-mm-long segments are available for examination from each heart. Results of studies that used this approach in patients with UAP, AMI, and SCD are summarized in Table 2 (2). Of 4016 5-mm segments studied in the 80 patients, 38% were narrowed 76% to 100% in cross-sectional area by plaque alone (controls 3%), 34% were narrowed 51% to 75% (controls 3%), 34% were narrowed 26% to 50% (controls 22%), and 20% were narrowed 25% or less (controls 31%). Similar degrees of narrowing by plaque alone in all 4 categories of narrowing were

Table 2 Amount of Cross-Sectional Area Narrowing in Each 5-mm Segment of the Four Major (Right, Left Main, Left Anterior Descending, and Left Circumflex) Epicaridal Coronary Arteries by Atherosclerosis Plaques in Subjects with Fatal Coronary Artery Disease

Subgroup	Patients (n)	Mean age (yr)	Number of 5-mm segments	Percentage of segments narrowed				Mean score
				0%–25%	26%–50%	51%–75%	76%–100%	
Sudden coronary death	31	47	1564	7%	23%	34%	36%	2.98
Acute myocardial infarction	27	59	1403	5%	23%	38%	34%	3.01
Unstable angina pectoris	22	48	1409	11%	12%	29%	48%	3.12
Total	80	51	4106	7%	20%	34%	38%	3.02
Control	40	52	1849	31%	44%	22%	3%	1.97

observed in the groups with AMI and SCD; patients with UAP had significantly more severe coronary narrowing than the other 2 groups.

Thus, in general, patients with fatal UAP have more extensive severe narrowing by plaque alone of the 4 major epicardial coronary arteries than patients with either AMI or SCD, and patients with UAP compared with the other 2 groups have significantly higher frequencies of severe narrowing of the left main coronary artery. In all coronary subsets, however, the atherosclerotic plaque was diffuse, involving to some degree every 5-mm-long segment in all 4 major coronary arteries.

II. COMPOSITION OF CORONARY ATHEROSCLEROTIC PLAQUES IN THE THREE CORONARY SUBSETS

Until recent years (3,4), no detailed information was available concerning the composition of atherosclerotic plaques in the epicardial coronary arteries of patients with fatal coronary events. Kragel et al. (3,4), with the use of a computerized morphometry system, traced the various components of atherosclerotic plaques in histologic sections prepared from 1438 5-mm segments of the 4 major epicardial coronary arteries in 37 patients with fatal coronary artery disease (UAP in 10, AMI in 15, and SCD in 12 patients). The results are summarized in Table 3. The dominant component of the coronary atherosclerotic plaques in all 3 subsets of patients was *fibrous tissue*, comprising

Table 3 Mean Composition of Coronary Arterial Atherosclerotic Plaques in the Four Major Epicardial Arteries

Components of plaque	Mean percentage of plaques containing various components in the major coronary arteries (1438 segments)		
	Unstable angina pectoris (n = 10)	Acute myocardial infaction (n = 15)	Sudden coronary death (n = 12)
Dense fibrous tissue	35	46	29
Loose fibrous tissue	1	3	3
Cellular fibrous tissue	52	32	50
Calcium	4	4	8
Pultaceous debris	4	8	4
Foam cells	0	1	0
Foam cells and lymphocytes	3	4	6
Inflammatory infiltrates without significant number of foam cells	1	2	1

about 80% of the plaques in each subset; extracellular *lipid* (pultaceous debris) and *calcium* each made up approximately 5% of the plaques, and several miscellaneous components comprised the remainder of the plaques. The cellular component of the fibrous tissue occupied a larger portion of plaque in the patients with UAP and SCD, and the acellular (dense) component of fibrous tissue occupied a larger portion of the plaque in the group with AMI. In all 3 subsets, the amounts of dense fibrous tissue increased as plaque size increased (or as lumen size decreased), and the amount of cellular fibrous tissue decreased as plaque size increased.

III. AMOUNTS OF LUMINAL NARROWING AND COMPOSITION OF PLAQUES IN ENDARTERECTEMY SPECIMENS OF THE RIGHT CORONARY ARTERY IN PATIENTS HAVING CORONARY BYPASS

The hitherto described observations were in patients with fatal coronary artery disease. Is the amount of coronary narrowing and the composition of the plaques similar or different than that of patients with symptomatic but nonfatal myocardial ischemia? One means to potentially answer this question is to study the amounts of narrowing and the composition of plaques of endarterectomy specimens of the right coronary artery in patients having coronary artery bypass grafting (CABG). Study of over 100 endarterectomy specimens of the right coronary artery excised at the time of CABG has disclosed neither significant differences in the amounts of luminal narrowing by plaque nor the composition of plaque in the endarterectomy specimens compared to the findings in the right coronary artery in the patients studied at necropsy with fatal coronary artery disease.

These observations suggest that there is little to no differences in the amounts of coronary narrowing by plaque or in plaque composition in patients with symptomatic myocardial ischemia severe enough to warrant CABG and in patients with fatal myocardial ischemia. Relatively little change appears to occur between the symptomatic nonfatal myocardial ischemic state and the fatal myocardial ischemic state.

IV. FREQUENCY AND TYPES OF ACUTE LESIONS IN THE MAJOR CORONARY ARTERIES IN THE THREE CORONARY SUBSETS

In recent years considerable effort has been directed toward understanding the acute changes in plaque and lumina that may be responsible for the development of UAP, AMI, and SCD. From angiographic, angioscopic, and autopsy studies, it has been speculated that plaque rupture and hemorrhage with overlying intraluminal thrombus, which are the acute lesions usually responsible for AMI, are also responsible for UAP and possibly SCD. Kragel et al. (5) examined 3101 5-mm segments of 268 epicardial coronary arteries from 67 patients with fatal coronary events (UAP in 14, AMI in 31, and SCD in 21 patients). The results of these detailed studies are summarized in Table 4. The frequency of *intraluminal thrombus* was similar in the groups with UAP and SCD (29% in each) and significantly lower than that in the group with AMI (69%). The thrombus was nonocclusive in all patients with UAP and in 5 of 6 patients with SCD but was nonocclusive in only 4 of 22 patients with AMI. The composition of the nonocclusive and occlusive thrombi also was different—that is, the nonocclusive thrombus consisted mainly of platelets and the occlusive thrombus, mainly of fibrin. Of the 32 patients with thrombus, plaque rupture was found in association with thrombus in 17 (53%): in none of the 4 with UAP, in 2 of 6 with SCD, and in 15 (83%) of 22 with AMI. Among the 15 patients with thrombus unassociated with plaque rupture, hemorrhage into the plaque at the site of thrombus was found in 7: in 3 of 4 patients with UAP, in 2 of 6 with SCD, and in 2 of 32 with AMI.

Plaque rupture was found in 33 (49%) of 67 patients. Its frequency was insignificantly different. In the groups with UAP (36% [5 of 14]) and SCD (19% [4 of 21]) in both groups the frequency was significantly lower than in the group with AMI (75% [24 of 32]).

Table 4   Frequency of Acute Coronary Lesions and Multiluminal Channels at
Autopsy in Patients with Unstable Angina Pectoris, Sudden Coronary Death, and
Acute Myocardial Infarction

Coronary subset	No. of patients	Coronary arteries		
		Thrombus	Plaque rupture	Plaque hemorrhage
Unstable angina pectoris	14	4 (29%)[*]	5 (36%)[*]	3 (21%)[*]
Sudden coronary death	21	6 (29%)[*]	4 (19%)[*]	4 (19%)[*]
Acute myocardial infarction	32	22 (69%)[†]	24 (75%)[†]	20 (63%)[†]
Total	67	32 (48%)	33 (49%)	27 (40%)

[*] Versus [†] in same vertical column = $P < .02$.

Plaque hemorrhage was observed in 27 (40%) of 67 patients, and its
frequency was significantly lower in the groups with UAP (21% [3 of 14])
and SCD (19% [4 of 21]) compared with that in the group with AMI (63%
[20 of 32]). Plaque hemorrhage was associated with plaque rupture or intraluminal thrombus in 20 (74%) of 27 patients with plaque hemorrhage: in 4 of 14
with unstable angina, in 4 of 21 with sudden death, and in 13 of 32 with AMI.

Multiple small-vascular channels were present in 60 (90%) of 67 patients and with an insignificantly different frequency in each of the 3 groups
of patients. The frequency of multiluminal channels in each 5–mm-long segment of coronary artery was significantly higher in the group with UAP (12%
[66 of 572]) than in either the SCD (7% [72 of 999]) or the AMI groups (7%
[107 of 1530]).

Several angiographic studies (6–10) have identified either intraluminal
filling defects consistent with thrombus or specific morphologic lesions (eccentric narrowings with irregular borders) in patients with UAP, and these
defects have been used to distinguish such patients from those with stable
angina. Comparison of postmortem angiographic and histologic findings (11),
however, in patients with coronary artery disease (not necessarily UAP) has
shown that these irregular eccentric lesions may represent not only sites of
intraluminal thrombus but also plaque rupture, plaque hemorrhage, or organized thrombus. In addition, 3 angioscopic studies (12–14) have identified
intraluminal thrombus and ulceration or rupture of plaque in patients with
UAP. On the basis of these studies, it has been widely speculated that the
lesion responsible for the development of UAP is an ulcerated plaque over
which nonocclusive intraluminal thrombus develops.

Before accepting that this hypothesis is indeed true for all or most patients with UAP, the limitations of the previous studies (6–14) need to be considered. Interpretation of the significance of the eccentric irregular lesions seen angiographically in patients with UAP is based largely on the work of Levin and Fallon (11), who compared postmortem coronary anteriograms and histologic sections of coronary artery narrowings in 39 patients who died either after coronary artery bypass surgery or of consequences of AMI. (Because the trauma of bypass surgery may be associated with plaque rupture or plaque hemorrhage or both, patients who had undergone this procedure were excluded from the study of Kragel et al. [5]). Levin and Fallon (11) identified 38 narrowings that had irregular borders or intraluminal lucencies by angiography. Of these, 8 (21%) were acute or organizing nonocclusive thrombi overlying atherosclerotic plaque, 6 (16%) were nonocclusive thrombi overlying sites of plaque rupture or hemorrhage, 10 (26%) were sites of plaque hemorrhage or rupture without thrombus, 6 (16%) contained recanalized thrombus (presumably multiluminal channels), and 21% showed narrowing of the segment by plaque without any complicating acute lesion. More than a third of the irregular eccentric lesions studied, therefore, showed no acute lesion that would account for the abrupt change in symptoms in the setting of UAP. In the study of Kragel et al. (5), plaques containing multiluminal channels, although common to all groups of patients, were seen with the greatest frequency in the group with UAP.

When interpreting results of angiographic or angioscopic studies in patients with UAP, it is assumed that these patients did not have left ventricular necrosis (AMI) at the time of study, an assumption that may or may not be true. Guthrie et al. (15) studied 12 patients with UAP who died shortly after coronary artery bypass surgery. At autopsy, 4 of the 12 patients had AMI that histologically appeared to have occurred before the operation, and AMI was not suspected clinically in any of the 4 patients. Therefore, when studying living patients it may be difficult to determine whether the patients have pure UAP or a combination of UAP and AMI.

Information regarding coronary artery morphology in patients with UAP is scant, difficult to obtain, and difficult to interpret for several reasons. UAP is rarely fatal, and those patients who do die during the period of UAP usually have had coronary angioplasty or a bypass procedure performed or have had an AMI shortly before death. In patients with AMI preceded by UAP, intracoronary lesions may not be representative of those occurring in patients with UAP not complicated by AMI.

Information regarding acute coronary lesions in patients who died shortly after coronary artery bypass surgery has been provided in several studies. Guthrie et al. (15) described 12 patients and Roberts and Virmani (16) described 19 patients with UAP who died shortly after coronary bypass surgery.

In both studies the frequency of intraluminal thrombus was low (8% and 12%, respectively) when patients with AMI were excluded. In a separate report, Virmani and Roberts (17) described the frequency of extravasated erythrocytes and fibrin in the plaque of 17 of 22 patients with UAP. Plaque hemorrhage (erythrocytes with or without fibrin) was identified in 94% of their patients. It is likely that surgical manipulation of the epicardial coronary arteries was responsible for the plaque hemorrhage in many of these patients.

In a study of UAP with fatal outcome, Falk (18) provided information regarding the frequency of acute lesions in the epicardial coronary arteries of patients with SCD, UAP, and AMI. He described autopsy findings in 25 patients, all of whom died of acute coronary thrombosis within 24 hours after the onset of acute symptoms. Of the 24 patients for whom clinical information was available, 15 clearly had UAP, 2 had an equivocal history of UAP, and 7 did not have UAP. Of these 25 patients, 15 had coagulative necrosis (AMI), which as determined histologically was compatible with an age of less than 24 hours. In these patients he described lamellar thrombi (21 of 25 patients, including 14 of 15 with UAP), 81% of which was associated with plaque rupture and hemorrhage. Neither the frequency of plaque rupture nor the number of thrombotic episodes differed between patients with and without UAP. Because all of these patients died suddenly (some with UAP and some with UAP complicated by AMI), the 3 ischemic syndromes cannot be analyzed individually.

Davies et al. (19) studied 90 patients who died suddenly outside the hospital within 6 hours of the onset of pain "or other symptoms." The data were presented in a report entitled, "Intramyocardial platelet aggregation in patients with unstable angina suffering sudden ischemic cardiac death." Of their 90 patients, 36 (45%) had chest or arm pain at some time in the 2 weeks preceding death. The history of chest pain was obtained by a coroner's police officer from the next of kin who had been living with the patient. Thus, the history was not obtained from the patient or by a physician. None of the 90 patients had been admitted to a hospital with increasing chest pain. There was no information on any patient regarding the presence or absence of chest pain at rest. Thus, in none of the 90 patients was the type, location, or severity of the pain known. Nevertheless, these patients were considered by the authors to have had UAP. Autopsies in the 90 patients disclosed the following: 31 (30%) had nonocclusive intracoronary thrombus; 22 (24%) had SCD associated with "regional coagulative necrosis" (AMI); and 23 (25%) had nontransmural necrosis. Of the 36 patients with chest or arm pain at some time in the 2 weeks before death, 35 had plaque rupture identified in one of the major epicardial coronary arteries. Of the 54 patients without chest pain in the 2 weeks before death, 51 had plaque rupture. Thus, whether the patients in that study had UAP is unknown. Some probably did have UAP, but some clearly had AMI and most would have fulfilled most investigators' definitions of SCD. Diagnosing UAP in persons not admitted to the hospital and whose history was obtained by a nonphysician is difficult, to say the least.

Multiluminal vascular channels were present in 90% of the 67 patients studied by Kragel et al. (5). Most likely they represented organized thrombus (the consequence of a previous nonfatal thrombotic event) and were usually at a site where the lumen was severely narrowed by plaque. Multiluminal channels were observed in a significantly higher percentage of the 5-mm coronary segments in the patients with UAP compared with those with either SCD or AMI.

The lower frequency of plaque rupture and occlusive thrombus in the groups with UAP and SCD compared with the frequency in the group with AMI may be a reflection of differences in plaque composition among these groups. Likewise, the similarity in the frequency of these acute coronary lesions in patients with UAP and SCD may be a reflection of the similarity in plaque composition in these 2 groups. As described earlier, in all 3 types of patients the mean percentage of dense fibrous tissue, calcific deposits, and pultaceous debris increased with increasing degrees of luminal narrowing, and the mean percentage of cellular fibrous tissue decreased. Severely narrowed segments in the group with AMI (those narrowed > 75% in cross-sectional area) contained significantly more pultaceous debris and significantly less calcium and cellular fibrous tissue than similarly narrowed segments in the groups with UAP and SCD. Because occlusive thrombus is seen almost exclusively in association with rupture of a lipid-rich plaque, the greater the amount of pultaceous debris, the greater the frequency of plaque rupture and occlusive thrombus.

V. AMOUNTS OF CORONARY LUMINAL NARROWING BY THROMBUS VERSUS AMOUNTS OF NARROWING BY UNDERLYING ATHEROSCLEROTIC PLAQUE IN TRANSMURAL AMI

Brosius and Roberts (20) studied at necropsy 54 patients with a first transmural AMI (no myocardial scars) and coronary arterial thrombi. They examined histologic sections of epicardial coronary arteries that contained thrombi to determine if the amount of luminal narrowing caused by thrombi was comparable to that produced by underlying atherosclerotic plaques, and they also determined the amount of luminal narrowing by plaques immediately proximal and immediately distal to the thrombi. The 54 coronary arteries in the 54 patients were narrowed 33% to 98% in cross-sectional area (mean 81%) by underlying atherosclerotic plaque alone at the site of the thrombus (occlusive in 47 and nonocclusive in 7), from 26% to 98% (mean 75%) within the 2-cm segments proximal to the thrombus, and from 43% to 98% (79%)

within the 2-cm segments distal to the thrombus. Of the 54 arteries studied, 52 (96%) were narrowed 76% to 98% in cross-sectional area by atherosclerotic plaque alone at or immediately proximal to distal to the thrombus, and 26 (48%) were narrowed 91% to 98% by plaque alone. The thrombi were 0.1 to 6.0 mm^2 (mean 1.4 mm^2) in cross-sectional area, and the underlying atherosclerotic plaques were 3.0 to 21.0 mm^2 (mean 8.7). Thus, among these necropsy patients with transmural AMI, coronary thrombi occurred at sites already severely narrowed by atherosclerotic plaque.

Several studies have indicated that thrombi, when present in a coronary artery in necropsy patients with AMI, most often are found in the more proximal portions of the major epicardial coronary arteries. The study by Brosius and Roberts (20) confirmed this observation, at least in regard to the 2 major branches of the left main coronary artery; but the authors also found thrombi to be more proximal in the case of nonocclusive thrombi than occlusive thrombi. Among the 47 patients with occlusive thrombi, the distance from the origin of the coronary artery to the proximal portion of the thrombus averaged 3.2 cm, and among the 7 patients with nonocclusive thrombi, 1.4 cm. Of the 28 patients with occlusive thrombi in either the left anterior descending or left circumflex coronary artery, this distance averaged 2.1 cm (range 0 to 6 cm), and with the right coronary artery, 4.8 cm (range 0.5 to 15.5 cm). Thus, thrombi in the right coronary artery tend to be in the middle third more often than the proximal third.

The length of coronary thrombi in necropsy patients with fatal AMI has been described by several investigators. Of 91 patients studied by Sinapius (21), the average coronary thrombus was 2.0 cm long. Of 12 patients studied by Earhardt and colleagues (22), the average coronary thrombus was 2.7 cm long. Among the 54 patients with a first AMI, studied by Brosius and Roberts (20), the average coronary thrombus was 1.6 cm long; the occlusive thrombi were longer than the nonocclusive thrombi (1.8 cm vs. 0.7 cm). Also, occlusive thrombi in the right coronary arteries tended to be longer than those in the left anterior descending and left circumflex coronary arteries (2.4 cm vs. 4 cm and 1.1 cm). Because the right and left anterior descending coronary arteries in adults are just over 10 cm long on the average and the left circumflex is usually at most 6 cm long, the actual length of a coronary artery occupied by thrombus is small, and in no patient was the entire length of a coronary artery occupied by thrombus. In the right coronary artery in the study by Brosius and Roberts (20), there was a weak but significant positive correlation between the length of an occlusive thrombus and the duration of survival of patients between time of AMI and death. This relation suggests that thrombi may lengthen or "grow" with time.

In 7 of 13 patients studied by Brosius and Roberts (20), the left circumflex coronary artery with a thrombus was also the dominant posterior artery, i.e., the artery that crossed the crux of the heart and supplied the artery to the atrioventricular node. (The left circumflex coronary artery is the dominant posterior artery in about 10% of the population.) Thus, the left circumflex appears to be more prone to thrombus formation when it is the dominant posterior artery.

Finally, not all thrombi occupy the entire residual lumen of a coronary artery. In 7 of the 54 patients (13%) studied by Brosius and Roberts (20), the coronary thrombus was nonocclusive. It occupied on an average only 7% of the cross-sectional area of the coronary arteries (range 2% to 24%) and was an average of 0.7 cm long. These nonocclusive thrombi probably have little if any capacity to interfere with coronary arterial blood flow. These thrombi, of course, could have been occlusive initially and shrunk as the interval increased between onset of myocardial ischemia and death.

VI. SIZES OF THE CORONARY ARTERIES IN THE THREE CORONARY SUBSETS

The amount of blood that can flow down an artery is dependent on many factors including the degree of cross-sectional area narrowing and the size of the artery. A large artery and a small artery can be similarly narrowed in cross-sectional area, and yet the area through which blood can flow in the large artery obviously is greater than the area through which blood can flow in the smaller artery. Roberts and Roberts (23) measured at autopsy by video-planimetry the area enclosed by the internal elastic membrane in the proximal 1 cm of the right, left anterior descending, and left circumflex coronary arteries in 20 patients with UAP, in 23 with AMI, and 19 with SCD. The results are summarized in Table 5. The patients with UAP had the smallest coronary arteries (mean cross-sectional area of each of the 60 arteries = 6.0 mm^2) and the smallest hearts (mean weight 386 g). The patients with AMI and SCD had similar-size coronary arteries (mean area 7.6 mm^2) and similar-size hearts (mean weight 471 g). The 31 control subjects with fatal cancer and normal or nearly normal-size hearts (mean weight 309 g) had the smallest coronary arteries (mean area 5.0 mm^2). The 16 control subjects with aortic valve disease had the largest hearts (mean weight 730 g) and the largest coronary arteries (mean area 9.6 mm^2).

Thus, significant differences are observed in the mean cross-sectional areas of the 3 major epicardial coronary arteries between patients with UAP and patients with either AMI or SCD. These differences result primarily from differences in heart weight. The anatomic determinant of myocardial oxygenation, therefore, is cross-sectional area narrowing, because the size of the epicardial coronary arteries is proportional to heart weight.

Table 5 Mean Cross-Sectional Area of the Right, Left Anterior Descending, and Left Circumflex Coronary Arteries and Heart Weight, Age, and Sex in Three Coronary Subsets and in Two Groups of Controls

Coronary subsets and control subjects	No. of patients	Male/ Female	Age (yr) Range (mean)	Heart weight (g) Range (mean)	Mean cross-sectional area (mm²) of right, LAD, and LC coronary arteries Range (mean)
Unstable angina pectoris	20	12/8	37–59 (49)	240–520 (386)	2.7–13.1 (6.0)
Acute myocardial infarction	23	17/6	33–82 (58)	310–720 (482)	3.6–11.9 (7.6)
Sudden coronary death	19	17/2	28–55 (54)	300–670 (459)	5.2–14.9 (7.7)
Cancer	31	17/14	26–74 (51)	135–470 (309)	2.0–9.1 (5.0)
Aortic valve disease	15	13/2	34–81 (56)	550–1050 (730)	7.1–14.9 (9.6)

LAD = Left anterior descending; LC = left circumflex.

VII. SUMMARY

The coronary atherosclerotic process in patients with either fatal or symptomatic myocardial ischemia is diffuse and extensive. Every 5–mn-long segment of the major epicardial coronary arteries is involved by atherosclerotic plaque. Some plaques, of course, are large, others are small, but the total amount of plaque present in the 4 major epicardial coronary arteries is extensive and diffuse. Although the plaques contain several components including intracellular and extracellular lipids, calcium, mucoid material, and fibrous tissue, the dominant component (about 80%) in the patients with fatal or symptomatic myocardial ischemia is fibrous tissue. Acute lesions such as thrombus, rupture of plaques, and hemorrhages into plaques probably are best viewed as complications of atherosclerosis rather than as primary and all-important lesions.

REFERENCES

1. Roberts WC. Qualitative and quantitative comparison of amounts of narrowing by atherosclerotic plaques in the major epicardial coronary arteries at necropsy in sudden death, transmural acute myocardial infarction, transmural healed myocardial infraction and unstable angina pectoris. Am J Cardiol 1989; 64:324–328.
2. Roberts WC, Kragel AH, Gertz SD, Roberts CS. Coronary arteries in unstable angina pectoris, acute myocardial infarction, and sudden coronary death. Am Heart J 1994; 127:1588–1593.
3. Kragel AH, Reddy SG, Wittes JT, Roberts WC. Morphometric analysis of the composition of atherosclerotic plaques in the four major epicardial coronary arteries in acute myocardial infarction and in sudden coronary death. Circulation 1989; 80:1747–1756.
4. Kragel AH, Red SG, Wittes JT, Roberts WC. Morphometric analysis of the composition of coronary arterial plaques in isolated unstable angina pectoris with pain at rest. Am J Cardiol 1990 6:562–567.
5. Kragel AH, Gertz SD, Roberts WC. Morphologic comparison of frequency and types of acute lesions in the major epicardial coronary arteries in unstable angina pectoris, sudden coronary death and acute myocardial infarction. J Am Coll Cardiol 1991; 8:801–808.
6. Cowley JM, DiSciasco G, Rehr RB, Vetrovec GW. Angiographic observations and clinical relevance of coronary thrombus in unstable angina pectoris. Am J Cardiol 1991; 108E-113E.
7. Gotoh K, Minamino T, Katoh O, et al. The role of intracoronary thrombus in unstable angina: angiographic assessment and thrombolytic therapy during ongoing anginal attacks. Circulation 1988; 77:526–534.
8. Ambrose JA, Winters SL, Stern A. Angiographic morphology and the pathogenesis of unstable angina pectoris. J Am Coll Cardiol 1985; 5:609–616.
9. Vetrovec GW, Leinba h R Gold HK, Cowley MD. Intracoronary thrombolysis in syndromes of unstable ischemia: angiographic and clinical results. Am Heart J 1982; 104:946–952.

10. Holmes DR, Hartzier GO, Smith HC, Fuster V. Coronary artery thrombosis in patients with unstable angina. Br Heart J 1981; 5:411–416.

11. Levin DC, Fallon JT. Significance of the angiographic morphology of localized coronary stenoses: histopathologic correlations. Circulation 1982; 66:316–320.

12. Hombach V, Hoher M, Kochs M, et al. Pathophysiology of unstable angina pectoris: correlations with angioscopic imaging. Eur Heart J 1988; 9:40–45.

13. Forrester JS, Litvack F, Grundfest W. A perspective of coronary disease seen through the arteries of living man. Circulation 1987; 75:505–513

14. Sherman CT, Litvack F, Grundfest W, et al. Coronary angioscopy in patients with unstable angina pectoris. N Engl J Med 1986; 315:913–919.

15. Guthrie RB, Vlodaver Z, Nicoloff DM, Edwards JE. Pathology of stable and unstable angina pectoris. Circulation 1975; 51:1059–1063.

16. Roberts WC, Virmani R. Quantification of cronary arterial narrowing in clinically isolated unstable angina pectoris: an analysis of 22 necropsy patients. Am J Med 1979; 67:792–799.

17. Virmani R, Roberts WC. Extravasated erythrocytes, iron, and fibrin in atherosclerotic plaques in coronary arteries in fatal coronary heart disease and their relation to intraluminal thrombus: frequency and significance in 57 necropsy patients and in 2958 five-mm segments of 224 major epicardial coronary arteries. Am Heart J 1983;105:788–797.

18. Falk E. Unstable angina with fatal outcome: dynamic coronary thrombosis leading to infarction and/or sudden death. Circulation 1985; 71:699–708.

19. Davies MJ, Thomas AC, Knapman PA, Hangartner JR. Myocardial platelet aggregation in patients with unstable angina suffering sudden ischemic cardiac death. Circulation. 1986; 73:418–427.

20. Brosius FC III, Roberts WC. Significance of coronary arterial thrombus in transmural acute myocardial infarction. A study of 54 necropsy patients. Circulation 1981; 3:810–816.

21. Sinapius D. Beziehungen Zwischen koronarthrombosen und myokardinfarkten. Dtsch Med Wochenschr 1972; 97:443.

22. Erhardt LR, Unge G, Boman G. Formation of coronary artery thrombi in relation to onset of necrosis in acute myocardial infarction in man. A clinical and autoradiographic study. Am Heart J 1976; 91:592.

23. Roberts CS, Roberts WC. Cross-sectional area of maximal portions of the three major epicardial coronary arteries in 98 necropsy patients with different coronary events. Relationship to heart weight, age and sex. Circulation 1980; 62:953–959.

12

Insulin Resistance and Atherosclerosis

Ronald B. Goldberg
University of Miami School of Medicine, Miami, Florida

I. INTRODUCTION

The report by Duff (1) in 1954 that insulin treatment increased atherosclerosis in an experimental diabetic rabbit model of atherosclerosis first raised concern that insulin might be atherogenic. The development of the insulin radio-immunoassay in the next decade led to the first observation in human subjects with coronary heart disease (CHD) that plasma insulin levels were elevated (2), and fueled the concept that hyperinsulinemia was a risk factor for athero-sclerosis. Then in 1973 the demonstration that hyperinsulinemia was associ-ated with resistance to insulin-mediated glucose uptake (3) focused attention on insulin resistance as a driving force for hyperinsulinemia and therefore for atherosclerosis (4). Despite intensive study, the nature of the relationship between hyperinsulinemia/insulin resistance and atherosclerosis is still poorly understood. Parallel research developments in the investigation of the rela-tionship between hyperinsulinemia/insulin resistance and type 2 diabetes has led to an improved understanding of how insulin resistance contributes to that disease (5), and efforts to improve insulin sensitivity in order to determine whether such treatment might prevent or ameliorate diabetes are now under way (6). The emergence of hyperinsulinemia/insulin resistance as a determi-nant of CHD in prospective observational studies (7), raises the question as to whether a similar approach might be needed for the prevention and treat-ment of atherosclerosis.

This review is intended to explore the nature of the relationship between insulin resistance and atherosclerosis. First, however, it is essential to define some commonly used terms in this area.

II. THE NATURE OF HYPERINSULINEMIA AND INSULIN RESISTANCE

The terms hyperinsulinemia or hyperinsulinism, and insulin resistance, are often used interchangeably to indicate a relationship between insulin and atherosclerosis usually without definition or qualification, and this contributes to considerable confusion in this area.

A. Hyperinsulinemia

Hyperinsulinemia simply means elevated plasma insulin levels. Since insulin assays have not been standardized because of differences in assay components and techniques, normal insulin concentrations cannot be defined (8); hyper-insulinemia is thus usually used to signify a value in the fasting state or after a glucose or other stimulus, greater than that found in normal, insulin-sensitive individuals. Rarely, hyperinsulinemia is caused by autonomous oversecretion of insulin by the β-cells of the pancreas as occurs, for example, in an insulinoma. Such hyperinsulinemia is clearly accompanied by hyperinsulinism, i.e. excess insulin action.

B. Insulin Resistance

The most frequent setting in which hyperinsulinemia is found is in states associated with reduced sensitivity to insulin action or insulin resistance. Insulin resistance was originally identified in certain subjects with diabetes whose hyperglycemia responded less well to insulin than did an insulin-sensitive group (9). Thus insulin resistance was originally and still is generally defined as a loss of sensitivity to the action of insulin on glucose metabolism although we now appreciate that the majority of individuals with insulin resistance do not have diabetes.

1. Definition of Insulin Resistance

Insulin action in vivo is usually measured by an exogenous insulin infusion (10,11), or a glucose infusion to stimulate endogenous insulin (12). The former approach includes the euglycemic-insulin clamp technique, which assesses the amount of glucose required to maintain euglycemia in the presence of a physiologic or supraphysiologic constant insulin infusion (10) or the steady-state plasma glucose measurement (SSPG) obtained during a constant insulin and glucose infusion, with endogenous insulin suppressed using somatostatin (11). Measurement of endogenous insulin action is performed by a glucose infusion (sometimes aided by tolbutamide) with computer modeling of the plasma glucose response to the endogenous insulin released (minimal model), providing a measure of insulin sensitivity (12). Thus insulin resistance when actually measured, usually refers to a dose related action of insulin on glucose metabolism located mainly in skeletal muscle—the major site of insulin-mediated glucose uptake, relative to that in normal weight, physically active, young adults. There is evidence, however, that reduced sensitivity of several metabolic targets to insulin action other than glucose metabolism is present in many insulin resistance states (e.g., adipose tissue lipolysis [13], amino acid uptake [14], lipoprotein lipase activity [15]).

2. Causes of Insulin Resistance

Insulin resistance is a frequent finding in the general population where it is influenced by ethnicity (16), gender (17), and age (18). It is estimated that 15% to 25% of individuals have a reduction of insulin sensitivity approximating that in type 2 diabetes (4,19). Obesity (20), reduced physical activity (21), pregnancy (22), and cigarette smoking (23) are known acquired determinants of insulin resistance. In addition, high-fat diets may contribute to insulin resistance as well (24). Inherited causes of insulin resistance are believed to be important in the development of essential hypertension (25), type 2 diabetes (19), and possibly the polycystic ovary syndrome (26).

At the molecular level, defects in insulin action leading to insulin resistance are being identified at each step along the complex pathway by which insulin acts, beginning at the insulin receptor through to the enzymes and transcription factors that are altered by insulin (27). Although this research effort is still in its infancy, it is clear that all insulin resistance is not the same; thus the insulin resistance of obesity appears to be characterized by reduced insulin receptor number and affinity (20), while insulin resistance in type 2 diabetes is clearly dominated by as yet poorly defined abnormalities in the postreceptor pathways of insulin action (27). It is expected that a whole range of molecular causes of insulin resistance will be found, considering the complexities of intracellular insulin action.

C. The Relationship Between Hyperinsulinemia and Insulin Resistance

Prospective and cross-sectional studies of insulin secretion and insulin resistance in subjects at various stages in the evolution of type 2 diabetes have demonstrated the complexity of the relationship between hyperinsulinemia and insulin resistance (19,28,29). The development of insulin resistance is accompanied by pancreatic β-cell hypersecretion of insulin to produce hyper-insulinemia. The stimulus to the β-cells is still unknown, but has been postu-lated to include rising glucose (30) or free fatty acid (FFA) (31) levels that may result from the defective regulation of glucose and FFA metabolism occurring as a result of insulin resistance. This implies that the development of insulin resistance would precede that of hyperinsulinemia. However, this is not necessarily so. For example, it has been proposed that the hyperinsuline-mia found in individuals with central obesity results from reduced hepatic extraction of insulin due to excess FFA flux from the expanded abdominal fat depot to the liver (32). This leads to subsequent downregulation of insulin receptors as a result of chronic hyperinsulinemia (20).

It is generally felt that hyperinsulinemia is compensatory for the insulin resistance (4,19,30) and is proportional to it, provided the β-cell can maintain its high insulin output. Beta-cell failure is characterized by a falling insulin secretory capacity in response to a glucose stimulus, by a fall in the proportion of mature insulin in relation to its precursor proinsulin leading to an overes-timation of insulin by immunoassay, and by an impairment of glucose toler-ance culminating in the development of diabetes. Chronic hyperglycemia is now known to induce insulin resistance as well—an apparently reversible phenomenon, known as glucose toxicity (30). Thus the correlation between fasting insulin levels and insulin resistance is greatest in individuals with normal glucose tolerance and becomes weaker in subjects with impaired glucose tolerance and diabetes, in whom the association between postglucose insulin levels and insulin resistance is lost completely (33). At best, fasting insulin levels account for no more than 60% to 70% of the variance of insulin resistance (33) (less in some studies), so that even in this situation there are other factors that have an important effect on insulin levels.

D. Hyperinsulinemia, Insulin Resistance, and Obesity

The relationship among hyperinsulinemia, insulin resistance, and atheroscler-osis is tightly bound up with central obesity although it is not dependent on it (34). High fasting insulin levels are linked with obesity and its central distribution, as are measures of insulin resistance (34,35). In addition, obesity is correlated with cardiovascular risk factors (36) and with CHD events (37). Enlarged fat cells in abdominal fat deposits are resistant to insulin's antilipo-lytic action (34) and more responsive to lipolytic hormones than in the glu-teal-femoral region (38). As a result there is an increased FFA flux into the liver which is thought to interfere with hepatic and peripheral insulin action (39) and hepatic clearance of insulin (32), resulting in hyperinsulinemia and insulin resistance. Evidence has also been obtained that increased testosterone and reduced sex hormone-binding globulin may promote central obesity, contributing to the typical gender-related differences in body fat distribution and cardiovascular risk (40). Obesity is thus an important determinant of hyperinsulinemia and insulin resistance. In addition, obesity may contribute independently to atherosclerosis risk as will be discussed below.

E. Pathophysiologic Aspects of the Hyperinsulinemia/Insulin Resistance—Atherosclerosis Relationship

1. Hyperinsulinemia

A key controversy in this area relates to whether hyperinsulinemic, insulin-resistant individuals exhibit excessive insulin action along atherogenic pathways or not. Proponents of this point of view emphasize that associations between hyperinsulinemia with cardiovascular risk factors such as dyslipidemia, hypertension, central obesity, and also with CHD events in epidemiologic studies, could imply a cause-and-effect relationship. In support of this is the demonstration in animal models and in isolated cell culture systems, that insulin acts on vascular tissues and influences hemostasis, in addition to its metabolic effects (41).

2. Hyperproinsulinemia

The insulin precursors proinsulin, and des 31, 32 proinsulin normally comprise about 10% of circulating insulin-like molecules, and have no more than 10% of the action of insulin. Concern that they might be linked to atherosclerosis initially arose from a study using recombinant proinsulin in human subjects in which an excess of CHD events occurred (42). In addition, insulin-resistant subjects secrete relatively more insulin precursor molecules, particularly in the presence of a failing β-cell (43). Since most insulin immunoassays cross-react with insulin, the possibility arises that the association between hyperinsulinemia and atherosclerosis might reflect hyperproinsulinemia. Epidemiologic surveys (44,45) experimental studies have provided some support for this thesis. However, other studies have not confirmed that proinsulin has a specific effect (46,47) and the availability of immunoassays specific for insulin has demonstrated that insulin alone has predictive value for CHD (7).

3. Insulin Resistance

The arguments against these points of view are that hyperinsulinemia and hyperproinsulinemia in clinical and epidemiologic studies represent markers for insulin resistance (48), and that it is insulin resistance which is more directly linked to atherosclerosis. There is as yet little evidence of excess insulin action in hyperinsulinemic, insulin-resistant individuals, and the experimental data are difficult to fit with the clinical situation. Indeed there is more evidence for reduced net insulin action in subjects with insulin resistance (49), raising the possibility that the increased risk for atherogenesis in these individuals might be a consequence of relative (or absolute) insulin deficiency and its effects on metabolism, hemostasis, and the vascular wall.

Whether insulin resistance actually leads to an activation of atherogenic pathways is still unclear. Like hyperinsulinemia, insulin resistance has been linked to the development of certain cardiovascular risk factors, particularly dyslipidemia and hypertension. It is difficult to conceive that defective glucose regulation in insulin-resistant normoglycemic individuals could be responsible for these abnormalities. On the other hand, the excessive release of FFA as a result of resistance to the action of insulin in the adipocyte could be an important determinant of widespread metabolic and structural abnormalities (50–52).

Most clinical studies investigating the relationship between insulin resistance and atherosclerosis in human subjects have measured fasting insulin levels only as a putative marker for insulin resistance. They will be discussed here as such, and with the caveats expressed above. Recently, in efforts to more accurately quantify this relationship, actual measurements of insulin resistance have been performed. In such instances the term *insulin resistance* will be used as defined above. The term *hyperinsulinemia/insulin resistance* will be used to signify the broadest possible connection between hyperinsulinemia and/or insulin resistance and atherosclerosis without implying a specific pathogenetic relationship. Studies of the hyperinsulinemia/insulin resistance-atherosclerosis relationship will be reviewed in three sections: observational studies of CHD occurrence; hyperinsulinemia/insulin resistance and cardiovascular risk factors; and insulin and the arterial wall.

III. HYPERINSULINEMIA/INSULIN RESISTANCE AND OBSERVATIONAL STUDIES OF CHD

A. Studies with Clinical or Electrocardiographic CHD Endpoints

The concept that hyperinsulinemia is a risk factor for human atherosclerosis was derived originally from two cross-sectional studies (2,53) and strengthened by the publication in 1979 and 1980 of three prospective clinical trials: the Helsinki Policeman Study (54), the Busselton Study (55), and the Paris Prospective Study (56). These trials found that fasting (56) or postoral glucose insulin levels (54–56) in European men without known glucose intolerance were positively predictive of atherosclerotic events in multivariate analyses. Subsequent to these reports, the Caerphilly Prospective Study (57) and the Multiple Risk Factor Intervention Trial (MRFIT) (58) have provided only qualified support in men, and the Gothenberg (59), Kuopic (60), Rancho Bernardo (61), San Luis Valley (62), and Pima Indian (63) studies did not find any association. In the Caerphilly trial, triglycerides accounted for the insulin effect and in MRFIT an association could be demonstrated only in men with apoprotein E3/2 phenotype rather than the usual E3/3. Recently the Quebec Cardiovascular Study in men demonstrated a strong, independent predictive value of fasting insulin levels for CHD events (7).

The Quebec Cardiovascular Study is important for two reasons. First it is the only trial in which an assay specific for insulin was used. Thus the Quebec study demonstrated that the predictive value of insulin for CHD did not depend on proinsulin. Second, this study performed more detailed lipoprotein measurements then any other prospective trial, and found that insulin and apoprotein (apo) B had largely independent and synergistic predictive value for CHD events. In men with elevated insulin and apo B values (top tertile) the odds ratio for CHD was 11.0. The investigators concluded that hyperinsulinemia may increase the risk of CHD through alteration of metabolic processes other than dyslipidemia.

Until the recent report of the Atherosclerosis Risk in Communities (ARIC) Study (64), no prospective trials had demonstrated an association between insulin and CHD in women (55,60–63). One cross-sectional study in women demonstrated an association between insulin levels and CHD (65) while another did not (66). ARIC found in a biracial community study that fasting insulin predicted CHD risk in women but not men in multivariate analysis. There were unfortunately too few black subjects to do subgroup analyses in this trial. In addition, there have been four prospective trials in subjects with either impaired glucose tolerance or established type 2 diabetes in which no association was found between insulin and CHD (67–69). In none of these studies were measures of insulin resistance performed.

These conflicting results indicated that the association between hyperinsulinemia and atherosclerosis is not a simple one. On the one hand there are sufficient positive data to incriminate hyperinsulinemia as a possible risk factor in men in some populations. However, there clearly are confounding factors. Studies in which insulin was not shown to be associated with CHD tended to include elderly subjects. It is possible that aging depletes the population of high-risk hyperinsulinemic subjects, although insulin resistance increases with age (18). McKeigue has proposed that undernutrition and poor health, two important determinants of mortality in the aging population may have been insufficiently controlled for and thus contributed to confounding of the insulin-atherosclerosis relationship (48). Another explanation relates to the close associations between hyperinsulinemia and several cardiovascular risk factors such as dyslipidemia, hypertension, and central obesity, which when taken into account often weaken the insulin-atherosclerosis relationship (57–60). This raises the possibility that these cardiovascular risk factors may be more proximate to atherogenesis than is hyperinsulinemia. Finally, insulin resistance may be more closely linked to atherosclerosis than hyperinsulinemia, which, as discussed earlier, is an imperfect marker for insulin resistance (33).

B. Studies of Subclinical or Clinical Atherosclerosis Using Angiography and B-Mode Ultrasound

The studies above utilized clinical or ECG endpoints that reflect the presence of advanced coronary atherosclerosis which may be complicated by potential confounding factors related to the CHD event. In an attempt to link hyper-insulinemia/insulin resistance more closely to the atherosclerotic vasculature itself, several investigators have examined the relationship between insulin levels or actual measurements of insulin resistance and the state of the vasculature using angiography or B-mode ultrasound.

The first report that insulin resistance is associated with asymptomatic atherosclerosis was published in 1991 by Laakso (70), who used the euglycemic clamp method to study insulin sensitivity in 30 nonobese subjects with asymptomatic carotid or femoral atherosclerosis compared to controls. No significant difference in insulin levels was found in the two groups, but those with atherosclerosis had a significantly reduced glucose response to insulin, signifying insulin resistance. Since this first report, subsequent studies have generally confirmed this finding. Using coronary angiography, fasting insulin levels were found to correlate with the severity of coronary disease in nondiabetic individuals, but not in a group consisting mainly of subjects with impaired glucose tolerance or diabetes (71). In a more carefully selected group of subjects with normal glucose tolerance, subjects with obstructive coronary disease had significantly higher SSPG levels after insulin infusion, signifying reduced sensitivity to insulin, than did subjects with normal coronary arteries (72). In addition, the SSPG level correlated with the coronary atherosclerosis score, suggesting a dose-effect relationship. Of interest in a study by the same group was the finding that subjects with vasospastic angina (no fixed coronary obstruction) had the same loss of insulin sensitivity compared to controls as did those with obstructive disease (73). Insulin resistance has been suggested to contribute to altered microvascular function in several vessel beds (74,75), and an increased clustering of cardiovascular risk factors such as diabetes and hypertension has been noted in individuals with so-called microvascular angina.

B-mode ultrasound of the carotid arteries used to quantitate intimal-medial thickness (IMT) has been shown to correlate with both carotid and coronary atherosclerosis (76,77). Using this technique, ARIC study investigators found that fasting insulin levels correlated with carotid wall IMT in 6474 men and women, although it contributed very modestly to the variance in wall thickness (78). The Insulin Resistance Atherosclerosis Study (IRAS) examined the relationship between insulin sensitivity using the minimal model method (12) and carotid wall IMT in a large triethnic group of men and women who were characterized into groups with normal glucose tolerance (n = 637), impaired glucose tolerance (n = 315), and diabetes (n = 445) (79). Significant inverse associations were found between insulin sensitivity and carotid wall IMT in non-Hispanic whites and in Hispanics but not in African-Americans. The lack of association between insulin and atherosclerosis in African-Americans has parallels with a lack of association between insulin resistance and blood pressure (80) as well as type 2 diabetes (81) in this ethnic group, and is currently unexplained. Adjustment for major cardiovascular risk factors, as well as adiposity, glucose tolerance, and insulin levels had only a marginal effect on the association in non-Hispanic whites, but accounted for the association in Hispanics.

It was concluded that insulin resistance was quantitatively correlated with atherosclerosis in whites that was only in part related to measured cardiovascular risk factors. This suggested that other effects, for example involving hemostasis (82), as well as putative direct effects of insulin resistance on the vessel wall might be operative. Similar associations between insulin resistance and carotid wall IMT have now been described in Italian (83), Swedish (84), and Japanese (85) men. Furthermore, in a group of subjects with ischemic stroke, reduced insulin sensitivity was evident only in those who had suffered an atherothrombotic event, compared to patients with lacunar or embolic strokes, as well as a control group (86).

Finally, in the only negative study of this type reported, fasting insulin levels did not predict the development of femoral plaques assessed ultrasonographically 8 years later, in a group of young Finnish men with normal glucose tolerance. This contrasted with the positive predictive value found for total and low density lipoprotein (LDL) cholesterol, apo B, glucose, and blood pressure (87). Insulin sensitivity measured at study end also did not correlate with femoral atherosclerosis. Although the study had several design limitations, and the participants were much younger than in any other trial and were not obese, hypertensive, or glucose-intolerant, the authors concluded that neither insulin levels nor insulin resistance appeared to have a significant role in femoral atherosclerosis.

This recent series of studies in which direct measurements of insulin sensitivity were performed have strengthened the notion that it is insulin resistance more than hyperinsulinemia that represents the principle determinant in the relationship with atherosclerosis. In addition, some of these studies suggest that this relationship is a graded one, and reflects both the influence of the cardiovascular risk factors commonly associated with insulin resistance and effects independent of these.

IV. HYPERINSULINEMIA/INSULIN RESISTANCE AND CARDIOVASCULAR RISK FACTORS

A. Clustering of Cardiovascular Risk Factors

In search of a meaning for the association between hyperinsulinemia and CHD, Reaven (4) was among the first to recognize that hyperinsulinemia/insulin resistance was common to a cluster of cardiovascular risk factors which he termed Syndrome X, and which he proposed represented a link between hyperinsulinemia/insulin resistance and CHD. Since then this syndrome of insulin resistance has been expanded, based on demonstrated associations with hyperinsulinemia/insulin resistance, to include central or visceral obesity, small dense LDL, increased plasminogen activator inhibitor-1 (PAI-1), increased fibrinogen, decreased sex hormone binding globulin, postprandial lipemia, microalbuminuria, and hyperuricemia. Since each of these variables has been related by investigators to CHD, several potential pathways by which insulin resistance might influence atherosclerosis could be identified (88).

Clustering of many of these cardiovascular risk factors within individuals more often than would be predicted by chance was not a new observation, having been originally proposed to be linked to "android obesity" in the 1950s by Vague (89). The close association between obesity and hyperinsulinemia/insulin resistance makes it very difficult to distinguish between the role of these two factors in the genesis of cardiovascular risk factor clustering. Analysis of the ARIC data indicates that risk factor clusters show graded, independent associations with both fasting hyperinsulinemia and central obesity (90). Thus although central obesity may be one important determinant of insulin resistance and increased CHD risk, insulin resistance does not necessarily require the presence of obesity for expression of its association with parameters of the insulin resistance syndrome. In a recent study of children, adolescents, and young adults from Finland, baseline insulin levels were higher in individuals who subsequently developed clustering of high triglycerides, low high-density lipoprotein (HDL) cholesterol, and high systolic blood pressure (91). Similar findings have been obtained in the Bogalusa Heart Study (92). These data suggest that genetic factors may play a role in the clustering of cardiovascular risk factors with hyperinsulinemia. There also appear to be population differences between the prominence of the association between insulin versus central obesity and cardiovascular risk factors (93–94). In addition, clustering tends to increase with aging (95).

B. Association Between Hyperinsulinemia/Insulin Resistance and Cardiovascular Risk Factors

In this section the extent to which hyperinsulinemia/insulin resistance could be playing a causal role in relation to atherosclerosis through an effect on cardiovascular risk factors will be reviewed.

1. Glucose Intolerance

Glucose intolerance is a major risk factor for atherosclerotic vascular disease (96). The determinants of this increased risk are still not well understood, although subjects with impaired glucose tolerance and diabetes have an increased prevalence of the cardiovascular risk factors associated with insulin resistance. These include hypertriglyceridemia, low HDL, increased small, dense LDL, increased postprandial lipemia, hypertension, microalbuminuria, increased fibrinogen, and increased PAI-1 (97). Since insulin resistance is a necessary contributor to glucose intolerance, and predates it by many years, it has been proposed to contribute both to the genesis of type 2 diabetes and the associated macrovascular disease (98). The frequency of cardiovascular risk factors in diabetes and thus the atherogenic milieu may be further enhanced by the concomitant presence of hyperglycemia itself (99). As pointed out above, hyperglycemia worsens insulin resistance (30), as well as having independent atherogenic effects (100).

Although subjects with type 2 diabetes are relatively insulin-deficient, insulin-treated subjects have peripheral hyperinsulinemia which could theoretically have deleterious effects if excess insulin action is in fact atherogenic. However, several prospective studies of insulin-treated diabetic subjects have shown no significant increase in cardiovascular risk factors or cardiovascular events compared to less intensive treatments (101).

2. Central Obesity

Central obesity has recently attracted renewed attention as a risk factor for CHD (102). As discussed above, central obesity is an important cause of insulin resistance and, as will be discussed below, may well contribute independently of insulin resistance to dyslipidemia and hypertension (103) and therefore to atherosclerosis. However, there is little evidence to suggest that insulin resistance is a determinant of obesity, and the relationship between obesity and cardiovascular disease will therefore not be considered further here.

3. Dyslipidemia

The term *dyslipidemia* was developed to explain the frequent association between hypertriglyceridemia and reduced HDL-cholesterol concentrations with or without elevated LDL-cholesterol or -apo B levels. Hyper-insulinemia/insulin resistance has been linked with dyslipidemia because of its associations with hypertriglyceridemia, low HDL, and, more recently, small, dense LDL.

a. Hypertriglyceridemia

Insulin Resistance as a Cause of Hypertriglyceridemia. It has been known for many years that fasting insulin and triglyceride levels were closely correlated, and that the presence of obesity added to the effect seen in lean individuals (104,105). Subsequently an inverse association was discovered between insulin levels and HDL-cholesterol concentrations, but no relationship between insulin and LDL-cholesterol levels has been demonstrated (106, 107). It was initially proposed that hyperinsulinemia together with raised FFA led to an increase in VLDL production (108), based on early work in the perfused rat liver (109). Subsequent emphasis has focused more on the role of an increased flux of FFA to the liver and less on hyperinsulinemia.

Although FFAs were known to be increased in prediabetic and diabetic states (110), their importance to the development of hypertriglyceridemia was less clear in normoglycemic individuals. It is now appreciated that the insulin-triglyceride association reflects an interrelationship between underlying insulin resistance and abnormalities in triglyceride-rich lipoprotein metabolism operative in both normal and glucose intolerant subjects (111), and that the mechanism for increased VLDL production involves increased FFA flux in the liver to boost VLDL-triglyceride and -apo B synthesis and secretion (112). In addition, at least in obese subjects, this may be associated with a reduction in adipose tissue lipoprotein lipase (LPL) activity (113). Insulin normally controls hepatic and intestinal triglyceride production and clearance by suppressing adipose tissue lipolysis (114) and apo B (115) and apo C-III production (116), as well as by enhancing LPL activity (117). Hence resistance to insulin could lead to abnormalities in both fasting and postprandial triglyceride metabolism as a result of reduced effective insulin action. Recent interest in postprandial lipemia has been stimulated by evidence of its independent risk factor role for CHD (118), as well as data that this phase of triglyceride metabolism is abnormal both in hyperinsulinemic, normoglycemic men (119) and in subjects with type 2 diabetes (120), probably due to lipoprotein removal defects.

All these mechanisms probably operate in type 1 diabetic subjects who have absolute insulin deficiency, and are likely to be important in type 2 diabetic individuals where net effective insulin action is likely to be reduced rather than increased. However, their role is less clear in those with insulin resistance and normal glucose tolerance. First, it has long been held that the associations between hyperinsulinemia and atherosclerosis reflect excess insulin action (41) despite the fact that there is little direct evidence for this. In addition, as pointed out above, insulin has an inhibitory effect on VLDL production (112,115). Furthermore patients with an insulinoma, which produces definite hyperinsulinism, have normal triglyceride levels (121). Steiner has proposed that chronic hyperinsulinemia leads to expanded hepatic fatty acid stores which may provide substrate for VLDL-triglyceride synthesis (122). However, it is likely that chronic hyperinsulinemia reflects chronic insulin resistance rather than chronic hyperinsulinism. In addition, it does not appear that intrahepatic lipolysis is influenced by insulin (123).

Second and perhaps more important is the demonstration that elevated FFA may a priori induce insulin resistance and hyperinsulinemia by interfering with insulin-mediated glucose uptake, enhancing hepatic gluconeogenesis and hepatic glucose production, and stimulating β-cell insulin secretion (124), while at the same time increasing hepatic apo B and triglyceride production (115). Thus primary disorders of FFA metabolism may cause both hyperinsulinemia, insulin resistance, and hypertriglyceridemia, making it impossible using measurements of insulin sensitivity to distinguish between primary and secondary insulin resistance and their respective metabolic roles.

Primary Disorders of FFA Metabolism Cause Insulin Resistance and Hypertriglyceridemia. There is increasing evidence that primary disorders of FFA metabolism may produce insulin resistance secondarily. As already mentioned, it has been proposed that the enlarged, lipolytically active, visceral fat depot characteristic of individuals with central or upper body obesity increases portal FFA flux, which interferes with hepatic insulin extraction causing hyperinsulinemia (32). It has also been demonstrated that obese individuals produce excess tumor necrosis factor-α (TNF-α) from adipocytes (125) and muscle (126). TNF-α is a cytokine that impairs insulin-mediated glucose uptake, reduces adipose LPL activity, increases lipolysis (126), and increases hepatic lipogenesis (127). These data imply that obesity can provoke insulin resistance and hypertriglyceridemia in parallel rather than in the conventionally accepted sequential mode (19).

Another line of research in obesity is directed to the role of the adipocyte hormone leptin, which induces satiety at the hypothalamic level as fat mass increases (128). There is evidence that leptin contributes to the homeostasis of body fat by activating the sympathetic nervous system as well (129). This could explain the increased adrenergic drive that is well described in obesity, but could also contribute both to increased activation of lipolysis through β-adrenergic receptors and to resistance to insulin. Finally, Sniderman has assembled evidence to show that some dyslipidemic individuals may have a primary defect in the pathway regulating post-LPL reesterification of FFA in adipose tissue leading to an increased FFA flux to the liver and insulin resistance (130).

These considerations demonstrate the complexity underlying the insulin-triglyceride relationship. They also bring a new perspective as to why hyperinsulinemia and insulin resistance are characteristic of many hypertriglyceridemic states, whether these are studied as disease entities—e.g., type IIb hyperlipidemia (131), familial combined hyperlipidemia (132), familial dyslipidemic hypertension (133), "endogenous hypertrglyceridemia" (104)— or identified from the population based on arbitrarily defined cutpoints for hypertriglyceridemia (105–107). Thus primary defects in the insulin action pathway may be the driving force for hypertriglyceridemia and its associated lipoprotein abnormalities such as in type 2 diabetes; alternatively, insulin resistance may be a secondary, induced abnormality in subjects with altered FFA and triglyceride metabolism such as in obesity, capable of aggravating the primary defect. In either case, the presence of insulin resistance would predispose to glucose intolerance which is frequently present in hypertriglyceridemic individuals (134). According to this thesis therefore, insulin resistance may be both a cause and a marker of defective lipid and lipoprotein metabolism, and by extension, of atherosclerosis.

b.   Reduced HDL

The inverse association between hyperinsulinemia and reduced HDL concentrations (106,107) is less well understood, but has also been demonstrated to be associated with reduced insulin sensitivity (135,136). Since triglyceride concentrations are inversely related to HDL levels and their metabolic pathways are linked, the relationship between insulin resistance and reduced HDL has been considered to reflect disordered triglyceride metabolism. Proposed mechanisms leading to reduced HDL concentrations include decreased LPL activity in association with hypertriglyceridemia which leads to a reduced flow of triglyceride-rich lipolysis products to HDL (137). In addition, raised VLDL-triglyceride is thought to lead to excess triglyceride exchange with HDL mediated by cholesteryl ester transfer protein (CETP) to produce a triglyceride-enriched HDL, which is converted by the action of hepatic lipase to a small, rapidly degraded form of HDL (138).

However, using the euglycemic insulin clamp technique it was demonstrated that even individuals with isolated low HDL, i.e., without conventionally-defined hypertriglyceridemia, are insulin-resistant (139). In addition, evidence that hepatic lipase (140) and CETP (141) activities are increased in insulin-resistant and -deficient states, raises the question as to whether the genesis of low HDL is necessarily dependent upon hypertriglyccridcmia, or whether both abnormalities reflect changes in key enzymatic and synthetic activities in lipid and lipoprotein metabolism that are perturbed in the insulin resistant state.

c. Small, Dense LDL

Although LDL-cholesterol levels do not correlate with insulin levels or insulin sensitivity, the close association between hypertriglyceridemia and an LDL size and density pattern characterized by a preponderance of the small, dense LDL subclass (phenotype B), has directed attention to the possibility that this LDL pattern is linked to insulin resistance. Factors thought to be important in the genesis of small dense LDL include increased CETP-catalyzed triglyceride-cholesteryl ester exchange between VLDL and LDL (142), and hepatic lipase-induced hydrolysis of LDL-triglyceride (143), which, as discussed above, may be common to the insulin resistant state. LDL size has in fact been demonstrated to be correlated with insulin sensitivity in healthy men independently of their body weight in those with triglyceride values above the median for the study population (120 mg/dl) but not in those with lower triglyceride levels, suggesting a threshold rather than a graded effect (144). Like low HDL, increased small, dense LDL and hypertriglyceridemia could reflect parallel effects of insulin resistance on important, rate-limiting steps in lipoprotein metabolism, namely, increased VLDL levels, and increased hepatic lipase and CETP activity.

d. Insulin Resistance, Dyslipidemia, and Atherosclerosis

Given the widespread documentation of the association of hyperinsulinemia or insulin resistance with hypertriglyceridemia and/or reduced HDL concentrations, it would appear that some form of insulin resistance is present in many if not most dyslipidemic subjects. Factors such as age, gender, ethnicity, body fat content and distribution, and lifestyle factors such as physical activity and cigarette smoking all may influence insulin sensitivity and thus affect the associated dyslipidemia. This is not to say that insulin resistance is the primary cause of all dyslipidemia. Clearly, genetic factors such as heterozygous LPL deficiency (145) are important. However, the finding of a dyslipidemic pattern must suggest the presence of insulin resistance.

It seems clear that increased triglycerides, reduced HDL, increased postprandial lipemia, small dense LDL, and hyperapobetalipoproteinemia comprise a dyslipidemic syndrome with increased risk for atherosclerosis (146). The close association between insulin resistance and dyslipidemia provides an important pathway linking insulin resistance and atherosclerosis because of the established relationship between dyslipidemia and atherosclerotic vascular disease. Although insulin sensitivity was not measured in the Quebec Heart Study, the results indicated that the predictive power for CHD of fasting insulin was largely independent of the effect of apo B, LDL size, or the LDL/HDL ratio (7). This suggests that dyslipidemia is only one pathway through which insulin resistance is linked to atherosclerosis

4. Hypertension

Although initial reports indicated that insulin levels were correlated with blood pressure and appeared to predict its appearance (147–149), several studies showed no such associations (150–152). The reason for this discrepancy may be partly related to ethnicity or to obesity, since no association could be found between insulin and blood pressure in obese African-Americans and Pima Indians. Unlike dyslipidemia, the presence of obesity seems to reduce the likelihood of finding an association between insulin and blood pressure (153). Using measurements of insulin resistance, several investigators have confirmed associations between insulin resistance and blood pressure in lean individuals, but usually not in obese subjects (80,154–156). In an analysis of the frequency and the associative clustering of five cardiovascular risk factors considered part of the insulin resistance syndrome in the ARIC study (hypertriglyceridemia, low HDL, diabetes, hyperuricemia, and hypertension), hypertension, although by far the most frequent risk factor, appeared to be the least specific to the syndrome (90). This suggests that insulin resistance may play a role only in selected subgroups with hypertension, and that pathways unrelated to insulin resistance are relatively more important in the genesis of hypertension in comparison with dyslipidemia.

The mechanisms by which hyperinsulinemia/insulin resistance might cause hypertension have focused principally on three areas of importance in the pathogenesis of essential hypertension—sodium retention, increased sympathetic drive, and peripheral vasoconstriction.

a.   Hyperinsulinemia and Hypertension

The traditional view is that hyperinsulinemia might be a causal factor in the genesis of hypertension. Evidence that insulin is antinatriuretic (157) and that acute insulin infusion in humans causes increased sympathetic nervous system activity (158), led to the proposal that hyperinsulinemia itself may be playing a causative role. Support for this theory was obtained using chronic insulin infusions, which causes hypertension in certain rat strains (159), but not in dogs (160), and the demonstration in cell culture experiments that insulin has a mitogenic, proliferative action on smooth muscle cells (161). However, the effect of insulin on sodium retention is short-lived (162), and the increased sympathetic activity is accompanied by a direct, vasodilatatory effect of insulin (163). Indeed, it has been suggested that the increase in sympathetic activity and even the salt-retention produced by an insulin infusion are responses to vasodilatation (164). In addition, the appropriateness of the rat insulin infusion model for human hypertension has been seriously questioned (164). Furthermore there is no evidence that insulin at concentrations found in obese, insulin-resistant individuals can cause smooth muscle proliferation in vivo. Finally there are no data indicating that the hyperinsulinemia associated with insulin resistance leads to excessive insulin action in vivo. Thus, there is no direct evidence in humans that hyperinsulinemia causes hypertension directly.

b. Insulin Resistance and Hypertension

The possibility that insulin resistance may be etiologically linked to the genesis of hypertension in some cases may be a more plausible theory and is based on the idea that there is attenuation of the vasodilatory effects of insulin leading to raised peripheral vascular resistance (165). Insulin-induced cellular uptake and metabolism of glucose leads to activation of $Na^+K^+ATPase$ followed by attenuation of calcium influx (165); insulin also increases endothelium-dependent nitric oxide synthesis and cyclic guanosine monophosphate production, which reduces the sensitivity of contractile proteins to calcium (166). Thus calcium-dependent vascular smooth muscle relaxation is strongly promoted by the action of insulin on glucose metabolism and appears to reflect the physiological action of insulin to promote glucose uptake in skeletal muscle (167). Reduced sensitivity of these pathways to insulin action could explain the blunting of insulin-induced vasodilatation and muscle sympathetic stimulation in insulin-resistant animals and humans (164,167). In this regard insulin-resistant rodents have been demonstrated to exhibit increased intracellular calcium concentrations (165). In addition, obese nondiabetic as well as type 2 diabetic individuals have impaired endothelium-dependent nitric oxide production or release (168). The mechanism for this is unknown, but could result from increased FFA-inhibiting nitric oxide synthase activity (169).

However, there is evidence that cardiac output and blood flow to many tissues, including the kidney, are increased in obese, insulin-resistant humans and dogs in contrast to the usual observations of decreased cardiac output and reduced peripheral and renal blood flow in experimental models of hypertension caused by vasoconstriction (170). These studies argue against insulin resistance-induced peripheral vasoconstriction as a mechanism for essential hypertension. It has also been proposed that hypertension might induce insulin resistance as a result of vasoconstriction leading to decreased substrate delivery to muscle (171). This now appears unlikely since renovascular hypertension which is associated with marked vasoconstriction is not associated with insulin resistance (172).

Thus at both epidemiologic and mechanistic levels, the nature of the link between hyperinsulinemia/insulin resistance and hypertension remains elusive. Obesity is associated with increased sympathetic activity, which could play a role in the overweight hypertensive individual but again hyperinsulinemia/insulin resistance does not seem to play a direct role.

5. *Hemostasis*

Clinical and epidemiological surveys of subjects with hyperinsulinemia/insulin resistance have demonstrated significant positive associations between the levels of the key determinant of fibrinolysis-plasminogen activator inhibitor type 1 (PAI-1), fasting insulin levels, central obesity measures, triglyceride levels, and blood pressure (82). In addition, hypercoagulability and reduced fibrinolytic activity are often seen in association with hypertriglyceridemia (173). PAI-1 correlates with the risk of CHD, and it has therefore been proposed that elevated insulin levels associated with the insulin resistance syndrome may contribute to atherogenesis by reducing fibrinolytic activity (174). Evidence in support of this proposal has been obtained in studies of cultured hepatocytes in which it was demonstrated that both insulin and proinsulin increase PAI-1 production at relatively high concentrations (175, 176). In addition, in intact rabbits, acute infusions of insulin or proinsulin in pharmacologic concentrations, raised plasma PAI-1 levels (45).

However, acute insulin infusions in normal human subjects do not cause an increase in PAI-1 levels (177), and, as emphasized earlier, it has yet to be demonstrated that the hyperinsulinemia in insulin-resistant individuals translates into increased insulin action. Attention has therefore been directed to the possibility that it is insulin resistance rather than hyperinsulinemia that is linked to increased PAI-1 activity. Although direct measurements of insulin sensitivity have demonstrated a strong inverse association with PAI-1 activity in univariate analyses, several studies (178,179), though not all (173), have indicated that after correction for obesity and triglyceride levels, there was no independent relationship between insulin sensitivity and PAI-1 levels. Recent human studies have in fact demonstrated that PAI-1 is produced in human adipose tissue (180) and that the correlation between PAI-1 and insulin levels may be mediated by an expanded visceral fat depot (181) or by elevated free fatty acid (182) or by VLDL (183). Thus once again, it appears that central obesity may be the hub at the center of the insulin resistance syndrome wheel (103).

V. INSULIN RESISTANCE AND THE ARTERIAL WALL

Early work suggested a direct effect of insulin on atherogenesis in animal models (41). This has led to the idea that the hyperinsulinemia associated with insulin resistance might be an atherogenic mediator. The demonstration that insulin has vasculogenic effects has helped to strengthen this notion. However, the absence of evidence for excess insulin action in hyperinsulinemic insulin resistant subjects, the difficulties inherent in extrapolating from animal and cell culture experiments to insulin resistant human subjects, and the recent focus on insulin resistance rather than hyperinsulinemia as the link with atherosclerosis, suggest the need for a critical reevaluation of the notion that insulin is itself atherogenic

A. Animal Models of Atherosclerosis

The original experiments by Duff in the alloxan-diabetic rabbit are often quoted to indicate support for the notion that insulin is directly atherogenic. These workers demonstrated that insulin treatment retarded the development of atherosclerosis (as well as the degree of lipemia) in the cholesterol-fed rabbit (1). Earlier observations had shown that the typical atherogenic response to cholesterol-feeding in these animals was inhibited when insulin deficient diabetes was induced in these hyperlipemic animals by alloxan treatment (184). Studies in the modern era (185) indicate that severely insulin deficient rabbits develop severe lipemia due to the accumulation of very large, triglyceride-rich lipoproteins that are probably unable to effectively penetrate the arterial wall, providing a possible explanation for the apparent "protective" effect of diabetes in animals given atherogenic diets. Thus the apparent deleterious effect of insulin treatment is ironically more likely ascribable to its antilipemic action, for this would allow the lipoproteins of the cholesterol-fed rabbit to be metabolized, become smaller, and once again be able to induce atherogenesis. It should also be emphasized that these are short-duration experiments using an animal model of atherosclerosis that differs in many ways from atherogenesis in humans. In addition, the presence of diabetes in this model purporting to show a protective effect of diabetes against atherosclerosis significantly complicates interpretation and has to be viewed with skepticism, given all the evidence for a deleterious effect of diabetes in humans.

Cruz's work, which is quite often quoted, is another example of data that require reinterpretation in the modern era. In this study (186) crystalline insulin (1 U/kg) was infused daily into the right femoral artery of alloxan-diabetic dogs—animals notoriously resistant to atherosclerosis—for up to 28 weeks. Examination of the right femoral artery demonstrated increased arterial cholesterol (487 ± 32 versus 401 ± 37 mg/100 Gm, $P < 0.012$) and total fatty acids (9.88 ± 1.4 versus 2.26 ± 0.33 Gm/100 Gm, $p < 0.001$), as well as an increased muscle content of total fatty acids (but not cholesterol) compared to that found in the control left leg. The arteries and arterioles in the right leg were noted to show proliferative changes and thickening of the media, whereas these changes were not noted on the left side. The dog experiments employed infusions of large concentrations of insulin directly into an artery. In addition, the major change in the regional arterial wall and muscle was not cholesterol deposition, but total fatty acids i.e. triglyceride accumulation—

a well known consequence of insulin's lipogenic action, and one that is not clearly atherogenic. The histological changes reported were proliferative in nature and typical atherosclerotic lesions were not noted.

In a similar but cleaner experiment, peripheral hyperinsulinemia was induced in pancreatectomized dogs with pancreatic autografts that drained into the iliac vein. The hyperinsulinemic dogs were found to have increased arterial and muscle triglyceride levels, but no mention was made of arterial cholesterol deposition or plaque formation (187).

Based on these results in experimental animals it would appear that the argument that insulin is directly atherogenic in vivo is weak and needs confimation in the modern context.

B. Cell Culture Studies

Traditional theories of atherogenesis have stressed the importance of cholesterol ester deposition in arterial wall cells, as well as smooth muscle proliferation in the genesis of the atherosclerotic plaque. Older studies that have documented an increase in cellular lipid deposition without specifying that this lipid is cholesterol, have limited value given the well known action of insulin on triglyceride synthesis. However, there have been several recent reports that insulin can modulate cellular cholesterol metabolism so as to enrich cells with sterol (188). Treatment of cultured cells with insulin has been shown to increase sterol synthesis (189), induce LDL receptors (190), and inhibit HDL-mediated removal of cellular cholesterol (191). These are relatively low-affinity responses to insulin and appear to be mediated by the interaction of insulin with the IGF-1 receptor (188). Furthermore, they have been conducted mainly in fibroblasts, which do not accumulate significant amounts of cholesterol. Thus these effects likely reflect the growth factor activity of insulin, and it is unknown whether they occur in macrophages, the precursors of foam cells. Nor is it clear that the hyperinsulinemia present in insulin-resistant individuals is sufficient to activate the IGF-1 receptor.

As mentioned above, insulin has been shown to produce a proliferative response in vascular smooth muscle cells. This phenomen has been interpreted to represent a potential atherogenic effect of insulin (41). However, this response often requires supraphysiological doses of insulin and does not appear to be sustained, and there is no evidence that it occurs in subjects with insulin resistance. Furthermore, recent developments in atherogenesis research emphasize the important role in clinical atherosclerosis of the cholesterol-filled plaque that has a weak fibrous cap. Such plaques have a high propensity to rupture and thus to initiate thrombus formation. It may therefore be possible that a robust smooth muscle proliferative response is more likely to yield a more stable plaque and thus render atherothrombosis less likely.

In summary, the experimental data suggesting that insulin has a direct atherogenic effect must be considered weak and insufficient to support the hypothesis that the hyperinsulinemia of the insulin-resistant state is directly atherogenic. Further work is clearly needed in this area.

VI. ISSUES IN THE PREVENTION AND TREATMENT OF INSULIN RESISTANCE

As this review has demonstrated, the relationship between inulin resistance and atherosclerosis is an extremely complex one. Though a relationship undoubtedly exists, the evidence that insulin resistance or the associated hyperinsulinemia has a direct etiologic role in atherosclerosis remains uncertain. The data are perhaps strongest in relation to the development of dyslipidemia, although even in this area obesity remains an important confounder. Clearly insulin resistance plays a critical role in the etiopathogenesis of type 2 diabetes, but even in this setting its direct involvement in atherosclerosis is unclear. Thus it is entirely possible that hyperinsulinemia/insulin resistance is merely a marker of a pro-atherogenic state.

There is unquestionably substantial value in having a novel marker for atherosclerosis which might improve our ability to predict the risk for this disease at an early stage. However, the measurement of insulin sensitivity is tedious and impractical for clinical purposes. This means that until more specific information is obtained regarding the linkages between reduced insulin sensitivity and pathways of atherogenesis, the only simple measure available is the fasting insulin level or some derivative of it. Although most insulin assays crossreact with proinsulin, this does not seem likely to influence its predictive value in subjects with normal glucose tolerance; in subjects with abnormal glucose tolerance where proinsulin levels may be significantly raised, the fasting insulin value is less reliably correlated with insulin resistance and therefore less useful. However, as has been pointed out, the insulin assay has an extremely large interassay variation, and is therefore not standardizable in its current form. Its use has therefore been restricted to research studies where control values are specifically developed for its particular applications. For these reasons it is premature to recommend that clinicians use fasting insulin measurements as a method for detecting insulin resistance except under well-controlled and well-defined circumstances.

Despite the uncertainties regarding the role and measurement of insulin resistance as an etiologic/risk factor for atherosclerosis, there is unanimity regarding the importance of lowering excess body weight and increasing physical activity in reducing atherosclerosis risk. Both of these measures will reduce insulin resistance (192) as they improve plasma lipids and lower blood pressure, although the contribution of the reduction in insulin resistance achieved by these means to improvements in lipid levels or blood pressure has not been ascertained. Nor can there be any argument concerning the need to introduce pharmacotherapy for dyslipidemia, hypertension, or diabetes promptly and, according to current recommendations, in subjects who fail to respond adequately to lifestyle modification. Whether pharmacotherapy should be more stringently introduced in subjects adjudged to be insulin-resistant will require testing in controlled clincical trials. However, it seems reasonable to attempt to avoid the use of drugs that aggravate insulin resistance such as β-blockers, thiazides, and perhaps niacin if there are alternatives. The absence of clinical trial data would place the first priority on treating the known CHD risk factor efficiently and dealing with insulin resistance as a secondary issue. Finally since obesity constitutes a major determinant of the insulin resistance syndrome, the question of whether to consider pharmacotherapy for weight reduction is currently limited by the paucity and dubious long-term safety of available medications. However, the introduction of safe and tolerable weight loss promoting agents will provide an additional approach to the treatment of the insulin resistance syndrome.

The development of pharmacologically active agents with insulin-sensitizing effects opens a new chapter on the therapeutics of insulin-resistant states. The biguanide metformin has been regarded as the first member of this class since it interferes with hepatic glucose production in diabetic subjects and thereby lowers insulin levels (192). However, it is not a true sensitizer of insulin action. The thiazolidinedione class of drugs, which have been found to act at the genomic level to improve insulin action (193), are insulin sensitizers. Although not indicated for the treatment of insulin resistance in individuals with normal glucose tolerance, experience with their use is being obtained in the treatment of insulin-resistant diabetes, where they have been found to be effective in reducing hyperglycemia, as well as lowering insulin levels. In addition, in some studies reduction in blood pressure and triglycerides have been reported. The only marketed thiazolidinedione, troglitazone, is also being tested along with metformin in the Diabetes Prevention Program, a randomized, controlled clinical trial, to determine whether the emergence of type 2 diabetes in subjects with IGT can be prevented or delayed through the use of these drugs. One of the secondary aims of the trial is to assess whether cardiovascular risk factors and carotid IMT respond to drug therapy. This trial should provide valuable information on the parallel effects of improvements in insulin sensitivity in relation to measures of atherosclerosis and atherosclerosis risk factors. Drugs of this type may also be useful in improving our understanding of the relationship between insulin resistance and atherosclerosis. However, the broader application of these agents to the treatment of insulin resistance in individuals with normal glucose tolerance must await a clearer understanding of the role of insulin resistance in promoting atherosclerosis.

REFERENCES

1. Duff GL, Brechin DJH, Findelstein WE. The effect of alloxan diabetes on experimental cholesterol atherosclerosis in the rabbit. IV. The effect of insulin therapy on the inhibition of atherosclerosis in the alloxan-diabetic rabbit. J Exp Med 1954; 100:371–380.
2. Peters N, Hales CN. Plasma insulin concentrations after myocardial infarction. Lancet 1965; 1:1144 1145.
3. Olefsky JM, Farquhar JW, Reaven GM. Relationship between fasting insulin level and resistance to insulin-mediated glucose uptake in normal and diabetic subjects. Diabetes 1973; 22:507–513.
4. Reaven GM. Role of insulin resistance in human disease. Diabetes 1988; 37: 1595–1607.
5. DeFronzo RA. The triumvirate: beta cell, muscle, liver: a collusion responsible for NIDDM. Diabetes. 1988; 37:667–687
6. Eastman RC, Cowie CC, Harris MI. Undiagnosed diabetes or impaired glucose tolerance and cardiovascular risk. Diabetes Care 1997; 20:127–128.
7. Desprès J-P, Lamarche B, Mauriège P, et al. Hyperinsulinemia as an independent risk factor for ischemic heart disease. N Engl J Med 1997; 334:952–957.
8. Robbins DH, Andersen L, Bowsher R, et al. Report of the American Diabetes Association's Task Force on Standardization of the Insulin Assay. Diabetes 1996; 45:242–256.
9. Himsworth H. Diabetes mellitus: a differentiation into insulin-sensitive and insulin-insensitive types. Lancet 1936; 1:127–130.
10. DeFronzo RA, Tobin JD, Andres R. Glucose clamp technique: a method for quantifying insulin secretion and resistance. Am J Physiol 1079; 237:E214–E223.
11. Nagulesparan M, Savage PJ, Unger RH, et al. A simplified method using somatostatin to assess in vivo insulin resistance over a range of obesity. Diabetes 1979; 28:980–983.
12. Bergman RN, Finegood DT, Ader M. Assessment of insulin sensitivity in vivo. Endocr Rev 1985; 6:45–86.
13. Chen Y-DI, Golay A, Swislocki AM, et al. Resistance to insulin suppression of plasma free fatty acid concentrations and insulin stimulation of glucose uptake in non-insulin dependent diabetes. J Clin Endocrinol Metab 1987; 64:17–21.
14. Suzuki M, Ikebuchi M, Shinozaki K, et al. Mechanism and clinical implications of insulin resistance syndrome. Diabetes 1996; 45 (Suppl 3):S52–S54.
15. Eckel RH. Lipoprotein lipase: a multifunctional enzyme relevant to common metabolic diseases. N Engl J Med 1989; 320:1060–1068.
16. Haffner SM, Howard G, Mayer E, et al. Insulin sensitivity and acute insulin response in African-Americans, non-Hispanic whites, and Hispanics with NIDDM: the Insulin Resistance Atherosclerosis Study. Diabetes 1997; 46:63–69.

17. Laws A, Hoen HM, Selby JV, et al. Differences in insulin suppression of free fatty acid levels by gender and glucose tolerance status. Relation to plasma triglyceride and apolipoprotein B concentrations. Arterioscler Thromb Vasc Biol 1997; 17:64–71.

18. DeFronzo RA. Glucose intolerance and aging. Diabetes Care 1981; 4:493–501.

19. DeFronzo RA, Ferrannini E. Insulin resistance. A multifaceted syndrome responsible for NIDDM, obesity, hypertension, dyslipidemia, and atherosclerotic cardiovascular disease. Diabetes Care 1991; 14:173–194.

20. Kolterman OG, Insel J, Saekow M, et al. Mechanisms of insulin resistance in human obesity. Evidence for receptor and post-receptor defects. J Clin Invest 1984; 65:1872–1884.

21. Koivisto VA, Soman V, Conrad P, et al. Insulin binding to monocytes in trained athletes: changes in the resting state and after exercise. J Clin Invest 1979; 64; 1011–1015.

22. Kuhl C, Hornnes PJ, Andersen O. Etiology and pathophysiology of gestational diabetes mellitus. Diabetes 1985; 34(suppl 2):66–70.

23. Rönnemaa T, Rönnemaa EM, Puukka P, et al. Smoking is independently associated with high plasma insulin levels in non-diabetic men. Diabetes Care 1996; 19:1229–1232.

24. Storlein LH, Jenkins AB, Chisholm DJ, et al. Influence of dietary fat composition on development of insulin resistance in rats. Relationship to muscle triglyceride and 3-3 fatty acids in muscle phospholipid. Diabetes 1991; 40:280–289.

25. Ferrannini E, Buzzigoli G, Bonadonna R, et al. Insulin resistance in essential hypertension. N Engl J Med 1987; 317:350–357.

26. Dunaif A, Segal KR, Shelley DR, et al. Evidence for distinctive and intrinsic defects in insulin action in polycystic ovary syndrome. Diabetes 1992; 41:1257–1266.

27. Kruszynska YT, Olefsky JM. Cellular and molecular mechanisms of non-insulin dependent diabetes mellitus. J Invest Med 1996; 44:413–428.

28. Lillioja S, Mott D, Zawadski JK, et al. Impaired glucose tolerance as a disorder of insulin action: longitudinal and cross-sectional studies in Pima Indians. N Engl J Med 1988; 318:1217–1225.

29. Polonsky KS. The beta cell in diabetes: from molecular genetics to clinical research. Diabetes 1995; 44:705–717.

30. DeFronzo RA, Bonnadonna RC, Ferrannini E. Pathogenesis of NIDDM. Diabetes Care 1992; 15:318–368.

31. Unger RH. Lipotoxicity in the pathogenesis of obesity-dependent NIDDM: genetic and clinical implications. Diabetes 1995; 44:863–870.

32. Svedberg J, Björntorp P, Smith U, et al. Free fatty acid inhibition of insulin binding, degradation and action in isolated rat hepatocytes. Diabetes 1990; 39: 570–574.

33. Laakso M. How good a marker is the insulin level for insulin resistance? Am J Epidemiol 1993; 137:959–965.

34. Nabulsi AA, Folsom AR, Heiss G, et al. Fasting hyperinsulinemia and cardiovascular disease risk factors in non-diabetic adults: stronger associations in lean versus obese subjects. Metabolism 1995; 44:914–922.

35. Krotkiewski M, Björntorp P, Sjöstrom L, et al. Impact of obesity on metabolism in men and women: importance of regional adipose tissue distribution. J Clin Invest 1983; 72:1150–1162.
36. Peiris AN, Sothman MS, Hoffman RG, et al. Adiposity, fat distribution and cardiovascular risk. Ann Intern Med 1989; 110:867–872.
37. Larrson B, Svärdsudd K, Welin L, et al. Abdominal adipose tissue distribution, obesity and risk of cardiovascular disease and death: a 13–year follow-up of participants in the study of men born in 1913. Br Med J 1984; 288:1401–1404.
38. Salans LB, Knittle JL, Hirsch J. The role of adipose tissue size and adipose tissue sensitivity in the carbohydrate intolerance of human obesity. J Clin Invest 1968; 47:153–165.
39. Evans DJ, Murray R, Kissebah AH. Relationship between skeletal muscle insulin resistance, insulin-mediated glucose disposal, and insulin-binding: effects of obesity and body fat topography. J Clin Invest 1984; 74:1515–1525.
40. Evans DJ, Hoffman RG, Kalkhoff RK, et al. Relationship of androgenic activity of body fat topography, fat cell morphology, and metabolic aberrations in premenopausal women. J Clin Endocrinol Metab 1983; 57:304–310.
41. Stout RW. Insulin and atheroma. Diabetes Care 1990; 13:631–634.
42. Galloway JA, Hooper SA, Spradlin CT, et al. Biosynthetic human proinsulin: review of chemistry, in vitro and in vivo receptor binding, animal and human pharmacology studies, and clinical trial experience. Diabetes Care 1992; 15:666–692.
43. Ward WK, LaCava EC, Pacquette TL, et al. Disproportionate elevation of immunoreactive proinsulin in type 2 (non-insulin-dependent) diabetes mellitus and in experimental insulin resistance. Diabetologia 1987; 30:698–702.
44. Nagi DK, Hendra TJ, Ryle AJ, et al. The relationships of concentrations of insulin, intact proinsulin and 32–33 split proinsulin with cardiovascular risk factors in type II (non-insulin dependent) diabetic subjects. Diabetologia 1990; 33:532–537.
45. Nordt TK, Sawa H, Fujii S, et al. Induction of plasminogen activator inhibitor type-1 (PAI-1) by proinsulin and insulin in vivo. Circulation 1995; 91:764–770.
46. Haffner SM, Mykkännen L, Stern MP, et al. Relationship of proinsulin and insulin to cardiovascular risk factors in nondiabetic subjects. Diabetes 1993; 42:1297–1302.
47. Bävenholm P, Proudler A, Tornvall P, et al. Insulin, intact and split proinsulin, and coronary artery disease in young men. Circulation 1995; 92; 1422–1429.
48. McKeigue P, Davey G. Associations between insulin levels and cardiovascular disease are confounded by comorbidity. Diabetes Care 1995; 18:1294–1298.
49. Pei D, Chen Y-DI, Hollenbeck CB, et al. Relationship between insulin-mediated glucose disposal by muscle and adipose tissue lipolysis in healthy volunteers. J Clin Endocrinol Metab 1995; 80:3368–3372.
50. Byrne CD, Wareham NJ, Day NE, et al. Decreased non-esterified fatty acid suppression and features of the insulin resistance syndrome occur in a sub-group of individuals with normal glucose tolerance. Diabetologia 1995; 38:1358–1366.
51. Hennig B, Shasby DM, Spector AA. Exposure to fatty acid increases human low density transfer across cultured endothelial monolayers. Circ Res 1985; 57:776–780.

52. Pronai L, Hiramatsu K, Saigusa Y, et al. Low superoxide scavenging activity associated with enhanced superoxide generation by monocytes from male hypertriglyceridemia with and without diabetes. Atherosclerosis 1991; 90:39–47.

53. Nikkilä EA, Miettenen TA, Vesenne MR, et al. Plasma insulin in coronary heart disease: response to oral and intravenous glucose and to tolbutamide. Lancet 1965; 1:508–511.

54. Pyörälä K. Relationship of glucose intolerance and plasma insulin to the incidence of coronary heart disease: results from two population studies in Finland. Diabetes Care 1979; 2:131–141.

55. Welborn TA, Wearne K. Coronary heart disease incidence and cardiovascular mortality in Busselton with reference to glucose and insulin concentrations. Diabetes Care 1979; 2:154–160.

56. Ducimetiere P, Eschwege E, Papoz L, et al. Relationship of plasma insulin levels to the incidence of myocardial infarction and coronary heart disease mortality in a middle-aged population. Diabetologia 1980; 19:205–210.

57. Yarnell JWG, Sweetnam PM, Marks V, et al. Insulin in ischemic heart disease: are associations explained by triglyceride concentrations? The Caerphilly Prospective Study. Br Heart J 1994; 71:293–296.

58. Orchard TJ, Eichner J, Kuller LH, et al. Insulin as a predictor of coronary heart disease: interaction with apo E phenotype: a report from MRFIT. Ann Epidemiol 1994; 4:40–45.

59. Welin L, Eriksson H, Larsson B, et al. Hyperinsulinemia is not a major coronary risk factor in elderly men: the study of men born in 1913. Diabetologia 1992; 35:766–770.

60. Kuusisto J, Mykkänen L. Pyörälä K, et al. Hyperinsulinemic microalbuminuria: a new risk indicator for coronary heart disease. Circulation 1995; 91:831–837.

61. Ferrara A, Barrett-Connor E, Edelstein SL, et al. Hyperinsulinemia does not increase the risk of fatal·cardiovascular disease in elderly men and women without diabetes: the Rancho Bernardo Study, 1984 to 1991. Am J Epidemiol 1994; 140:857–869.

62. Rewers M, Shetterley SM, Baxter J, et al. Insulin and cardiovascular disease in Hispanics and non-Hispanic whites (NHW): the San Luis Valley Diabetes Study. Circulation 1992; 85:865.

63. Liu QZ, Knowler WC, Nelson RG, et al. Insulin treatment, endogenous insulin concentration, and ECG abnormalities in diabetic Pima Indians: cross-sectional and prospective analyses. Diabetes 1992; 41:1141–1450.

64. Folsom AR, Szklo M, Stevens J, et al. A prospective study of coronary heart disease in relation to fasting insulin, glucose and diabetes. The Atherosclerosis Risk in Communities (ARIC) Study. Diabetes Care 1997; 20:935–942.

65. Rönnemaa T, Laakso M, Pyörälä K, et al. High fasting plasma insulin is an indicator of coronary heart disease in non-insulin-dependent diabetic patients and non-diabetic subjects. Arterioscler Thromb 1991; 11:80–90.

66. Modan M, Or J, Karasik A, et al. Hyperinsulinemia, sex and risk of atherosclerotic cardiovascular disease. Circulation 1991; 84:1165–1175.

67. Jarrett RJ, McCartney P, Keen H, et al. The Bedford Survey: ten year mortality rates in newly diagnosed diabetics, borderline diabetics and normoglycemic controls and risk indices for coronary heart disease in borderline diabetics. Diabetologia 1982; 22:79–84.

68. Fontbonne A, Eschwege E, Cambien F, et al. Hypertriglyceridemia as a risk factor of coronary heart disease mortality in subjects with impaired glucose tolerance or diabetes: results from the 11–year follow-up of the Paris Prospective Study. Diabetologia 1989; 32:300–304.

69. Uusitipa MIJ, Niskanen LK, Siitonen O, et al. 5–year incidence of atherosclerotic vascular disease in relation to general risk factors, insulin level, and abnormalities in lipoprotein composition in non-insulin-dependent diabetic and nondiabetic subjects. Circulation 1990; 82:27–36.

70. Laakso M, Sarlund H, Salonen R, et al. Asymptomatic atherosclerosis and insulin resistance. Arterioscler Thrombosis 1991; 11:1068–1076.

71. Tomono S, Kato N, Utsugi T, et al. The role of insulin in coronary atherosclerosis. Diab Res Clin Prac 1994; 22:117–122.

72. Shinozaki K, Suzuki M, Ikebuchi M, et al. Demonstration of insulin resistance in coronary artery disease documented with angiography. Diabetes Care 1996; 19:1–7.

73. Shinozaki K, Suzuki M, Ikebuchi M, et al. Insulin resistance associated with compensatory hyperinsulinemia as an independent risk factor for vasospastic angina. Circulation 1995; 92:1749–1757.

74. Dean JD, Jones CJH, Hutchison SJ, et al. Hyperinsulinemia and microvascular angina ("syndrome X"). Lancet 1991; 337:456–457.

75. Sax FL, Cannon RO, Watson RM, et al. Forearm flow in patients with Syndrome X: evidence of a generalized disorder of vascular tone. N Engl J Med 1987; 317:1366–1370.

76. Craven TE, Ryu JE, Espeland MA, et al. Evaluation of the associations between carotid artery atherosclerosis and coronary artery stenosis: a case control study. Circulation 1990; 82:1230–1242.

77. Howard G, Ryu JE, Evans GW, et al. Extracranial carotid atherosclerosis in patients with and without transient ischemic attacks and coronary artery disease. Arteriosclerosis 1990; 10:714–719.

78. Folsom AR, Eckfeldt JH, Weitzman S, et al. Relation of carotid artery wall thickness to diabetes mellitus, fasting glucose and insulin, body size, and physical activity. Atherosclerosis Risk in Community (ARIC) Study Investigators. Stroke 1994; 25:66–73.

79. Howard G, O'Leary DH, Zaccoro D, et al. Insulin sensitivity and atherosclerosis. Circulation 1996; 93:1809–1817.

80. Saad MF, Lillioja S, Nyomba BL, et al. Racial differences in the relation between blood pressure and insulin resistance. N Engl J Med 1991; 324:733–739.

81. Chaiken RL, Banerji MA, Huey H, et al. Do blacks with NIDDM have an insulin resistance syndrome? Diabetes 1993; 42:444–449.

82. Hamsten A, Eriksson P, Karpe F, et al. Relationships of thrombosis and fibrinolysis to atherosclerosis. Curr Opin Lipidol 1994; 5:382–389.

83. Bonora E, Tessari R, Micciolo R, et al. Intimal-medial thickness of the carotid artery in non-diabetic and NIDDM patients. Diabetes Care 1997; 20:627–631.
84. Agewall S, Fagerberg B, Attvall S, et al. Carotid artery wall intima-media thickness is associated with insulin-mediated glucose disposal in men at high and low coronary risk. Stroke 1995; 26:956–960.
85. Suzuki M, Shinozaki K, Kanazawa A, et al. Insulin resistance as an independent risk factor for carotid wall thickening. Hypertension 1996; 28:593–598.
86. Shinozaki K, Naritomi H, Shimizu T, et al. Role of insulin resistance associated with compensatory hyperinsulinemia in ischemic stroke. Stroke 1996; 27:37–43.
87. Kekalainen P, Sarlund H, Farin P, et al. Femoral atherosclerosis in middle-aged subjects: association with cardiovascular risk factors and insulin resistance. Am J Epidemiol 1996; 144:742–748.
88. Desprès J-P, Marette A. Relation of components of insulin resistance syndrome to coronary disease risk. Curr Opin Lipidol 1994; 5:274–289.
89. Vague J. The degree of masculine differentiation of obesities: a factor determining predisposition to diabetes, atherosclerosis, gout and uric calculous disease. Am J Clin Nutr 1956; 4:20–34.
90. Schmidt MI, Watson RL, Duncan BB, et al. Clustering of dyslipidemia, hyperuricemia, diabetes, and hypertension and its association with fasting insulin and central and overall obesity in a general population. Metabolism 1996; 45: 699–706.
91. Raitakari OT, Porkka KVK, Rönnemaa T, et al. The role of insulin in clustering of serum lipids and blood pressure in children and adolescents. The Cardiovascular Risk in Young Finns Study. Diabetologia 1995; 38:1042–1050.
92. Bao W, Srinivasan SR, Wattigney WA, et al. Persistence of multiple cardiovascular risk factor clustering related to Syndrome X from childhood to young adulthood. The Bogalusa Heart Study. Arch Int Med 1994; 154:1842–1847.
93. Haffner SM, Valdez RA, Hazuda HP, et al. Prospective analysis of the insulin resistance syndrome (syndrome X). Diabetes 1992; 41:714–722.
94. Zimmet PZ, Collins VR, Dowse GK, et al. Is hyperinsulinemia a central characteristic of a chronic cardiovascular risk factor clustering syndrome? Mixed findings in Asian Indian, Creole and Chinese Mauritians. Diabetic Med 1994; 11:388–396.
95. Laakso M, Rönnemaa T, Mykkänen L, et al. Insulin resistance syndrome in Finland. J Cardiovasc Risk Factors 1993; 3:44–45.
96. Kannel WB, McGee DL. Diabetes and cardiovascular disease: Framingham study. JAMA 1979; 241:2035–2038.
97. Proceedings of the 15th International Diabetes Federation Satellite Symposium on "Diabetes and Macrovascular Complications." Diabetes 1996; 45(suppl 3):S1–S141.
98. Haffner SM, Stern MP, Hazuda HP, et al. Cardiovascular disease risk factors as predictors in confirmed prediabetic individuals: does the clock for coronary heart disease start ticking before the onset of clinical diabetes? JAMA 1990; 263:2893–2896.
99. Uusitupa MIJ, Niskanen LK, Siitonen O, et al. Ten-year cardiovascular mortality in relation to risk factors and abnormalities in lipoprotein composition in type 2

(non-insulin-dependent) diabetic and non-diabetic subjects. Diabetologia 1993; 36:1175–1184.

100. O'Brian R, Timmins K. The role of oxidation and glycation in the pathogenesis of diabetic atherosclerosis. Trends Endocrinol Metab 1994; 5:329–334.

101. Colwell JA. Intensive insulin therapy in type II diabetes. Diabetes 1996; 45(suppl 3):S87–S90.

102. Garrison RJ, Hoggins MW, Kannel WB. Obesity and coronary heart disease. Curr Opin Lipidol 1996; 7:199–202.

103. Hopkins PN, Hunt SC, Wu LL, et al. Hypertension, dyslipidemia and insulin resistance: links in a chain or spokes on a wheel? Curr Opin Lipidol 1996; 7:241–253.

104. Reaven GM, Lerner RL, Stern MP, et al. Role of insulin in endogenous hypertriglyceridemia. J Clin Invest 1967; 46:1756–1767.

105. Bagdade JD, Bierman EL, Porte D Jr. Influence of obesity on the relationship between insulin and triglyceride levels in endogenous hypertriglyceridemia. Diabetes 1971; 20:664–672.

106. Orchard TJ, Becker DJ, Bates M, et al. Plasma insulin and lipoprotein concentrations: an atherogenic association. Am J Epidemiol 1983; 118:326–337.

107. Zavaroni I, Dall'Aglio E, Alpi O, et al. Evidence for an independent relationship between plasma insulin and concentration of high density lipoprotein cholesterol and triglyceride. Atherosclerosis 1985; 55:259–266.

108. Tobey TA, Greenfield M, Kraemer F, et al. Relationship between insulin resistance, insulin secretion, very low density lipoprotein kinetics and plasma triglyceride levels in normotriglyceridemic men. Metabolism 1981; 30:165–171.

109. Topping DL, Maye PA. Insulin and non-esterified fatty acids. Acute regulators of lipogenesis in perfused rat livers. Biochem J 1982; 204:433–439.

110. Reaven GM, Greenfield MS. Diabetic hypertriglyceridemia. Evidence for three clinical syndromes. Diabetes 1981; 30(suppl 2):66–75.

111. Yki-Järvinen H, Taskinen M-R. Interrelationships between insulin's antilipolytic and glucoregulatory effects and plasma triglycerides in non-diabetic and diabetic patients with endogenous hypertriglyceridemia. Diabetes 1988; 37:1271–1278.

112. Lewis GF, Uffelman KD, Szeto LW, et al. Interaction between free fatty acids and insulin in the acute control of very low density lipoprotein production in humans. J Clin Invest 1995; 95:158–166.

113. Eckel RH. Lipoprotein lipase: a multifunctional enzyme relevant to common metabolic diseases. N Engl J Med 1989; 320:1060–1068.

114. Bonnadonna RC, Groop LC, Zych K, et al. Dose dependent effect of insulin on plasma free fatty acid turnover and oxidation in humans. Am J Physiol 1990; 259:E736–E750.

115. Sparks CE, Sparks JD, Bolognino M, et al. Insulin effects on apolipoprotein B lipoprotein synthesis and secretion by primary cultures of rat hepatocytes. Metab Clin Exp 1986; 35:1128–1136.

116. Chen M, Breslow JL, Weihua L, Leff T. Transcriptional regulation of the apoC-III gene by insulin in diabetic mice: correlation with changes in plasma triglyceride levels. J Lipid Res 1994; 35:1918–1924.

117. Yki-Järvinen H, Taskinen M-R, Koivisto VA, et al. Response of adipose tissue lipoprotein lipase activity and serum lipoproteins to acute hyperinsulinemia in man. Diabetologia 1984; 27:364–369.

118. Havel RJ. Post-prandial hyperlipidemia and remnant lipoproteins. Curr Opin Lipidol 1994; 5:102–109.

119. Schrezenmeir J, Keppler J, Fenselau S, et al. The phenomenon of a high triglyceride response to an oral lipid load in healthy subjects and its link to the metabolic syndrome. Ann NY Acad Sci 1993; 683:302–314.

120. Chen Y-D, Reaven DM. Intestinally derived lipoproteins: metabolism and clinical significance. Diabetes Metab Rev 1991; 7:191–208.

121. O'Brien T, Young WF Jr, Palumbo PJ, et al. Hypertension and dyslipidemia in patients with insulinoma. Mayo Clin Proc 1993; 68:141–146.

122. Steiner G. Hyperinsulinemia and hypertriglyceridemia. J Intern Med 1994; 236 (suppl 736):23–26.

123. Wiggins D, Gibbons GF. The lipolysis/esterification cycle of hepatic triacylglycerol. Its role in the secretion of very-low-density-lipoprotein and its response to hormones and sulfonylureas. Biochem J 1992; 284:457–462.

124. Boden G. Role of fatty acids in the pathogenesis of insulin resistance and NIDDM. Diabetes 1997; 45:3–10.

124. Crespin SR, Greenbough WB, Steinberg D. Stimulation of insulin secretion by long-chain free fatty acids. J Clin Invest 1973; 52:1979–1984.

125. Hotamisligil GS, Arner P, Caro JF, et al. Increased adipose tissue expression of tumor necrosis factor-α in human obesity and insulin resistance. J Clin Invest 1995; 95:2409–2415.

126. Saghizadeh M, Ong JM, Barvey WT, et al. The expression of TNF-α by human muscle. Relationship to insulin resistance. J Clin Invest 1996; 97:1111–1116.

127. Feingold KR, Grünfeld C. Tumor necrosis factor-α stimulates hepatic lipogenesis in the rat in vivo. J Clin Invest 1987; 80:184–190.

128. Considine RV, Sinha MK, Heiman ML, et al. Serum immunoreactive-leptin concentrations in normal-weight and obese humans. N Engl J Med 1996; 334:292–295.

129. Ezzell C. Fat times for obesity research: tons of new information, but how does it all fit together? J NIH Res 1995; 7:39–43.

130. Cianflone K, Maslowska M, Sniderman AD, et al. Impaired response of fibroblasts in patients with hyperapobetalipoproteinemia to acylation stimulation protein. J Clin Invest 1990; 85:722–730.

131. Karhapää P, Voutilainen E, Malkki M, et al. Obese men with type IIb hyperlipidemia are insulin resistant. Arterioscler Thromb 1993; 13:1469–1475.

132. Bredie SJH, Tack CJJ, Smits P, et al. Nonobese patients with familial combined hyperlipidemia are insulin resistant compared to their nonaffected relatives. Arterioscler Thromb Vasc Biol 1997; 17:1465–1471.

133. Hunt SC, Wu LL, Hopkins PN. Apolipoprotein, low density lipoprotein subfraction, and insulin associations with familial combined hyperlipidemia: study of Utah patients with familial dyslipidemic hypertension. Arteriosclerosis 1990; 10:520–530.

134. Olefsky JM, Farquhar JW, Reaven GM. Reappraisal of the role of insulin in hypertriglyceridemia. Am J Med 1974; 57:551–560.

135. Abbott WGH, Lillija S, Young AA, et al. Relationships between plasma lipoprotein concentrations and insulin action in an obese hyperinsulinemic population. Diabetes 1987; 36:897–904.

136. Laakso M, Saarlund H, Mykkänen L. Insulin resistance is associated with lipid and lipoprotein abnormalities in subjects with varying degrees of glucose tolerance. Arteriosclerosis 1990; 10:223–231.

137. Patsch JR, Prasad S, Gotto AM Jr, et al. High density lipoprotein$_2$: relationship of the plasma levels of this lipoprotein species to its composition, to the magnitude of postprandial lipemia, and to the activities of lipoprotein lipase and hepatic lipase. J Clin Invest 1987; 80:341–347.

138. Miesenbock G, Patsch JR. Postprandial hyperlipidemia: The search for the atherogenic lipoprotein. Curr Opin Lipidol 1992; 3:196–201.

139. Karhapää P, Voutilainen E, Laakso M, et al. Isolated low HDL cholesterol. An insulin-resistant state. Diabetes 1994; 43:411–417.

140. Knudsen P, Eriksson J, Lahdenperä, et al. Changes of lipolytic enzymes cluster with insulin resistance syndrome. Diabetologia 1995; 38:344–350.

141. Dullart RPF, Cluiter WJ, Dikkeschei LD, et al. Effect of adiposity on plasma lipid transfer activities: a possible link between insulin resistance and high density lipoprotein metabolism. Eur J Clin Invest 1994; 24:188–194.

142. Caslake MJ, Packard CJ, Series JJ, et al. Plasma triglyceride and low density lipoprotein metabolism. Eur J Clin Invest 1992; 22:96–104.

143. Zambon A, Austin MA, Brown BG, et al. Effect of hepatic lipase in LDL in normal men and those with coronary heart disease. Arterioscler Thromb 1993; 13:147–153.

144. Mykkänen L, Haffner SM, Rainwater DL, et al. Relationship of LDL size to insulin sensitivity in normoglycemic men. Arterioscler Thromb Vasc Biol 1997; 17:1447–1453.

145. Babirak SP, Brown, Brunzell JD. Familial combined hyperlipidemia and abnormal lipoprotein lipase. Arterioscler Thromb 1992; 12:1176–1183.

146. Grundy SM. Small LDL, atherogenic dyslipidemia and the metabolic syndrome. Circulation 1997; 95:1–4.

147. Modan M, Halkin H, Almog S, et al. Hyperinsulinemia: a link between hyperinsulinemia, obesity and glucose intolerance. J Clin Invest 1986; 75:809–817.

148. Ferrannini E, Haffner SM, Stern MP, et al. High blood pressure and insulin resistance: influence of ethnic background. Eur J Clin Invest 1991; 21:280–287.

149. Wing RR, Bunker CH, Kuller LH, et al. Insulin, body mass index, and cardiovascular risk factors in premenopausal women. Arteriosclerosis 1989; 9:479–484.

150. Dowse GK, Collins VR, Alberti KGMM, et al. Insulin and blood pressure levels are not independently related in Mauritians of Asian Indian, Creole or Chinese origin. J Hypertens 1993; 11:297–307.

151. Mbanya JCN, Thomas TH, Wilkinson R, et al. Hypertension and hyperinsulinemia: a relation in diabetes but not essential hypertension. Lancet 1988; 1:733–734.

152. Ferrannini E, Buzzigoli G, Bonnadonna R, et al. Insulin resistance in essential hypertension. N Engl J Med 1987; 317:350–357.

153. Haffner SM. Epidemiology of hypertension and insulin resistance syndrome. J Hypertens 1997; 15(suppl 1):S25–S30.

154. Laakso M, Saarlund H, Mykkänen L. Essential hypertension and insulin resistance in non-insulin dependent diabetes. Eur J Clin Invest 1989; 19:518–526.

155. Mykkänen L, Haffner SM, Rönnemaa T, et al. Relationship of plasma insulin concentration and insulin sensitivity to blood pressure. Is it modified by obesity? J Hypertens 1996; 14:399–405.

156. Bonora E, Moghetti P, Zebere M, et al. β-cell secretion and insulin sensitivity in hypertensive and normotensive obese subjects. Int J Obesity 1990; 14:735–742.

157. DeFronzo RA. The effect of insulin on renal sodium metabolism. Diabetologia 1981; 21:165–171.

158. Landsberg L, Krieger DR. Obesity, metabolism and sympathetic nervous system. Am J Hypertens 1989; 2:1255–1325.

159. Brands MW, Hildebrandt DA, Mizelle HL, et al. Sustained hyperinsulinemia increases arterial pressure in conscious rats. Am J Physiol 1991; 260:R764–R768.

160. Brands MW, Mizelle HL, Gaillard CA, et al. The hemodynamic response to chronic hyperinsulinemia in conscious dogs. Am J Hypertens 1991; 4:164–168.

161. Stout RW, Bierman EL, Ross R. Effect of insulin on the proliferation of cultured primate arterial smooth muscle cells. Circ Res 1991; 36:319–327.

162. Hall JE, Brands MW, Mizelle HL, et al. Chronic intrarenal hyperinsulinemia does not cause hypertension. Am J Physiol 1991; 260:F663–F669.

163. Anderson EA, Balon TW, Hoffman RP, et al. Insulin increases sympathetic activity but not blood pressure in borderline hypertensive humans. Hypertension 1992; 19:621–627.

164. Hall JE, Brands MW, Zappe DH, et al. Insulin resistance, hyperinsulinemia, and hypertension: causes, consequences, or merely correlations? Proc Soc Exp Biol Med 1995; 208:317–329.

165. Sowers JR. Insulin resistance and hypertension. Mol Cell Endocrinol 1990; 74: C87–C89.

166. Steinberg HO, Brechtel G, Johnson A, et al. Insulin-mediated skeletal muscle vasodilatation is nitric oxide dependent. J Clin Invest 1994; 94:1172–1179.

167. Hall JE, Brands MW, Zappe DH, et al. Cardiovascular actions of insulin: are they important in long-term blood pressure regulation? Clin Exp Pharmacol Physiol 1995; 22:689–700.

168. Steinberg HO, Chaker K, Leaming R, et al. Obesity/insulin resistance is associated with endothelial dysfunction. J Clin Invest 1996; 97:2601–2610.

169. Stepniakowski KT, Goodfriend TL, Egan BM. Fatty acids enhance vascular alpha-adrenergic sensitivity. Hypertension 1995; 25:774–778.

170. Hall JE, Brands MW, Dixon WM, et al. Obesity-induced hypertension: renal function and systemic hemodynamics. Hypertension 1993; 22:292–299.

171. Baron AD, Brechtel-Hook G, Johnson A, et al. A possible link between insulin resistance and blood pressure. Hypertension 1993; 21:129–135.

172. Mark AL, Anderson EA. Genetic factors determine the blood pressure response to insulin resistance and hyperinsulinemia: a call to refocus the insulin hypothesis of hypertension. Proc Soc Exp Biol Med 1995; 208:330–336.

173. Simpson HCR, Meade TW, Stirling Y, et al. Hypertriglyceridemia and hyper-coagulability. Lancet 1983; 1:786–790.

174. Juhan-Vague I, Alessi MC, Vague P. Increased plasma plasminogen activator inhibitor 1 levels. A possible link between insulin resistance and atherothrombosis.

175. Kooistra T, Bosma PJ, Töns HAM, et al. Plasminogen activator inhibitor 1: biosynthesis and mRNA levels are increased by insulin in cultured human hepatocytes. Thromb Haemost 1989; 62:723–728.

176. Nordt TK, Schneider DJ, Sobel BE. Augmentation of the synthesis of plasminogen activator inhibitor type-1 by precursors of insulin: a potential risk factor for vascular disease. Circulation 1994; 89:321–330.

177. Potter Van Loon BJ, de Baart ACW, Radder JK, et al. Acute exogenous hyperinsulinemia does not result in elevation of plasma plasminogen activator inhibitor 1 concentrations in humans. Fibrinolysis 1990; 4:93–94.

178. Mykkännen L, Rönnemaa T, Marniemi J, et al. Insulin sensitivity is not an independent determinant of plasma plasminogen activator inhibitor-1 activity. Arterioscler Thromb 1994; 14:1264–1271.

179. Cigolini M, Targher G, Seidell JC, et al. Relationships of plasminogen activator inhibitor-1 to anthropometry, serum insulin, triglycerides and adipose tissue fatty acids in healthy men. Atherosclerosis 1994; 106:139–147.

180. Alessi, MC, Peiretti F, Morange P, et al. Production of plasminogen activator inhibitor 1 by human adipose tissue. Possible link between visceral fat accumulation and vascular disease. Diabetes 1997; 46:860–867.

181. Shimomura I, Funahashi T, Takahashi M, et al. Enhanced expression of PAI-1 in visceral fat: possible contributor to vascular disease in obesity. Nature Med 1996; 2:800–803.

182. Bastard JP, Bruckert E, Robert JJ, et al. Are free fatty acids related to plasma plasminogen activator inhibitor 1 in android obesity? Int J Obesity 1995; 19:836–838.

183. Stiko-Rahm A, Wiman B, Hamsten A, et al. Secretion of plasminogen activator inhibitor 1 from cultured human umbilical vein endothelial cells is induced by very low density lipoprotein. Arteriosclerosis 1990; 10:1067–1073.

184. Duff GL, McMillan G. The effect of alloxan diabetes on experimental cholesterol atherosclerosis in the rabbit. I. The inhibition of experimental cholesterol atherosclerosis in alloxan diabetes. II. The effect of alloxan diabetes on the retrogression of experimental cholesterol atherosclerosis. J Exp Med 1949; 89:611–629.

185. Nordestgaard BG, Zilversmit DB. Large lipoproteins are excluded from the arterial wall in diabetic cholesterol-fed rabbits. J Lipid Res 1988; 29:1491–1500.

186. Cruz AB Jr, Amatuzio DS, Grande F, et al. Effect of intraarterial insulin on tissue cholesterol and fatty acids in alloxan diabetic dogs. Circ Res 1961; 9:39–43.

187. Falhot K, Cutfield R, Alejandro R, et al. The effects of hyperinsulinemia on arterial wall and peripheral muscle metabolism in dogs. Metabolism 1985; 34:1146–1149.

188. Oram JF. Can insulin promote atherogenesis by altering cellular cholesterol metabolism? J Lab Clin Med 1995; 126:229–230.

189. Krone W, Greten H. Evidence for post-transcrptional regulation by insulin of 3–hydroxy-3–methylglutaryl coenzyme A reductase and sterol synthesis in human mononuclear leucocytes. Diabetologia 1984; 26:366–369.

190. Chait A, Bierman EL, Albers JJ. Low density lipoprotein receptor activity in cultured human skin fibroblasts: mechanism of insulin-induced stimulation. J Clin Invest 1979; 64:1309–1319.
191. Oppenheimer MJ, Sundquist K, Bierman EL. Downregulation of high density lipoprotein receptor activity in human fibroblasts by insulin and IGF-1. Diabetes 1989; 38:117–122.
192. Torjeson PA, Birkeland KI, Anderssen SA, et al. Lifestyle changes may reverse development of the inulin resistance syndrome. Diabetes Care 1997; 20:26–31.
193. Bailey CJ. Metformin revisited: its actions and indications for use. Diabetic Med 1988; 5:315–320.
194. Saltiel AR, Horikoshi H. Thiazolidinediones are novel insulin-sensitizing agents. Curr Opin Endocrinol Diabetes 1995; 2:341–347.

Index

About the Editor

JOHN C. LAROSA is a Professor in the Department of Medicine, Adjunct Professor in the Department of Biostatistics and Epidemiology in the School of Public Health and Tropical Medicine, and Chancellor of Tulane University Medical Center, New Orleans, Louisiana. The author or coauthor of over 180 professional papers and book chapters, he is a Fellow of the American College of Physicians and the American Heart Association's Councils on Arteriosclerosis and Geriatric Cardiology, and a member of the American Medical Association and the American Society of Internal Medicine, among other organizations. Dr. LaRosa, certified by the American Board of Internal Medicine, received the M.D. degree (1965) from the University of Pittsburgh, Pennsylvania.